# Multiple Sclerosis: A Self-Care Guide to Wellness

*Second Edition*

Nancy J. Holland, EdD, RN, MSCN
Vice President, Clinical Programs
National Multiple Sclerosis Society
New York, New York
*and*

June Halper, MSCN, ANP, FAAN
Executive Director, Gimbel Multiple Sclerosis Center
Executive Director, Consortium of Multiple Sclerosis Centers
Executive Director, International Organization of MS Nurses
Teaneck, New Jersey

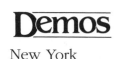

**Demos**

New York

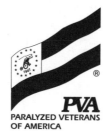

**PVA**
PARALYZED VETERANS
OF AMERICA

D1119626

Demos Medical Publishing, LLC. 386 Park Avenue South, New York, NY 10016, USA

Library of Congress Cataloging-in-Publication Data

Holland, Nancy J.
  Multiple sclerosis : a self-care guide to wellness / Nancy J. Holland and June Halper. — 2nd ed.
    p. cm.
  Includes index.
  ISBN 1-932603-07-7 (pbk. : alk. paper)
  1. Multiple sclerosis—Popular works. 2. Self-care, Health. I. Halper, June. II. Title.
  RC377.H65 2005
  616.8'34—dc22

                                       2004030482

# Dedication

In memory of Labe C. Scheinberg, MD and Pamela F. Cavallo, MSW, ACSW.

Dr. Labe C. Scheinberg passed away on February 21, 2004. Dr. Scheinberg had a brilliant mind, quick wit, and a sensitivity to the needs of others. He was a pioneer in MS care and research, and was well known for his knowledge of science and literature. He led the fight against MS in symptomatic management including psychosocial and spiritual care. Dr. Scheinberg is missed today and will be missed by future generations of patients, families, and the MS team.

Pamela Cavallo (1947–2001) was the former Director of the Clinical Programs Department of the National Multiple Sclerosis Society. Her entire career focused on ways to help people with MS and their families have better quality of life. She implemented her vision with programs aimed at people with MS and their families to end the devastating effects of this disease.

# Acknowledgments

WE WOULD LIKE TO THANK many people for their encouragement and support in this project: Thomas E. Stripling, Elinor Tucker, and Jim Angelo of the Paralyzed Veterans of America for their dedication to the fight against MS; Dr. Vivian Beyda of the United Spinal Association for always seeking new ideas; the National Multiple Sclerosis Society, the Consortium of Multiple Sclerosis Centers, and all organizations seeking to help people with MS and their families; our own families for their patience and support; and last, but not least, Dr. Diana M. Schneider of Demos Medical Publishing, for her wit, wisdom, and sharp pencil that have helped make MS publications widely available during the past decade.

# Contributors

**John Booss, MD**
National Director of Neurology
Department of Veterans Affairs
VA Connecticut Health Care System
West Haven, Connecticut
Professor of Neurology and Laboratory
    Medicine
Yale University School of Medicine
New Haven, Connecticut

**Pamela F. Cavallo, MSW, ACSW
    (deceased)**
Director, Clinical Programs
National Multiple Sclerosis Society
New York, New York

**Thomas D. Davies, AIA**
Architect
Annapolis, Maryland
Consultant Architect
Paralyzed Veterans of America
Washington, DC

**Frederick W. Foley, PhD**
Associate Professor of Psychology
Yeshiva University
Albert Einstein College of Medicine
Bronx, New York
Director, Neuropsychology and
    Psychosocial Research
Gimbel Multiple Sclerosis Center
Holy Name Hospital
Teaneck, New Jersey

**Debra Frankel, MS, OTR**
Senior Associate
Health Services Research and Evaluation
Abt Associates Inc.
Cambridge, Massachusetts
Senior Consultant
National Multiple Sclerosis Society
New York, New York

**Susan Goodman, MA, RD, CDN, CDE**
Dietitian
Brookdale Department of Geriatrics and
    Adult Development
Division of Experimental Diabetes and
    Aging
Mount Sinai School of Medicine
New York, New York

**Joseph B. Guarnaccia, MD**
Director, Multiple Sclerosis Treatment
    Center
Derby, Connecticut
Director, Multiple Sclerosis Center of Care
    New England
East Greenwich, Rhode Island
Assistant Clinical Professor
Department of Neurology
Yale University
New Haven, Connecticut

**Linda Guiod, RN, BA, BSN**
Vice President of Chapter Programs
National Multiple Sclerosis Society
Central New England Chapter
Waltham, Massachusetts

**June Halper, MSCN, ANP, FAAN**
Executive Director
Gimbel Multiple Sclerosis Center
Holy Name Hospital
Executive Director, Consortium of Multiple
    Sclerosis Centers
Executive Director, International
    Organization of MS Nurses
Teaneck, New Jersey

**Deborah Hertz, MPH**
National Director, Medical Programs
National Multiple Sclerosis Society
New York, New York

**Richard W. Hicks, PhD**
Former Director
The Huega Center
Edwards, Colorado

**Nancy J. Holland, EdD, RN, MSCN**
Vice President, Clinical Programs
National Multiple Sclerosis Society
New York, New York

**Brian Hutchinson, PhD**
President and Chief Executive Officer
The Huega Center
Edwards, Colorado

**Rosalind C. Kalb, PhD**
Director, Professional Resource Center
National Multiple Sclerosis Society
New York, New York

**Patricia Kennedy, RN, CNP, MSCN**
Nurse Practitioner
Rocky Mountain Multiple Sclerosis Center
Englewood, Colorado

**Nicholas G. LaRocca, PhD**
Director, Health Care Delivery and Policy
   Research Program
National Multiple Sclerosis Society
New York, New York

**Nancy T. Law, BA**
Vice President, Client Programs
National Multiple Sclerosis Society
Denver, Colorado

**Linda Lehman, MSN, RNCS, FNP**
Nanuet, New York

**Carol Peredo Lopez, AIA**
National Architecture Director
Paralyzed Veterans of America
Washington, DC

**Dorothy E. Northrop, MSW, ACSW**
National Director, Clinical Programs
National Multiple Sclerosis Society
New York, New York

**Beverly Noyes, PhD, LPC**
Director, Program and Staff Development
National Multiple Sclerosis Society
Denver, Colorado

**Margie O'Leary, MSN, RN, MSCN**
Clinical Research Nurse Director
Department of Urology
University of Pittsburgh
Pittsburgh, Pennsylvania

**Patricia A. O'Looney, PhD**
Director of Biomedical Research Programs
National Multiple Sclerosis Society
New York, New York

**Mary Ann Picone, MD**
Medical Director
Gimbel Multiple Sclerosis Center
Holy Name Hospital
Teaneck, New Jersey

**James H. Rimmer, PhD**
Professor, Department of Disability and
   Human Development
Director, National Center on Physical
   Activity and Disability
University of Illinois at Chicago
Chicago, Illinois

**Audrey Sorgen, PhD**
Denver, Colorado

**Thomas E. Stripling**
Director of Research, Education and
   Practice Guidelines
Paralyzed Veterans of America
Washington, DC

**Frances Tromp van Holst, OTR/L, CDRS**
Occupational Therapist
Certified Driving Rehabilitation Specialist
Department of Rehabilitation Medicine
University of Washington Medical Center
Seattle, Washington

**Teresa Valois, OTR/L, ATP, CDRS**
Manager, Assistive Technology
Provail
Seattle, Washington

# Preface

MULTIPLE SCLEROSIS is a disease of the central nervous system that has a far-reaching and variable impact on young adults; it can have profound physical, social, and psychological consequences for patients and their families. MS is a disease that has evolved from the mysterious "crippler of young adults" to, more recently, one that has generated a great deal of public interest due to highly publicized treatments, both conventional and unconventional.

Impairments in MS are the result of demyelination in the brain or spinal cord or both, and manifest themselves in mild sensory symptoms, weakness, fatigue, bowel or bladder dysfunction, tremor, incoordination, or paralysis. These impairments and their many manifestations can result in social, emotional, vocational, educational, and sexual disruptions. This book is designed to empower those affected by multiple sclerosis with updated information about MS care, available resources, and other valuable tools to remain well despite chronic illness. It is the second edition of a book that has proven valuable to people with MS who are impacted by the disease on a day-to-day basis.

The philosophy of each chapter is consistent with a phrase coined by the National MS Society: "Knowledge is power," and your authors and editors hope that each reader takes an active role in planning and implementing healthcare and self-care activities and acts as a consultant to his or her healthcare team. The goal of our work is to support the development of an MS Expert Person who is challenged by MS, but who can overcome problems with realistic and appropriate solutions.

Whether diagnosed for a few years or having lived with the disease for some time, the person with MS will find in this book many practical tips on self-care designed to promote maximum independence, well-being, and productivity. Despite the diagnosis, wellness *can* be achieved with knowledge and commitment.

This book was developed in partnership with and under the auspices of the Paralyzed Veterans of America, which has made a major and continuing commitment to multiple sclerosis care.

# Foreword

Since 1998, when Paralyzed Veterans of America (PVA) first published *Multiple Sclerosis: A Guide to Wellness*, great strides have been made in research findings and treatment options. For this reason, PVA is proud to present this newly updated edition of the "MS Wellness Guide," as it has come to be called.

Edited by Nancy J. Holland, RN, EdD, MSCN and June Halper, MSCN, ANP, FAAN, this second edition has been expanded to include new chapters on the promise of research, disease management, general health issues, managing financial resources, health insurance options, and community living options. Each of the other chapters has been updated and revised to reflect advances in the field and changing management strategies. The table of contents has been reorganized to facilitate finding information of special interest to the reader, and the appendix on "Helpful Resources" has been greatly expanded.

The new edition continues to focus on staying well in the presence of MS. Wellness is a concept that does not normally come to mind when we think about a disease. We usually think of diseases in terms of curable or incurable. But MS is a disease that—while incurable—*can* be managed and yields to many treatments and therapies. Although not cures, they can provide the patient with a great deal of control over his or her experience of well-being.

This book covers a broad spectrum of topics related to MS and its effects, focusing especially on the needs of those who have been living with the disease for some time. Practical tips on self-care are designed to promote maximum independence, well-being, and productivity. The objective is to emphasize that wellness can be achieved with knowledge and commitment.

PVA has been pleased to partner with Demos Medical Publishing in updating and producing this new edition. We are proud to see it take its place among the other books in the Demos catalog of reliable, practical guides on living with multiple sclerosis.

Randy Pleva
National President
Paralyzed Veterans of America

# About the Paralyzed Veterans of America

FOUNDED IN 1946, PVA is the only congressionally chartered veterans service organization dedicated solely to individuals with spinal cord injury or diseases. PVA has 34 local chapters around the country and represents over 21,000 members. Approximately 20 percent of PVA members have MS. To serve them better, PVA has published a number of books on MS, promoted the development of MS Centers of Excellence within the Department of Veterans Affairs and engaged with other organizations in vigorous efforts to promote MS program building.

The first "Wellness Guide" has been one of PVA's most popular publications. Through the partnership with Demos, PVA hopes to be able to reach an even wider audience.

# Contents

# Chapter 1

# An Overview of Multiple Sclerosis

Joseph B. Guarnaccia, MD and John Booss, MD

Mᴜʟᴛɪᴘʟᴇ sᴄʟᴇʀᴏsɪs (MS) is a disease of myelin, the insulating cover around the nerves of the central nervous system (CNS: brain, optic nerves, and spinal cord) (see Figure 1.1), that becomes damaged in MS. MS most commonly begins in young adulthood and affects about twice as many women as men. Although its initial symptoms vary greatly, certain patterns are typical: a previously healthy woman or less frequently, a man, 20 to 30 years old suddenly experiences neurologic symptoms. These symptoms may range from dimming of vision to numbness in the legs or body to dizziness or imbalance. Symptoms of this first attack (or exacerbation) usually remit (clear) or improve.

Four general patterns of disease course are diagnosed as MS (see Figure 1.2). *Relapsing-remitting* MS is a pattern of attacks (exacerbations) followed by partial or complete recovery from symptoms (remission). This relapsing/remitting pattern may give way to a pattern of progressive disability, called *secondary progressive* MS.

Some individuals rarely experience remission of symptoms. They have *primary progressive* MS, in which there is steady progression without remissions. A fourth pattern, recently defined, is *progressive-relapsing* MS. This is a chronic progressive course in which infrequent relapses occur.

The reasons for these differences in the course of MS are unknown. However, the relapsing-remitting pattern most typically affects young adults, especially women. Older individuals are more likely to have patterns of progressive MS. In these latter cases, onset is usually after age 40, and men and women are affected equally.

The multiple scars of MS (plaques) can be seen as pale, well-defined patches scat-

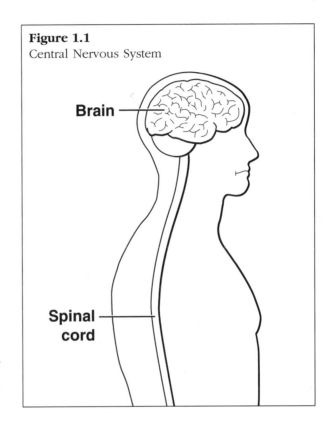

**Figure 1.1**
Central Nervous System

Brain

Spinal cord

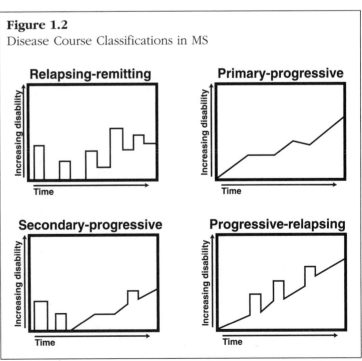

**Figure 1.2**
Disease Course Classifications in MS

**Relapsing-remitting**

Increasing disability / Time

**Primary-progressive**

Increasing disability / Time

**Secondary-progressive**

Increasing disability / Time

**Progressive-relapsing**

Increasing disability / Time

tered throughout the brain and spinal cord. They are located in the white matter, which contains a high percentage of *myelin*, an insulating material that covers sections of nerve cells that carry electrochemical messages from the nerve cells to "action" parts of the body, such as the eyes or the muscles in the hands or legs. Because many of these messages from the brain must travel relatively long distances, myelin is critical for impulse conduction (see Figure 1.3). In MS, myelin is the primary target of an attack by the body's immune system, although damage to the underlying nerve is now known to occur. Multiple sclerosis is an autoimmune (self-immune) disease, because the body's immune system mistakenly attacks healthy myelin.

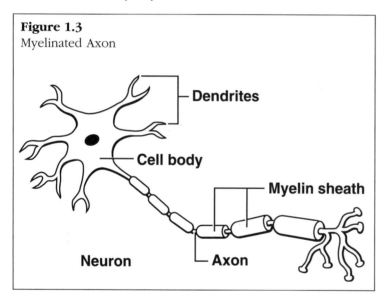

**Figure 1.3**
Myelinated Axon

Dendrites

Cell body

Myelin sheath

Neuron — Axon

## WHO GETS MULTIPLE SCLEROSIS?

For decades, medical scientists have sought clues to causes for the variable incidence of MS in different parts of the world. The disease is far more common in temperate zones than in the tropics. Zones with low, medium, and high risk for MS are roughly based on distances north and south of the equator. The north-south or south-north gradient occurs within countries as well. In the United States, for instance, MS is more

common in northern states than in southern states. Possible reasons for these variations are discussed in the next section.

However, whatever factors in high-risk zones predispose the development of MS, exposure to them during childhood or adolescence seems to have the greatest effect. If an individual moves after that critical period from a high-risk zone to a lower risk zone, or vice versa, the risk level of the original habitat applies. For example, a person who moves after adolescence from a temperate, high-risk zone to a tropical, low-risk zone will continue to have a higher risk of developing MS than the population in the tropical zone. What makes this observation intriguing is that MS does not usually begin in individuals until they reach their twenties and thirties—years or even decades after the period when MS is thought to originate.

Location alone does not account for all the variability, however. Multiple sclerosis is also more common in people of certain ethnic or racial backgrounds. Parts of the British Isles have the highest concentration of MS in the world, affecting one out of every hundred. Immigrants of Northern European descent have colonized other high-incidence areas of the world, including the United States and Canada. By contrast, MS is rare to nonexistent among African natives, Native Americans, and Laplanders in Scandinavia.

## IS MULTIPLE SCLEROSIS INHERITED?

Because people of similar ethnic or racial composition share certain inherited traits, genes may play an important role in MS. But MS is not a simple genetic disease; that is, it is not due to a defective gene that causes the disease on its own. However, some individuals may inherit a cluster of genes that increases their susceptibility to the disease.

Scientists are investigating genetic factors and how they contribute to the disease.

We know that certain genes control some aspects of immune system development and function. It is possible that those or other unidentified genes may *predispose* the immune system to attack CNS myelin.

In some families, more than one individual may have MS, although the chances of more than one family member developing the disease are still low, less than 5 percent. Even for identical twins, who have identical genes, the risk is still only about 30 percent that both twins will have MS.

## WHAT ELSE MAY BE IMPORTANT IN CAUSING MULTIPLE SCLEROSIS?

The combination of unidentified genes, geographic location, and an abnormal immune response to myelin has led scientists to consider that MS may be caused by a virus. Some viruses can infect the CNS, including, in rare instances, viruses that cause common childhood diseases. Polio, a once-common scourge that has been virtually eradicated in industrialized nations, was, like MS, more common in temperate climates than in the tropics. One hypothesis is that paralytic polio does not develop in the less stringent sanitary conditions and close living arrangements that are common in warmer climates and favor the occurrence of infections earlier in childhood, when maternal antibodies are still present and paralysis is much less likely.

The notion of an infectious cause of MS gained support when the disease emerged in the Faroe Islands, off the coast of England, after occupation by British troops during World War II. It has been speculated that dogs kept as pets by the British brought canine distemper or another virus to the island, exposing the native human inhabitants. However, no links to the canine distemper virus have been demonstrated.

Scientists have also speculated that MS results from altered immune response to one or more common viral infections, and that this abnormal response is more likely to occur when infection is acquired later in childhood. Many other viruses have been implicated and continue to be studied by researchers as possible causes of MS. One large study found that the disease was seven times more common in people who have had infectious mononucleosis, which is caused by the Epstein-Barr virus. But, however appealing the idea, there is no direct proof that any one virus causes the disease.

Other pieces of the puzzle remain unsolved as well. During their reproductive years, women are more susceptible to MS than men. Female hormones, such as estrogen and progesterone, significantly influence immune function. During pregnancy, women with MS seem to be relatively protected from neurologic attacks. However, the disease has a greater tendency to flare within the first six months of the postpartum period. These observations, however, are not absolute. A great majority of women successfully manage both pregnancy and the postpartum period.

Emotional stress, common infections such as colds or sinusitis, and trauma to the CNS also have been studied as possible causes both of MS and of periodic exacerbations. Except for the observation that common viral infections often precede exacerbations, no cause-and-effect relationship has been validated in scientifically controlled studies.

## WHAT IS UNLIKELY TO CAUSE MULTIPLE SCLEROSIS?

Some theories of the cause of MS are highly speculative. Many books and articles in the popular press have touted particular causes of MS and suggested inappropriate treatments based on unscientific theories. For example, exposure to mercury through dental fillings has been cited as a possible cause of MS; as a result, many people have asked their dentists to perform costly and inconvenient replacement of fillings. There is no scientific evidence to suggest such an approach.

Likewise, some medical authors have tried to show that diets rich in animal fats are important in causing and sustaining the disease, but their findings are not based on sound scientific studies. The National Multiple Sclerosis Society (NMSS) recommends the dietary guidelines published by the American Heart Association, in the absence of any compelling evidence linking MS to animal fat in the diet.

## HOW DOES MULTIPLE SCLEROSIS CAUSE SYMPTOMS?

The effects of MS occur because messages to and from the CNS fail to reach their targets properly. Why does this happen? As noted, myelin insulates nerves within the CNS. When myelin is lost, messages lose strength because they "leak out" at the places where myelin has been damaged or destroyed. Therefore, the messages either slow down or fail altogether. This accounts for the nerve's loss of function. Also, the demyelinated nerve itself becomes unstable and begins to initiate spontaneous nerve impulses. These impulses are experienced as pain, the sensation of "pins and needles," or abnormal movements (see Figure 1.4).

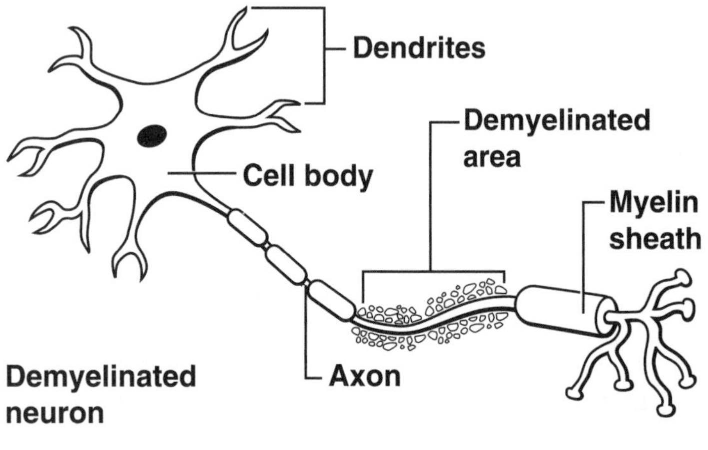

Physical symptoms may include loss of muscle strength, clumsiness, altered sensation, decreased sight, or reduced perception of the position of the body or limbs in space. More subtle symptoms include a mild decrease in mental acuity or memory, or mood swings. Plaques in the so-called "silent" areas of the brain do not cause outward symptoms. Remission of symptoms has been explained by reduced inflammation in the plaque and remyelination by the cells that make myelin, *oligodendrocytes*.

## COMMON SYMPTOMS OF MULTIPLE SCLEROSIS

Virtually any aspect of neurologic function can be affected by MS, but some symptoms, such as *optic neuritis* in a young person, are characteristic. Optic neuritis usually results in partial loss of vision in one eye because of inflammatory demyelination of the optic nerve. Vision may be blurred, and colors may be difficult to distinguish. Eye movement may be uncomfortable.

Double vision, another common symptom, is caused by plaques in the brainstem, the part of the brain directly above the spinal cord. Brainstem plaques may also cause vertigo, a sensation of spinning, or dizziness.

*Trigeminal neuralgia*, or tic douloureux, also occurs, although this condition is also common in individuals who do not have MS. Tic douloureux causes sharp, shooting pains in the face, usually precipitated by chewing or speaking.

The *cerebellum* is the part of the brain that controls balance and the rhythm of muscle movement. Involvement of the cerebellum and its connections may cause gait

**Figure 1.4**
Demyelinated Nerve

- Dendrites
- Demyelinated area
- Cell body
- Myelin sheath
- Demyelinated neuron
- Axon

instability, problems with hand coordination, or slurred speech.

The spinal cord is frequently affected by MS. Individuals sometimes experience a sharp, seemingly electrical sensation, called *L'hermitte's sign*, when they flex their necks. Plaques in the spine can cause a variety of symptoms, including numbness, weakness, bowel or bladder difficulty, or gait imbalance. Plaques in the brainstem or higher levels of the brain can also cause these symptoms, but the hallmark of MS involvement in the spinal cord is simultaneous involvement of both the right and left sides of the body.

In addition to muscle weakness, *spasticity* may also occur. This results when communication from the brain to the motor cells that directly control muscle movement in the spinal cord is interrupted and primitive spinal cord reflexes take over. Spastic weakness may cause difficulty in walking because considerable effort is needed to overcome stiffness in order to raise and propel the leg forward. However, spasticity is a boon when it partially compensates for muscle weakness by acting as a "splint" in walking, standing, or transferring.

The concept of spasticity also applies to bladder function. Individuals may experience a sudden urge to urinate and inability to hold their urine, even in public places. Other problems are retention of urine or difficulty initiating urination. (Bladder problems are addressed in detail in Chapter 7, "Bladder and Bowel Management.")

## HOW IS MULTIPLE SCLEROSIS DIAGNOSED?

None of the symptoms described so far occurs only in MS. Strokes, tumors, or infections can cause the same disabilities when they affect the same areas of the brain and spinal cord. Therefore, the diagnosis of MS requires the exclusion of other neurologic diseases. Diagnosing MS was a greater problem in the past, before physicians could produce sophisticated images of the brain and spinal cord and test other aspects of neurologic function. In the past, the diagnosis of MS relied primarily on a patient's medical history and a physical examination. Criteria for the diagnosis required at least two verified neurologic attacks, separated in time, and caused by damage in at least two different areas of the CNS. These criteria reflected the natural history of relapsing forms of MS. Progressive MS could be diagnosed, in the absence of another known neurologic condition, after a progressive worsening of neurologic symptoms over a six-month period.

These criteria have been modified in light of improved diagnostic tests. These tests include magnetic resonance imaging (MRI) of the brain, measuring nerve conduction through the CNS, and cerebrospinal fluid testing for abnormal proteins or cells. The earlier standard required evidence of multiple brain or spinal cord lesions by history and neurologic examination. Now these methods can be augmented with imaging and laboratory tests.

The diagnosis of MS should always be made or confirmed by a *neurologist*, a physician who specializes in diseases of the nervous system. It is wrong and potentially damaging to say that an individual has the disease in the absence of positive test results. However, positive test results should be corroborated by the patient's medical history, symptoms, and abnormal findings on physical examination.

MRI scans and other test results must be carefully interpreted in light of each person's history and examination. The plaques typical of MS have been found at autopsy in individuals who never reported symptoms of the disease during their lifetime. Furthermore, other neurologic diseases can mimic MS, and a skilled physician is required to differentiate among them. Equally important, the possibility of MS should be recognized in patients who have atypical symptoms, so that costly, unnecessary, or even potentially hazardous treatments are not given for an erroneously diagnosed condition.

## WHAT ARE THE TESTS FOR MULTIPLE SCLEROSIS?

### MAGNETIC RESONANCE IMAGING (MRI)

The most revolutionary advance in diagnosis of MS, as well as other diseases of the CNS, is imaging the brain and spinal cord by magnetic resonance. The MRI has revolu-

tionized the ability to diagnose MS, and it has emerged as a primary research tool as well (see Figure 1.5).

MRI scanning determines the progression of the disease by measuring the size and number of both "silent" and active plaques. The technique is especially useful in clinical studies of new therapies, because it allows unbiased investigators to compare disease activity and progression by comparing the MRI scans of treated and untreated individuals.

### EVOKED POTENTIALS

*Evoked potential tests* measure electrical transmissions in the CNS from the point of origin, such as the eye or ear, to the place in the brain where the message is received. The tests can measure visual, auditory, and other sensory perceptions.

The tests may consist of a changing visual pattern placed in an individual's field of sight, a series of clicks delivered to each ear, or a small electrical current delivered to the finger or toe. The diagnosis of MS is aided by these tests because demyelination in the CNS results in an increase in the amount of time needed to transmit electrical messages.

Evoked potentials are useful additions to other tests, particularly the MRI when the brain scan is normal. Although MRI scanning of the brain is very sensitive in detecting MS plaques, the technique is less precise in the spinal cord or optic nerve because they are smaller areas. Visual evoked potentials may be particularly helpful when demyelination in the optic nerve is not yet sufficient to cause visual complaints by individuals.

### CEREBROSPINAL FLUID EXAMINATION

*Cerebrospinal fluid* surrounds the brain and spinal cord and often reflects disease conditions in the CNS. In MS, certain abnormalities in the spinal fluid reflect the inflammatory nature of the disease. These abnormal-

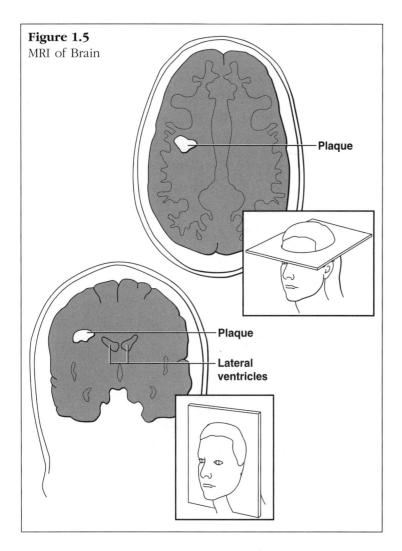

**Figure 1.5**
MRI of Brain

Plaque

Plaque

Lateral ventricles

ities include the presence of white blood cells, which are involved in inflammation, and the protein products of these cells. (White blood cells differ from red blood cells, whose function is to transport oxygen to tissues.)

In MS, the number of white blood cells in the spinal fluid may be mildly elevated, but a more characteristic finding is the presence of inflammatory proteins, called *antibodies* or *immunoglobulins*. The presence of these substances in spinal fluid, and their absence in the blood, indicates that they are being produced within the CNS. Both the amount (IgG index) and properties (oligoclonal bands) of these proteins indicate CNS inflammation, which is characteristic of MS.

## MULTIPLE SCLEROSIS AS A DISEASE OF THE IMMUNE SYSTEM

Normally, the immune system is able to distinguish between infectious organisms or foreign tissues (such as a transplanted organ), which are attacked or rejected, and the body's own organs or tissues, which are tolerated. How white blood cells perform these functions is a fascinating story. The process requires continual adaptation on the part of white blood cells to recognize—through receptors on their surfaces and in proteins they make—any disease-producing bacteria, virus, or fungus, and even the body's own cells that have become cancerous.

Scientists have learned to activate the immune system—through vaccination—to defend the body against potentially infectious challengers. The other side of immunity, however, is that these white blood cells sometimes misrecognize and cause damage to the body's own cells and proteins. White blood cells that act in this way must be destroyed or held in check. If the system breaks down, autoimmune disease may occur. The immune system is then said to have "lost tolerance" to a particular organ or tissue in the body. Restoration of this tolerance is the ultimate goal of any treatment for autoimmune disease.

In MS, tolerance is lost to myelin in the CNS. By a process that continues to be clarified at a rapid rate, white blood cells cross into the CNS and destroy myelin. Some white blood cells specifically misrecognize myelin, others make antibodies to myelin, and still others digest myelin. Moreover, in keeping with the natural system of checks and balances in immunity, other classes of white blood cells suppress the inflammatory attack.

The ability of scientists to produce an MS-like disease—called experimental allergic encephalomyelitis—in laboratory animals has been critical to understanding the immune process in general and MS in particular. This animal research has been instrumental in the development and testing of therapeutic interventions prior to clinical testing in humans with MS.

## DRUGS USED TO TREAT MULTIPLE SCLEROSIS

All accepted medical therapies (see Chapter 3 and Appendix C) used to ease or prevent attacks of MS or to slow its progress have an effect—either a suppressive or modifying effect—on the immune system. A good example are the *glucocorticosteroids*. When given by intravenous infusion at high doses for short periods of time, glucocorticosteroids have many actions, including the suppression of white blood cell functions. In MS, glucocorticosteroids are commonly used to treat exacerbations. Individuals who receive intravenous corticosteroids for optic neuritis have had improved visual outcomes. These medications have definite—if uncommon—risks, however, which should be discussed with the treating physician. In general, the risks and side effects of short courses of intravenous corticosteroids are minimal when compared with those of daily oral steroids taken over a long period of time.

Traditionally, long-term treatments for MS have suppressed immune function. Those that have been tested and are still used include azathioprine, cyclophosphamide, and methotrexate. Their use may slow disease progression, but individuals taking these drugs must be carefully monitored by their physicians because of the medical risks.

It was not until the advent of the beta interferons in 1993 that a relatively safe, non-toxic, long-term treatment for MS became available. The first drug of this type was *interferon beta-1b*, Betaseron®. Testing in a large clinical trial showed that interferon beta-1b could produce a 33 percent decrease in the number and reduce their severity. Its clinical efficacy was further supported by findings on MRI scans that the rate of new plaque formation was significantly reduced. Interferon beta-1b is administered by injection just beneath the skin every other day.

In 1996, a second beta interferon, *interferon beta-1a*, Avonex®, was approved for distribution. It is administered by injection into a large muscle once a week. The beta interferons are natural products of cells that participate in immunity. They have a number of modulating effects that tip the balance away from an immune attack.

A third drug is glatiramer acetate, Copaxone®. Glatiramer acetate is a mixture of four amino acids—the building blocks of protein—that have been shown to reduce neurologic exacerbations in individuals with relapsing/remitting disease. It is hypothesized to work either by binding receptors on T-lymphocytes that would otherwise bind myelin basic protein or by stimulating other subsets of T-lymphocytes that suppress activated cells.

In 2001, a second interferon beta-1a, Rebif®, was approved in the United States after being available for several years in Europe and Canada.

Beta interferons and glatiramer acetate offer two distinct advantages over general immune suppressants. First, they do not disturb general immunity to infections. Second, they have fewer side effects on other organ systems. They therefore appear to be safer to use over long periods of time. Disadvantages of the interferons are their frequent side effects, which include fever, chills, muscle aches, depression, and skin reactions at injection sites, particularly common at the beginning of treatment.

Glatiramer acetate is relatively free of these side effects. However, some individuals suffer occasional brief reactions immediately after an injection. These reactions, which consist of flushing, sensations of a rapid heartbeat, and shortness of breath, usually resolve within 5 or 10 minutes and are of no known threat to health.

Some individuals with rapidly progressive disease benefit from *cytotoxic* therapies. Mitoxantrone, one such chemotherapy, was FDA approved in 2000 for individuals with rapidly progressive MS. Presently under study is the effect of these drugs on preventing long-term disability in individuals who have relapsing/remitting and progressive MS, because the underlying immune process is not significantly changed in individuals with these types of the disease.

In 2005, Tysabri® (natalizumab) was approved by the FDA for relapsing forms of MS. Although encouraging early data resulted in "fast track" approval, one death and other related concerns led to the suspension of Tysabri®. This was a very disappointing event, and there is hope that analysis of the problems may one day lead to re-introduction of natelizumab.

## THE FUTURE OF MULTIPLE SCLEROSIS TREATMENTS

Restoring normal immune tolerance to myelin without disturbing other functions of the immune system is the ultimate goal of therapy. As more is understood about the natural mechanisms for establishing and maintaining this tolerance, new drugs will be designed to treat MS. Our knowledge of immune regulation is built partly on the tremendous strides made in this century in augmenting with vaccines the immune system's ability to fight infectious diseases that once were uniformly fatal or disabling. Strategies for treating MS and other autoimmune diseases, and for tolerating transplanted organs, may include vaccines to train the immune system not to react.

For individuals who are disabled from MS, there is hope that some day demyelination will be reversible or that myelin can be regenerated in the CNS. Scientists are investigating chemical substances that stimulate myelin growth and nerve repair, as well as the transplantation of myelin-producing cells to sites of damage. So far, most of this work is confined to animals, but it is anticipated that clinical trials will be performed on humans in the not-so-distant future.

The horizon for individuals with MS is brighter now than at any other time. The revolution in biotechnology has made modern treatments for MS possible and will continue to provide novel strategies for the development of newer and better therapies. People with MS, their families, and their care partners can look to the future with great optimism.

## Chapter 2
# Hope through Research
Patricia A. O'Looney, PhD

PROGRESS IN MULTIPLE SCLEROSIS (MS) research is being made at a remarkable rate. Twenty years ago, very little was known about the regulation of the immune system, and before the approval of Betaseron® in 1993, no therapy had ever proved capable of changing the underlying course of MS. Now five approved, disease-modifying drugs are available to treat individuals with MS. But the work in MS research is not over. Scientists are closer than ever to understanding the underlying cause of MS, and finding additional treatments for all forms of MS. Research efforts sponsored by the National Multiple Sclerosis Society (NMSS), the National Institutes of Health (NIH), private drug and biotechnology companies, and other MS agencies around the world are contributing to this progress.

## A SNAPSHOT OF MS

Multiple sclerosis is a chronic disease affecting the central nervous system (CNS: the brain, spinal cord, and optic nerves). It is not contagious, and it is rarely fatal, but it is unpredictable. The term "multiple sclerosis" literally means "many scars," referring to the hardened scars, or plaques, this disease leaves in many parts of the CNS tissue after damage has occurred.

Most researchers believe that MS involves a misguided immune-system attack against the myelin sheath, the fat and protein coating that insulates nerve fibers, and against myelin-making cells called *oligodendrocytes*. Nerve fibers themselves are also targets of the immune attack in MS, and ongoing research suggests that nerve fiber damage can occur early in the disease, and that this damage accounts for much of the progressive loss of function experienced by many with the disease. Damage and loss of nervous-system tissue leads to a disruption of nerve messages within the brain and spinal cord. Messages may not get properly through to outlying muscles and nerves, and incoming sensory messages may also get scrambled or disrupted. Nerve signal disruption leads to the many different symptoms of MS.

Multiple sclerosis can attack at any age, but it most often strikes adults in the prime of life, between the ages of 20 and 50. For reasons that are not yet clear, women develop MS at a rate two to three times that of men. Worldwide, an estimated 2 million people have MS.

MS is found more frequently among people in colder climates. Scientists don't understand why, but studies suggest that where a person was born and lived during his or her first 15 years strongly influences the likelihood of developing MS.

No one knows exactly what causes MS, although it is thought to be an "autoimmune disease," meaning the body's immune system attacks its own tissues. Although MS is not directly inherited, MS seems to occur after a person who has one or more hereditary factors (genes) that make him or her susceptible to the disease encounters something in the environment that serves as a trigger.

For years, researchers have been searching for evidence that a virus or other infectious agent could be the culprit, not necessarily by directly causing MS, but possibly by fouling up immune responses such that the body's brain and spinal cord tissues are mistaken for an appropriate immune target.

To understand the underlying mechanisms that cause MS and to shed light on how MS damage might be halted and repaired, researchers are gathering information on many different fronts. Some of the major approaches investigators are taking to understand MS include:

- Exploring *immune processes* underlying the destruction of myelin and nerve fibers in MS to understand how our complex immune systems normally work and what might trigger the immune system to attack the body's own tissues. New opportunities are opening up for exploiting natural chemicals that can turn the immune attack in MS off or on. New technology offers the possibility of finding ways to harness protective chemicals or block destructive ones.
- Studying *myelin-making cell*s (oligodendrocytes) and the nerve fibers they serve, including what makes myelin a target in MS and how to harness natural substances that stimulate myelin and nerve fiber repair.
- Investigating possible *infectious trigger(s)* for MS, which could possibly initiate the disease by altering immune responses.
- Searching for *genes* that cause susceptibility to MS, which may offer clues to the actual cause of MS. Several areas on various chromosomes have been identified as having possible links to susceptibility to MS and also to disease severity. The fact that more than one gene is involved in MS makes the undertaking more difficult, but opportunities and new technologies are ripe for exploring this area further.
- Searching for *new treatments* that will specifically halt myelin and nerve fiber destruction and leave the rest of the immune system intact. Researchers are also seeking ways to enhance myelin repair and better ways to treat symptoms, and are exploring the roles of rehabilitation and exercise.

- A recent growing awareness of *gender differences* in MS, and efforts focusing on what sex-based disparities can reveal about the cause and treatment of MS. Twice as many women as men get MS, yet men tend toward progressive MS and tend to have more severe disease. Sex hormones appear to influence the disease, and those influences are being explored to see whether they can be exploited to find new treatments for MS.
- Newer technologies enabling researchers to ask old questions in new ways. For example, investigators are focusing on MS *lesion pathology* (deciphering the damage wrought upon CNS tissues) for clues to the cause or causes of MS and to refine its treatment.

Investigators for an international study based at the Mayo Clinic (led by Luccinetti and Lassmann) called the MS Lesion Project have reported preliminary evidence for specific patterns of MS damage that form subtypes of the disease that do not match up with the clinical subtypes, such as the relapsing-remitting form. They are searching for noninvasive ways to identify who has which subtype, which may alter the way the disease is treated. These data provide further evidence for the possibility that different patterns of MS tissue damage in the brain may be responsive to different kinds of treatments.

In addition, magnetic resonance imaging (MRI) and other imaging techniques are helping us to understand MS pathology. They offer "windows" into the brain and allow noninvasive study of the disease course and the steps that underlie inflammation and tissue destruction. These technologies could lead to quicker clinical trials of promising drugs and a deeper understanding of the causes of MS.

## SEARCHING FOR BETTER TREATMENTS

Several drugs are currently being tested against MS, each taking a different approach to combat the disease.

- Tysabri® (natalizumab) is a monoclonal antibody that was removed from the marketplace due to one death and other drug-related issues. This introduces the need for serious caution with this group of agents.
- Some early-stage clinical studies are attempting to inhibit only immune cells that recognize myelin. In "peptide therapy," an altered fragment of the immune docking site, or T-cell receptor, is injected. A variation is *T-cell vaccination*, in which the person's own disease-causing T cells are removed and deactivated, then injected back into the body.
- Immune cells produce powerful messenger chemicals called *cytokines* (pronounced SY-toe-kines) that help regulate immune responses. Scientists are seeking ways to block harmful cytokines and enhance the activity of protective ones. For example, researchers at NIH and elsewhere are testing the ability of Zenapax® (daclizumab), an immune-modulating drug given by monthly intravenous (into the vein) infusions. Preliminary results recently reported in 16 individuals suggest that the drug may stabilize or even improve the clinical status of individuals with relapsing-remitting and secondary-progressive MS who had not benefited from other therapies. Zenapax is a monoclonal antibody that inhibits the ability of the cytokine interleukin-2 to stimulate destructive immune activity. The potential of this drug is being explored, alone and in combination with other immune-modulating drugs, in a Phase 2 clinical trial.
- As more is revealed about other steps along the pathway of the immune attack in MS, new targets along that pathway open up for potential therapy. For example, scientists are exploring how to increase the activity of so-called regulatory T cells that can shut down the immune attack. They are also looking at the involvement of immune B cells and the antibodies they produce and ways to block their destructive activity.
- Another approach to treatment is to stimulate *myelin repair* and *nerve regeneration*. In some ways, our bodies already know how to repair myelin because some repair does occur during the course of MS. As scientists uncover the natural chemicals and growth factors that facilitate these processes, new opportunities arise for stimulating the repair of myelin and nerve fibers destroyed by MS. Researchers are attempting to transplant progenitor cells capable of maturing into myelin-making cells or even nerve cells, and are exploring the best source of such cells and the best form of delivery. One source is the bone marrow, which opens up the intriguing possibility that a person's own bone marrow could be a source of replacement for brain and spinal cord cells.
- Literally dozens of combinations of available drugs are being tested to see if their effectiveness can be increased. This plays to the possibility that a "cocktail" of drugs that have different modes of action may assault the disease on more than one front, hopefully to stop the disease process. In addition, some drugs that are already available to treat other disorders are being tested to fight MS. These include the statin drugs, which are used for lowering cholesterol levels and have been shown to successfully fight MS in animal models, and also var-

ious chemotherapy and immune-suppressing agents used to fight rejection of transplanted tissues.

- Other agents are also under investigation for possible use in alleviating or managing MS symptoms. These include Fampridine (4-aminopyridine), which is being tested for its ability to temporarily speed nerve conduction and thereby improve some physical functions. Marijuana derivatives are being explored for relief of a variety of symptoms including spasticity and pain. The results of clinical tests have been difficult to analyze and there are potential long-term and short-term side effects that cause concern.
- Researchers are also investigating exercise and rehabilitation strategies, fatigue and sleep disorders, and cognitive changes such as memory loss and poor concentration, in order to understand the basic mechanisms and to identify the most effective therapeutic approaches.

## AN INTERNATIONAL EFFORT TO SPEED CLINICAL TRIALS

Imagine you have just been diagnosed with MS and your doctor says, "I see by your clinical profile that you will do well on medication 'X,' you will likely have one exacerbation two years from now, and in 10 years you will still retain your current physical abilities." It is the dream of those involved with the Sylvia Lawry Centre for MS Research (SLCMSR), an international collaboration launched by the Multiple Sclerosis International Federation, that such profiling will become available in the future by amassing and analyzing data from scores of MS clinical trials.

With more than 160 clinical studies ongoing worldwide, the data accumulated by investigators can become a valuable resource for understanding the course of MS

and for improving the design and conduct of clinical studies. Since it was established in February 2001, the SLCMSR has already collected information on 19,000 participants in 44 past MS studies, including clinical trials, natural history studies, and clinical data sets.

The Centre is located at the Technical University of Munich. Centre staff—largely statisticians and mathematicians—benefit from a Scientific Oversight Committee of MS experts. With data now in hand, the group is developing a database designed to answer questions that can only come from large numbers of patients, and aims to share its data with MS investigators worldwide.

In all these ways, the SLCMSR is helping to improve clinical studies in MS and speed the development of effective therapies for this disease.

## IMPROVING HEALTH CARE

If the cure for MS were found tomorrow, it would be meaningless if people who have the disease could not gain access to the treatment. Even today, with five drugs available that can help some people, and with physical therapy and exercise regimens that can help individuals maximize their capabilities, impediments can prevent people from getting the care they need.

Biomedical research in MS is aided and supported by research on healthcare delivery and policy, which can provide meaningful statistics and information for advocacy efforts aimed at improving quality of life for persons with this disease. The issues being studied include availability of health insurance, access to disease-modifying therapies, special needs of older individuals with MS, quality and standards of medical care, quality of nursing home facilities, and many more.

We now know more than ever before about the mechanisms underlying MS. As scientists uncover new facts about the disease, new research avenues open up for exploration. There has never been a more exciting time in the history of MS and never better prospects that a cure will be found.

# Chapter 3
# Disease Management
June Halper, MSCN, ANP, FAAN

THERE ARE DRUG treatments that reduce both the severity and duration of relapses in multiple sclerosis (MS). Three types of medications have this effect: *steroids*, routinely prescribed by some neurologists for acute exacerbations (or relapses); *immunomodulators* that are approved for relapsing forms of MS, two of which are also approved for progressive disease; and *immunosuppressants*, which are still viewed by some neurologists as experimental, although one is approved by the Food and Drug Administration (FDA) for worsening MS.

## STEROIDS

Corticosteroids are naturally occurring hormones in the human body. There are a variety of steroids including glucocorticoids, mineralcorticosteroids, androgens, and progestins. Of these, only the glucocorticoids are prescribed regularly to treat relapses in MS.

*Glucocorticoids* occur naturally in the body as cortisone and hydrocortisone. These hormones are produced by a pair of organs called the adrenal glands, which are situated next to the kidneys. The adrenal glands are organized into two discrete tissue types, somewhat confusingly called the medulla and cortex. These have nothing to do with their namesakes in the brain. Cortisone and hydrocortisone are produced in the adrenal cortex in response to the release of a regulatory hormone called *adrenocorticotrophic hormone* (ACTH), which is manufactured in both the pituitary gland in the brain and the adrenal cortex. ACTH is naturally secreted in response to a variety of stress factors including fear, anxiety, pain, exercise, infection, and very low levels of blood glucose.

During the mid-20th century, research determined that ACTH given intramuscularly induced recovery from MS exacerbations. More recently, either intravenous or oral steroid administration has become the preferred method prescribed for acute exacerbations of MS. The route of delivery (intravenous or oral) and the length of time that steroids are prescribed varies from physician to physician. You should discuss this issue with your doctor when you first begin your care for MS.

Steroids are not without side effects. Acne, weight gain, seizures, psychosis, depression, headaches, fatigue, facial hair, nausea, vomiting, and adrenal insufficiency can be very serious adverse events. Thus, the long-term use of steroids is not advised, nor is it effective in MS.

Steroids do not appear to have a beneficial effect on progressive forms of the disease. Trials have been done on monthly methylprednisolone use with *secondary progressive MS* (SPMS) and, although the results were equivocal, the degree of disability was not affected. SPMS is a course that changes over time to a worsening pattern with or without continued relapses. However, this study concluded that more work needed to be done to determine whether steroids might have a place in treating SPMS.

## IMMUNOMODULATORS: THE ABCR DRUGS

Perhaps the most effective treatments currently available today deal with the autoimmune component of MS and work by regulating aspects of the immune system. Avonex®, Betaseron®, Copaxone®, and

Rebif® have been approved to modify the disease in relapsing forms of MS; Betaseron® has been FDA-approved for use in people who have SPMS. Avonex® is being used for worsening MS in people presenting with a clinically isolated syndrome (CIS): one neurologic attack with MRI evidence of demyelination. A fifth drug, Novantrone® (mitoxantrone), has become available during the past few years for worsening multiple sclerosis. The interferons and Copaxone® are given by self-injection; Novantrone® is administered intravenously by nurses (or your physician).

## INTERFERON BETA TYPE I

Beta interferon (IFN-b) comes in two preparations: interferon beta-1a (Avonex® and Rebif®) and interferon beta-1b (Betaseron® in the U.S. and Betaferon® in Europe). Beta interferon is a naturally occurring biochemical in the human body and belongs to a group of biochemicals known as *interferons* (IFNs), which regulate the functioning of the immune system. The mechanism by which IFN-b functions is complex and not fully understood.

Beta interferon reduces the levels of another interferon, called interferon gamma (IFN-g), which is known to be associated with activating the disease process in MS. It appears to block certain white blood cells from attacking the myelin covering of the nerves in the brain and spinal cord. It also seems to stop a type of white blood cell, called a *T cell*, from releasing immune system signaling molecules (that would otherwise encourage inflammation). It also seems to interfere with the process of summoning new immune system cells to the site of inflammation.

All interferons can be self-administered: Betaseron® subcutaneously (under the skin) every other day; Rebif® subcutaneously three times a week; and Avonex® intramuscularly (into the muscle) once a week.

We know that MS is a very unpredictable disease and none of us knows what disease course a person will have from the outset. Based on the newest MS research, thought leaders believe that early treatment is extremely important. If MS continues to progress while you are using IFN-b, that doesn't mean the drug isn't working—it might have progressed faster if you hadn't been using it. In fact, studies imply this.

When research shows a benefit in the burden of new lesions shown on MRI between the people being treated with IFN-b as compared to a *placebo* group (those not receiving the drug) over the same period, it is very hard to tell whether it has worked fully for some people, partially for others, and not at all for the rest. This is because no one has any idea of what would have happened to any particular person without the drug. Unless the studies are extremely large, all that can be said is that the drug reduces *lesion load* (changes seen on MRI demonstrating loss of healthy tissue in the brain, spinal cord, or both) by an average over a certain period of time.

The interferons may not work for everyone and, indeed, some people seem to do very well with them whereas others do not. Research is currently underway to enable clinicians to predict "responders" versus "nonresponders" to treatment.

What IFN-b is *not*, is a cure for some people and not at all effective for others. The bottom line is that, even if it doesn't appear to be fully working for you, it may very well be helping modulate your disease.

The principle side effects of IFN-b use are flu-like symptoms—fever, night sweats, and muscle aches. These can be very unpleasant, but often subside after a few months and respond well to nonsteroidal medications such as ibuprofen, acetaminophen (Tylenol) or even low-dose steroids. Slowly increasing the dose (dose titration) has also been shown to be effective in reducing this side effect.

Liver toxicity (effect on blood liver function) has been noted in some patients, particularly at higher doses, although this problem is usually mild. Be sure to notify your doctor if you are experiencing new symptoms, whether they appear to be attributable to MS.

Depression has been described as another potential side effect and should be addressed by your healthcare team before you start interferon therapy.

*Injection site reactions* can also be a problem, and it is essential to rotate the injection site to reduce these. Briefly numbing the skin at the injection site with ice or anesthetic cream, site rotation, getting the drug to room temperature before injecting, and taking antihistamines before injecting may help. One of the difficulties many people face is having to inject themselves. Autoinjectors are available with Betaseron® and Rebif®. If injection becomes too great a challenge, people confronting this difficulty are advised to enlist an injection partner. Most people get over this "needle phobia" eventually with the proper support.

In one study in Europe, IFN-b was shown to reduce the relapse rate in SPMS by a statistically significant amount. However, two other similar studies failed to show statistically significant effects. It is known that relapse rate falls off during the course of the disease and that inflammatory activity is correlated with relapses. It is also believed that the mechanism of disease activity changes from an inflammatory one to a neurodegenerative one during the secondary progressive phase of the disease (SPMS). Based on these and other results, it seems likely that IFN-b is only effective at preventing inflammation and relapses and not effective in people with progressive courses without relapses.

COPAXONE®

Copaxone®, or glatiramer acetate, is a collection of synthetic peptide derivatives—the building blocks of protein—that are believed to work by modifying the body's immune response to myelin. As with IFN-b, its method of action is complex and is not fully understood. One theory proposes that, by flooding the body with the substances similar to those in proteins found in the myelin sheath, the drug acts as a decoy and draws some of the attack away from the brain and spinal cord.

Copaxone® is about equally effective as IFN-b in reducing relapses and MRI changes. It is injected subcutaneously on a daily basis. The most common problem that users have are injection site reactions that include itching and inflammation. These reactions can be alleviated by site rotation and by ensuring that the drug is at room temperature before injecting it. An autoinjector is available for administrating Copaxone®. Copaxone® comes in a prefilled syringe, as does Rebif® and Betaseron®. Avonex® is available as a prefilled product or one may prefer to reconstitute the powder and liquid. Betaseron® is available with a prefilled liquid (diluent) that is mixed with the powder.

A systemic reaction may *rarely* occur with Copaxone® involving flushing, chest and joint pains, weakness, nausea, anxiety, and muscle stiffness. This reaction tends to resolve after about a quarter of an hour without any treatment.

## IMMUNOSUPPRESSIVE TREATMENTS

While Betaseron®, Avonex®, Copaxone®, and Rebif® belong to a category of medications called immunomodulators (modulating or moderating the immune system), other medications exist that generally, and less specifically, suppress the immune system. Some are taken by mouth (azathio-prine, methotrexate), while others are administered intravenously (mitoxantrone, cyclophosphamide).

Novantrone® (mitoxantrone) belongs to the general group of medicines called *anti-neoplastics*. Prior to its approval for use in MS, mitoxantrone was used only to treat certain forms of cancer. It acts in MS by sup-pressing the activity of T cells, B cells, and macrophages that are thought to lead the attack on the myelin sheath and axons.

The use of Novantrone® for the treat-ment of MS has been evaluated in a series of European studies over a period of 10 years. In a recent randomized, placebo-controlled, multicenter clinical trial involving patients with secondary-progressive or progressive-relapsing disease, participants received 12 mg/m² of Novantrone® by short intravenous infusion once every 3 months for 24 months. Novantrone® was found to delay the time to first treated relapse and time to disability progression. It also reduced the number of treated relapses and number of new lesions detected by MRI.

Based on findings from these studies, the FDA approved Novantrone® in October 2000 for reducing neurologic disability and/or the frequency of clinical relapses (attacks) in:

- *Secondary progressive* MS (SPMS—dis-ease that has changed from relapsing-remitting to a progressive course).
- *Progressive relapsing* MS (PRMS—dis-ease characterized by a gradual increase in disability from onset with clear relaps-es along the way).
- *Worsening relapsing-remitting* MS (Worsening RRMS—disease character-ized by clinical attacks without complete remission, resulting in a stepwise wors-ening of disability).

Novantrone® has not been approved for the treatment of primary progressive MS (PPMS—characterized by progression from disease onset with no acute attacks or remissions). At this time, there is no FDA-approved therapy for PPMS.

The evaluation of cardiac output is nec-essary before treatment is started. The drug should be used only in those with normal cardiac function, once every 3 months, at a dose of 12 mg/m². Periodic cardiac monitor-ing is required throughout the treatment period.

The lifetime cumulative dose is limited to 140 mg/m² (approximately 8–12 doses over 2 to 3 years) because of possible effects on the heart. Because Novantrone® can increase the risk for infection by decreasing the num-ber of protective white blood cells, blood counts and liver function tests should be evaluated prior to each dose.

It is important that your doctor check your progress at regular intervals to make sure that this medicine is working properly and to check for unwanted side effects.

While being treated with this medication, and during the period following treatment, do not have any immunizations (vaccina-tions) with live virus vaccines without your doctor's approval. Novantrone® may lower your body's resistance to infection, making you susceptible to the infection that the immunization is designed to help you avoid. Neither you nor anyone in your household should take the oral polio vaccine.

If possible, avoid people with infections. Contact your physician if you think you are getting an infection, or if you get a fever or chills, cough or hoarseness, lower back or side pain, or painful or difficult urination.

When receiving Novantrone®, it is important for your physician to know if you are taking any cancer medications or are being treated with radiation therapy.

The presence of other medical prob-lems may affect the use of Novantrone®. Let your doctor know if you have any of the following:

- Chicken pox or recent exposure to it
- Herpes zoster (shingles)
- Gout or history of gout or kidney stones
- Heart disease
- Liver disease

The fluid for infusion is dark blue and may cause your urine to become blue-green in color for 24 hours after each administration. The whites of the eyes may also appear bluish in color.

You should tell your doctor if you are pregnant or intending to have children. This medicine may cause birth defects if either the man or woman is receiving it at the time of conception. A pregnancy test is recommended prior to each treatment for women of childbearing age. Many medications of this type can cause permanent sterility. Be sure you have discussed this with your physician before taking this medication.

Because Novantrone® is excreted in human milk, breast-feeding should be discontinued before a woman starts treatment.

A higher incidence of leukemia has been reported in cancer patients previously treated with chemotherapy who were then treated with Novantrone®; however, the dose used was higher than that prescribed for treating MS.

Side effects that may go away as your body adjusts to the medication and do not require medical attention unless they continue or are bothersome include nausea, temporary hair loss, and menstrual disorders in women. Side effects that should be reported to your physician as soon as possible include fever or chills, lower back or side pain, painful or difficult urination, swelling of feet and lower legs, black tarry stools, cough or shortness of breath, sores in mouth and on lips, and stomach pain.

## CONCLUSION

Currently, there is no cure for MS, but there are treatments that modify disease activity, slow the course of the disease, and alleviate its effects. A number of new treatments are in the research stage or in clinical trials. Some of these are very promising indeed, and the current mood in MS research is very optimistic. We can look forward to more effective treatments in the near future.

Chapter 4

# Fatigue

June Halper, MSCN, ANP, FAAN

FATIGUE IS ONE of the most common symptoms of MS, occurring in about 80 percent of people. Fatigue can significantly interfere with a person's ability to function at home and at work, and may be the most prominent symptom in a person who otherwise has minimal activity limitations. Fatigue is a primary cause of early departure from the workforce.

The characteristics of MS fatigue that make it different from fatigue experienced by persons without MS include:

- Generally occurs on a daily basis
- May occur early in the morning, even after a restful night's sleep
- Tends to worsen as the day progresses
- Tends to be aggravated by heat and humidity
- Comes on more easily and suddenly
- Is generally more severe than normal fatigue
- Is more likely to interfere with daily responsibilities

Researchers believe that fatigue in MS is caused by poor nerve conduction through demyelinated nerve fibers that increases the amount of energy needed to perform normal activities. For example, simple household tasks such as washing dishes or making a bed may require more energy for a person with MS than for someone without the disease. Standing for long periods, working at a task for a long time, or concentrating on one activity may be very difficult because of fatigue. We now know that fatigue in MS can have many causes and it is important to carefully assess your lifestyle, MS symptoms, and emotional outlook when determining why you are tired. There are many strategies to improve stamina and reduce fatigue using new medications, lifestyle modifications, and rehabilitation services at the core of improvement.

## TYPES OF FATIGUE

Most people experience fatigue after physical exertion or emotional stress. Many people feel sleepy early in the afternoon as part of their natural body rhythm, particularly after eating a large meal. This type of fatigue improves with rest and sleep and normal restoration of energy. MS fatigue is different and can lead to alterations in symptoms and reduced function. Fatigue in MS may or may not correlate with the disease course—a mildly affected person may have severe fatigue, an individual who uses a wheelchair may have amazing stamina, or a person may experience increased fatigue only during exacerbations.

Many thought leaders have identified several types of fatigue that are unique to MS:

- Fatigue caused by sleep deprivation or sleep disturbance (this can be due directly to MS or to poorly managed symptoms such as bowel or bladder)
- Fatigue caused by dietary factors (overeating, eating hot meals, or inadequate diet)
- Deconditioning fatigue (loss of muscle tone from lack of use)
- Fatigue of handicap (trying to function without appropriate assistance or assistive devices)
- Fatigue associated with depression

- Neuromuscular fatigue (due to overactivity and muscle strain)
- Side effects of medications (to manage symptoms or modify the disease itself)
- Fatigue that is directly associated with the disease.

## HOW TO MINIMIZE AND MANAGE THE DIFFERENT TYPES OF FATIGUE

*Sleep deprivation.* Normal fatigue in people with MS can be managed by getting adequate rest at night and by napping at strategic times during the day. If you are experiencing insomnia, talk to your physician about medications that will help you sleep. In addition, training programs are available to help you relax and sleep. Many of these programs are offered through local medical centers and may require a referral from your physician. If sleep deprivation is caused by frequent awakening to urinate (nocturia), bladder management should be pursued with your physician. Bladder management strategies are discussed in Chapter 7 in this book, and will assist those of you experiencing problems with elimination to have adequate rest and sleep. In addition, there has been recent evidence that MS can cause sleep disturbance. Therefore, it is important that you discuss your concerns with your physician for appropriate management.

*Dietary factors.* What you eat fuels your body with energy stores. It is important for you to eat a well-balanced diet to minimize fatigue and maximize function. Good nutrition will also contribute to your skin integrity, your mood, and elimination patterns. (Nutrition is discussed in detail in Chapter 15, "The Role of Nutrition in Multiple Sclerosis.")

*Deconditioning.* Deconditioning, or lack of activity and exercise, can lead to a loss of muscle tone and aerobic capacity. Aerobic capacity is your ability to sustain activity without becoming tired and unable to complete your task. With guidance from your doctor and your rehabilitation specialist, you can initiate individualized aerobic programs to counteract this type of fatigue (see Chapter 13, "Exercise Options and Wellness Programs").

*Fatigue of handicap.* Urinary symptoms, bowel problems, incoordination, weakness, spasticity, and diminished capacity for ambulation can force you to adopt less efficient, more energy-consuming approaches to routine activities. Compensating for symptoms may, in turn, result in increased fatigue. Your level of function can be increased if you use assistive devices, such as wheelchairs and motorized tricarts, that conserve your energy. This strategy is called effective energy expenditure.

*Depression.* Your feelings of fatigue may be worsened by underlying depression. Depression is recognized as a symptom of MS and can also occur if life becomes very difficult when you are dealing with the day-to-day challenges of the disease. If so, feelings of overwhelming tiredness or lassitude may be unrelated to your level of activity and more to your mood. In addition, depression can affect sleep, appetite, motivation, and participation in activities. Such feelings can occur in the morning, afternoon, or evening. They do not appear to occur at any particular time of day; in fact, when you are depressed, you may wake up feeling tired. If you feel that your fatigue is related to depression, ask your physician to discuss what medications you can take to improve your mood. In addition, psychotherapy, stress management, relaxation training, and support groups can help you deal with the complexities of your disease and the symptoms it can cause.

*Neuromuscular fatigue.* Neuromuscular (muscle tiredness) fatigue is not well understood, but it appears to be the result of the demyelinated nerve fibers using more energy to conduct nerve signals. More research is needed in this area. Physical therapy is particularly useful in improving gait efficiency, decreasing spasticity, and developing an ongoing wellness program for you to follow throughout the week.

Medications such as methylphenidate (Ritalin®), modafinil (Provigil®), amantadine, pemoline (Cylert®; limited use at this time due to reported problems with liver function), or fluoxetine (Prozac®) have been reported to work well for people with MS. Ask your physician about obtaining a prescription for one of these drugs that you can use in conjunction with one or more of the above-mentioned strategies.

In addition, positive experiences, moderate exercise, relaxation, and cooling your core body temperature may reduce your fatigue and increase your stamina. Cooling can be accomplished by taking a cool shower or bath, swimming in cool water, drinking iced fluids, and using an external cooling device. Another important strategy is the use of a wheeled walker with a basket and a seat, reachers in the kitchen, a lightweight wheelchair, or a motorized scooter to conserve your energy at appropriate times.

*Consult a physical therapist (PT) or an occupational therapist (OT).* A consultation with a rehabilitation specialist (PT or OT) may be helpful in managing your fatigue. PTs can assist you to increase your stamina, improve your balance, and make your walking safer and more efficient. OTs can help you devise a special program to conserve your energy. There may be activities to help you increase your level of function and assistive devices that can reduce the amount of energy you expend doing simple tasks.

*Rearrange your routine.* You may decide that your daily routine should be rearranged so that you have energy left for later in the day. The following tips can help:

- Do physically demanding activities at a time of day when you feel less tired.
- Allow time to rest and put up your feet.
- Set realistic daily goals for yourself.
- Save your energy for the things that are the most meaningful and rewarding to you.

It is extremely important that you get enough sleep and rest. You may need 8 or more hours each night. If your sleep is interrupted, you may want to evaluate your sleep patterns. Ask yourself the following questions:

- Do I awaken during the night to go the bathroom? If so, why is this happening? Do I need bladder management? Could I have an infection? (Remember that an infection can worsen the symptoms of MS, including fatigue.)
- Am I eating too late in the evening? (A full stomach digesting a meal can interrupt sleep.)
- Am I comfortable at night? Is my bedroom well ventilated? Is my bed suitable?

Because fatigue can also be caused by treatable medical conditions such as depression, thyroid disease, or anemia, or may occur as a side effect of various medications or be the result of inactivity, persons with MS should consult a physician if fatigue becomes a problem. A comprehensive evaluation can help identify the factors contributing to fatigue and develop an approach suited to the individual.

All of these factors play an important role in getting enough sleep. First evaluate, then correct any problems that could be

## FSS Questionnaire

During the past week, I have found that:

1. My motivation is lower when I am fatigued.
   Score    1    2    3    4    5    6    7

2. Exercise brings on my fatigue.
   Score    1    2    3    4    5    6    7

3. I am easily fatigued.
   Score    1    2    3    4    5    6    7

4. Fatigue interferes with my physical functioning.
   Score    1    2    3    4    5    6    7

5. Fatigue causes frequent problems for me.
   Score    1    2    3    4    5    6    7

6. My fatigue prevents sustained physical functioning.
   Score    1    2    3    4    5    6    7

7. Fatigue interferes with carrying out certain duties and responsibilities.
   Score    1    2    3    4    5    6    7

8. Fatigue is among my three most disabling symptoms.
   Score    1    2    3    4    5    6    7

9. Fatigue interferes with my work, family, or social life.
   Score    1    2    3    4    5    6    7

### Scoring your results:

Now that you have completed the questionnaire, simply add all the numbers you circled to get your total score.

### The FSS key:

A total score of less than 36 suggests that you may not be suffering from fatigue.
A total score of 36 or more suggests that you may need further evaluation by your physician.

### Your next steps:

This scale should not be used to make your own diagnosis. If your score is 36 or more, please share this information with your clinician.

Reprinted with permission from Krupp LB, LaRocca NG, Muir-Nash J, Steinberg AD. The fatigue severity scale applied to patients with multiple sclerosis and systemic lupus erythematosus. *Arch Neurol* 1989;46:1121–1123.

preventing you from getting the rest you need to lead a fulfilling life.

Fatigue is a complex symptom of MS that must be managed in order to promote an optimal quality of life. Set daily goals for yourself. Put energy into the things that are most meaningful and rewarding. Ask yourself questions such as, "Is walking 10 blocks more important than spending time with family and friends?" Then, follow through on the changes required to reduce this symptom.

## THE FATIGUE SEVERITY SCALE

The Fatigue Severity Scale (FSS) is a method of evaluating fatigue in MS and other conditions. The FSS is designed to differentiate fatigue from clinical depression, since both share some of the same symptoms. Essentially, the FSS consists of answering a short questionnaire that requires the subject to rate his or her own level of fatigue. The obvious problem with this measure is its subjectivity.

The FSS questionnaire on page 26 containing nine statements that attempt to explore severity of fatigue symptoms. The subjects are asked to read each statement and circle a number from 1 to 7, depending on how appropriate they felt the statement applied to them over the preceding week. A low value indicates that the statement is not very appropriate, whereas a high value indicates agreement.

# Chapter 5
# Pain Management
Mary Ann Picone, MD

PAIN IS AN OFTEN overlooked symptom in multiple sclerosis (MS)—one that many doctors don't associate with the disease. Pain is reported by people with both relapsing and progressive forms of MS. For many patients, pain may be the most debilitating aspect of the disease, affecting their ability to function and, therefore, their overall quality of life. Pain occurs in about 80 percent of those with MS; about 20 percent experience significant pain. Up to 15 percent suffer chronic pain and often seek relief from a chiropractor, a physical therapist, or an acupuncturist, in addition to a neurologist. Women are twice as likely to have pain symptoms as men.

One effect of MS is to hamper the nervous system's ability to shut out painful sensations. This results in an influx of information that is not wanted and often can't be controlled. For example, sensations known as *paresthesias* are often associated with MS. Paresthesias can be felt as burning, pressure, or pins-and-needles tingling. They can be merely annoying or very uncomfortable. Some people with MS cannot tolerate the touch of clothing on their skin.

Physical and emotional factors also can cause pain or make it worse. If an individual has a lot of physical or emotional problems, pain will be less tolerable than if the individual is basically happy. Chronic pain can, in turn, lead to depression.

If you are experiencing pain, you may worry that it indicates a worsening of your disease. This is not the case. The severity, location, and extent of pain bear little relationship to the extent or seriousness of MS. People who have MS are also subject to other medical conditions, such as migraine headaches, low back pain, arthritis, and cardiac or abdominal disease. Your pain may stem from sources other than MS and should always be investigated and treated by your physician.

## PAIN SYNDROMES

Several pain syndromes can affect those with MS (see Table 5.1). One type, *neuralgia*, can cause pain along specific nerve routes, usually the cranial nerves (nerves in the head), but it can strike throughout the body. Occasionally patients may complain of a tight bandlike sensation across the abdomen, and this can be secondary to demyelination lesions present in the thoracic spinal cord.

*Trigeminal neuralgia* is pain along the fifth cranial nerve and causes sharp jolting electrical sensations in the face (Figure 5.1). It can last a few seconds at a time, or it can last for hours. Some people suffer from stinging or burning sensations at points in the abdomen and chest, sometimes so severe as to cause limitation of movement.

## MEDICATIONS FOR MS-RELATED PAIN

Medications are usually successful in alleviating MS-related pain, but determining which drug at what dosage is right for you can be a time-consuming process that may take days and even weeks. Often, a trial-and-error period is involved, because some drugs can take weeks to deliver relief, while others must be taken in combination to be effective. Be patient, and take comfort in the fact that most MS-related pain is temporary, so treatment is generally short-term.

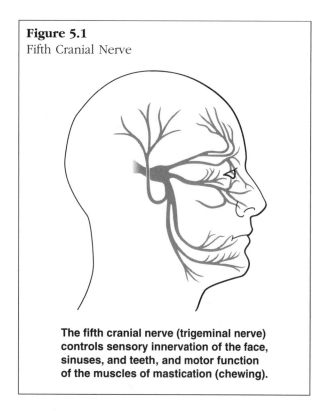

**Figure 5.1**
Fifth Cranial Nerve

**The fifth cranial nerve (trigeminal nerve) controls sensory innervation of the face, sinuses, and teeth, and motor function of the muscles of mastication (chewing).**

Baclofen, a drug that is usually taken orally, is very useful in treating spasticity and neuralgic pain. Tricyclic antidepressants, such as amitriptyline (Elavil®) and nortriptyline (Pamelor®), are also helpful. When using these drugs, physicians often start at a low dosage that is increased gradually until it is effective. Do not abandon a medication before you have given it sufficient time or reached a high enough dosage for it to work.

Both baclofen and tricyclic antidepressants work to calm excited nerve fibers and can be used in combination. With the tricyclic antidepressants, the most common side effects are dry mouth, fatigue, urinary hesitation, and weight gain.

Other drugs used in treating chronic pain include anticonvulsants, such as carbamazepine (Tegretol®), gabapentin (Neurontin®), clonazepam (Klonopin®), phenytoin (Dilantin®), divalproex (Depakote®), and most recently the newer anticonvulsants, oxcarbazepine (Trileptal®), levetiracetam (Keppra®), topiramate (Topamax®), and lamotrigine (Lamictal®). The dosage used to treat pain is often lower than that used to control seizures. Side effects of the anticonvulsants may include sleepiness and nausea. Liver dysfunction may also occur, which is detected by blood tests that monitor liver function. Lowered white blood cell counts can also be seen. Both liver function studies and blood counts should be monitored periodically. Nonsteroidal anti-inflammatory drugs can also be helpful in treating pain, but usually for only a short time due to concerns with gastrointestinal side effects. Often, especially with trigeminal neuralgia, which tends to have remissions, you can be on drugs intermittently and may not need preventive medication on a long-term basis. Creams such as capsaicin and topical anesthetic patches such as the Lidoderm® patch can be helpful on the skin in areas that experience pain.

## REHABILITATION PROGRAMS

Physical therapy is often effective in reducing back pain or spasticity. Swimming and other forms of aquatherapy are helpful. Ultrasound, massage, stretching, and gait training can reduce discomfort, treat injury, and improve function.

## PAIN MANAGEMENT THROUGH SURGERY

Severe spasticity in the lower extremities can be associated with pain. In these cases, benefit may be obtained from an intrathecal (within the spine) *baclofen pump*, which delivers tiny doses of baclofen directly into the spinal fluid by a surgically implanted pump. Morphine can also be delivered this way.

Nerve blocks (injections of local anesthetic into the inflamed nerve) can also be used.

**Table 5.1**

Origins of Pain in Multiple Sclerosis

| Origin | Where | Why | What Helps |
|---|---|---|---|
| Musculoskeletal pain | Sacral-tailbone area and hipbone | Immobility causes pressure on body | Swing legs back and forth, as in walking. |
| | Muscles, tendons, and ligaments | Keeping a limb in a fixed position "freezes" muscles so it becomes painful to change position | Change position frequently; practice a few minutes of physical therapy daily; sit in a rocking chair with feet supported at a 90-degree angle. |
| | Spasms in muscles | When there is spinal cord involvement, flexor spasms occur. | Try medication such as baclofen by mouth or implanted pump, tizanidine by mouth, or clonazepam by mouth. Move often to decrease the severity of spasms. |
| | | Sudden shortening of large muscles can result in cramps. | Keep a board at the foot of the bed; press ball of foot against it as soon as cramp occurs. Watch diet. Inadequate intake of potassium can cause muscle cramps. |
| Neurological pain | Burning or aching sensations in the limbs; tight or constrictive pain around the trunk | Defective conduction of nerve impulses in the spinal cord and brain results in abnormal sensations. | Apply warm compresses to the skin to relieve burning pain; use antidepressants such as amitriptyline to modify how the central nervous system reacts to pain. An anticonvulsive, gabapertin, may also help. Firmly wrap an Ace bandage over the area—but not over the face—to alter the sensation from pain to pressure, being careful that the bandage is kept loose enough to allow free circulation. |
| | Sharp pain in the face is called trigeminal neuralgia. | | Baclofen, carbamazepine, gabapentin, alone or in conjunction, have been used successfully. |

In severe cases of pain, surgery can be performed to cut some of the spinal sensory nerves. Called partial posterior rhizotomy, these surgical cuts are irreversible.

In summary, pain can be a significant symptom of MS. A combination of modalities often provides the best outcome. Physical therapy, emotional support, and drug therapy, along with a trusting relationship between patient and doctor, often prove the most helpful.

# Chapter 6
# Maintaining Joint Flexibility and Mobility
June Halper, MSCN, ANP, FAAN and Nancy J. Holland, EdD, RN, MSCN

Your body is made up of a series of bone junctions called *joints*. Their purpose is to provide motion within your body and to support or bear weight. Each joint is surrounded by muscles, tendons, ligaments, and a joint capsule. These provide stability to the joint.

The range of motion (or number of degrees of motion) of a joint is determined by the tightness of the ligaments, tendons, muscles, and joint capsule surrounding that joint. The looser or more flexible the structures, the more movement; the tighter the structures, the less movement. Generally, a person's everyday movements are enough to keep the joints loose and flexible, but weakness caused by multiple sclerosis (MS) can interfere with the full range of motion of the joints.

## IMPACT OF LOSS OF MOTION

If any of your joints—whether your hips, knees, or shoulders—are tight, you may find that the number of positions you can move into independently is limited. This, in turn, may limit the types of activities you can do for yourself.

Tightness in your trunk and legs can affect your sitting or standing posture, especially when one side of your body feels tighter than the other. This can lead to a curving or twisting of your back and can throw your balance off. It also can interfere with cleansing your groin and with positioning your legs during sex.

Decreased range of motion in your arms, legs, and trunk tends to increase pressure at localized points and to prevent pressure from being evenly distributed. This

localization of pressure significantly increases your risk of skin breakdown or pressure sores (called *decubiti*).

If you use a manual wheelchair, you may experience tightness in the anterior (front of the body) muscles of the shoulder, leading to a rounded shoulder posture. Careful stretching of these muscles and strengthening of the posterior (back of the shoulder) muscles are essential to improve your posture and maintain healthy, pain-free shoulders.

Range-of-motion exercises are the most basic element of an activity program for people with MS. Moving joints through their full range of motion even once a day will help to prevent development of contractures (frozen joints) and of permanently reduced range of motion of a particular joint. Maintaining the flexibility of your joints and of the structures around them will also decrease spasticity of your muscles.

Your physical or occupational therapist can design a series of range-of-motion exercises specifically for you. If you are not able to do these exercises by yourself, your therapist can teach you to instruct others to do the exercises with you. Remember, even if you are unable to do the exercises by yourself, it is important that they be done—daily.

When doing your range-of-motion exercises, allow plenty of time for your muscles and other structures to loosen and stretch. Try to hold a position for a slow count of 10. When you are moving your body, move slowly and smoothly. Then, as you hold the position, maintain a firm, but gentle pressure. Do not bounce your body, as this tends to encourage spastic muscles to tighten. Repeat each exercise 10 times.

## SELF-STRETCHING

The following are important points to remember when stretching:

- Never use excessive force when stretching. Use only enough force to allow the muscle fibers to stretch.
- Hold the position still. Don't bounce, especially if you have spasticity. Holding still allows your muscle fibers to relax and stretch. Bouncing increases the tension in muscles. Excessive force can result in fractures, torn or pulled muscles, or dislocated joints.
- Do your stretching program when you are least tired and when you have adequate time.
- Exercise in a cool environment.

## TYPES OF EXERCISES

The following series of range-of-motion exercises uses the SAM format, which describes the correct body position for you and your attendant, if you need assistance, and details the proper motions for you to perform the exercises safely. Remember 10-10-1. Hold for a slow 10 count, repeat 10 times, one session a day.

### SAM

**S:** Your starting position
**A:** Your attendant's or care partner's action and position
**M:** The actual movement

### HAND MOBILIZATION

**S:** Place your palm down, with your thumb and fingers relaxed.
**A:** Cup your hand in both hands, with attendant's right thumb and index finger holding one knuckle while the left thumb and index finger hold the next knuckle over.
**M:** Push one hand down gently on the knuckle it is holding while the other

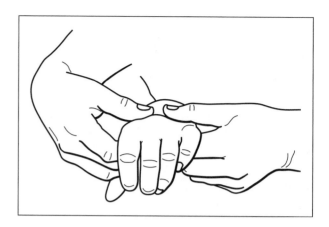

hand pushes up; then, reverse directions and move across your hand.

### FINGER ABDUCTION

**S:** Straighten your wrist and relax your fingers and thumb.
**A:** Holds adjacent fingers straight.
**M:** Spread fingers apart.

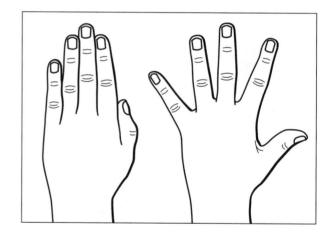

### FINGER EXTENSION

**S:** Relax your wrist and fingers.
**A:** Supports your forearm and keeps your

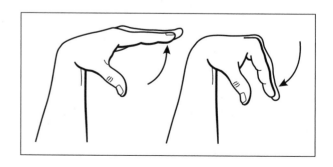

wrist bent down with one hand while the other hand cups your fingertips.

**M:** Bend your wrist straight down to your fingers; the movement should come from your knuckles and the joints of your fingers, not from your wrist.

### THUMB OPPOSITION

**S:** Place your palm up with your fingers and thumb relaxed.

**A:** Holds your thumb over your nail.

**M:** Touch the tip of your thumb to the base of your little finger.

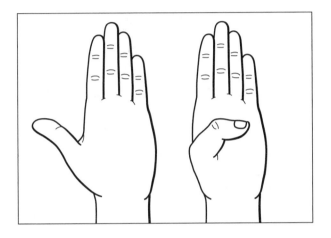

### THUMB ABDUCTION AND EXTENSION

**S:** Place your palm up with your fingers and thumb relaxed.

**A:** Stabilizes your palm with one hand while the other grasps your thumb; your attendant's thumb should be at the base of your thumb.

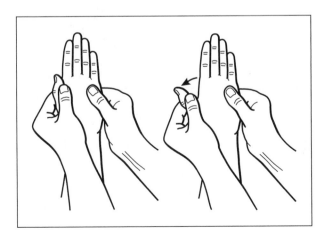

**M:** Move your thumb out and away from your palm as if you were hitchhiking.

### TRUNK BENDING

**S:** Lie on your back with your legs together and your knees slightly bent.

**A:** Kneels at your feet with both hands placed on your knees.

**M:** Bend your knees to your chest, stretching your back muscles.

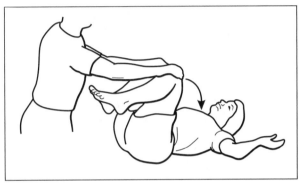

### TRUNK ROTATION

**S:** Lie on your back with your knees bent to your chest.

**A:** Kneels at your feet with both hands placed on your knees.

**M:** Rotate your knees and hips to one side; bring them as close to the bed as they will go; keep your shoulders flat on the bed.

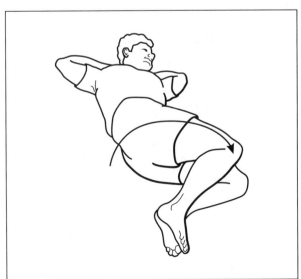

Chapter 6: Maintaining Joint Flexibility and Mobility    35

Your attendant may need to put one hand on your opposite shoulder to hold it down.

### Heel Cord (Gastrocnemius/Soleus)

**S:** Lie on your back with your knees straight.

**A:** Cups one hand on the inside of your heel, with the forearm pressed up against the ball of your foot.

**M:** Keeping your knee straight, attendant pulls down at your heel and presses up with the forearm, bending your foot toward your knee.

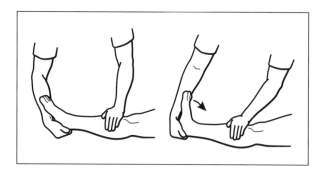

### Leg Rotation

**S:** Lie in bed with your legs straight and relaxed.

**A:** Places both hands on top of your thigh, or places one hand on top of your thigh and the other underneath your thigh.

**M:** Roll your knee in and out. Do not let your attendant's hands fall below your knee or there will be excessive stress to your knee.

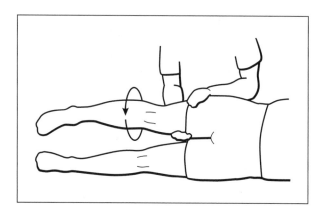

### Hip Flexion and Extension

**S:** Lie on your back with your toes pointing toward the ceiling, one knee bent toward your chest.

**A:** Places one hand on your bent knee and the other hand just above the knee of your straight leg.

**M:** Bend your bent leg further toward your chest, keeping your other leg straight on the bed.

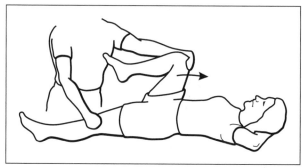

### Hip Extension

**S:** Lie on your side, not leaning forward or backward, with your upper leg slightly bent.

**A:** Kneels behind you, one arm cupping under your knee with your calf resting on the attendant's forearm and the other hand holding your pelvis in place.

**M:** Pull your leg straight back toward your attendant.

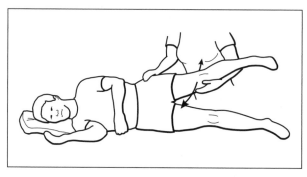

### Hip Abduction with Knees Bent

**S:** Lie on your back with your legs bent.

**A:** Kneels at your feet, with your feet between the attendant's knees to hold

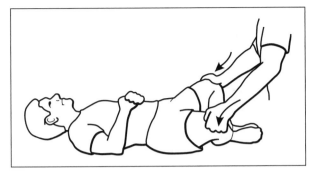

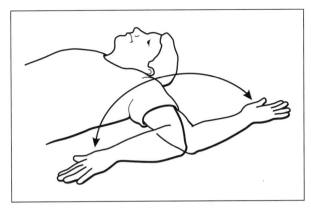

them in place, both hands placed on your knees.

**M:** Spread your knees apart and pull them down toward the bed, applying a firm, but not heavy pressure.

### SHOULDER EXTENSION

**S:** Sit in your chair or lie in bed on your side.

**A:** Stabilizes your shoulder with one hand while the other cups your arm near your elbow.

**M:** Bring your arm behind you as if you were going to reach into your rear pocket.

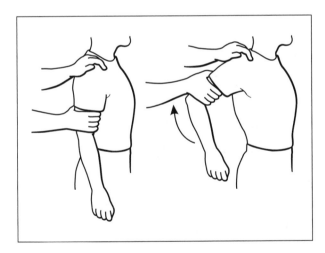

### SHOULDER ROTATION

**S:** Lie on your back with your arm out to your side at a 90-degree angle, and your elbow bent at a 90-degree angle.

**A:** Cups your elbow with one hand while the other supports your wrist and hand.

**M:** Rotate your hand to the bed toward your pillow and then down to the bed by

your hip. Keep your shoulder and elbow bent at a 90-degree angle.

### ABDUCTION

**S:** Lie on your back with your arm at your side and your palm up.

**A:** Supports your hand and wrist with one hand while the other cups your elbow.

**M:** Bring your arm out to your side and up to your head (similar to the movement in jumping jacks).

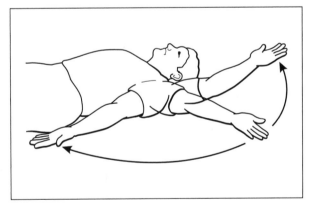

### FORWARD FLEXION

**S:** Lie on your back with your arm at your side, palm up.

**A:** Supports your wrist or hand with one hand while the other supports the back of your elbow.

**M:** Raise your arm up over your head, keeping your forearm in front of your elbow straight, as if you were raising your hand to ask a question.

### STRAIGHT LEG RAISE

**S:** Lie on your back with your legs straight and slightly apart.

**A:** Two positions are possible:

• Kneels between your legs, with one hand cupping your heel while the other hand holds the knee of the same leg. The attendant's knee may be resting lightly on your other thigh to stabilize your leg on the bed.

• Kneels between your legs, with your heel cord resting on the attendant's shoulder. One of the attendant's hands should be placed on that knee to keep it straight; the other hand should be on your other thigh to stabilize that leg on the bed.

**M:** Slowly raise your leg up, keeping your knee straight. Do not allow your leg to roll out. When your raised knee begins to bend slightly from the tension, ask your attendant to lower your leg slightly and hold. Do not move beyond the leg pointing straight up to the ceiling.

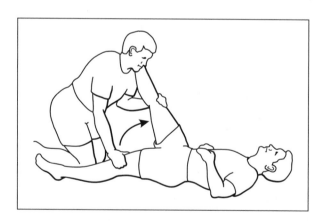

Please remind your care partner or attendant to use careful movements and to protect against stretching out or hurting his or her back!

### SUPINATION AND PRONATION

**S:** Lie on your back with your arm at your side and your elbow bent at a 90-degree angle.

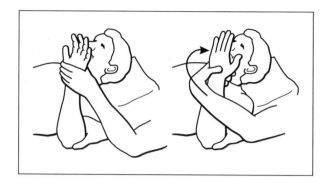

**A:** Supports your wrist and hand and stabilizes your arm just above your elbow.

**M:** Turn your palm up, then turn your palm down. Repeat, keeping your elbow straight.

### ELBOW FLEXION AND EXTENSION

**S:** Lie on your back with your arm straight at your side, palm up.

**A:** Supports your wrist and hand with one hand while the other stabilizes your upper arm.

**M:** Straighten your arm to its fullest, then bend your elbow, bringing your hand to your shoulder.

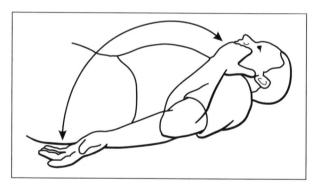

### SCAPULAR PROTRACTION

**S:** Lie on your side with your arm resting on your hip or behind your back.

**A:** Cups one hand on the front of your shoulder, with the other placed so that the pinkie side of the attendant's hand is next to your shoulder blade.

**M:** Applying a firm pressure backward on your shoulder, slide the other hand under your shoulder blade, lifting away from your back.

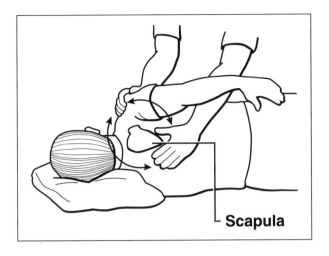

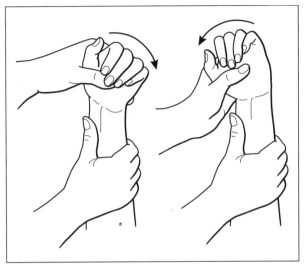

### SCAPULAR CIRCUMDUCTION

**S:** Lie on your side with your arm resting on your hip or behind your back.

**A:** Cups one hand on the front of your shoulder, with the other placed so that the web of the thumb meets with the angle of your shoulder blade.

**M:** Moving both hands circularly in the same direction, roll the shoulder blade slowly in a large circle.

### FINGER FLEXION

**S:** Bend your wrist up, keeping your fingers relaxed.

**A:** Supports your hand and wrist.

**M:** Gently bend your fingers toward your palm, being certain to keep your wrist cocked (bent) up.

**A:** Supports your hand with one hand while the other stabilizes your forearm.

**M:** Move your hand from side to side, not allowing your wrist to bend up or down.

### WRIST FLEXION AND EXTENSION

**S:** Relax your wrist and fingers.

**A:** Supports your forearm with one hand while the other hand clasps your palm, being certain that your fingers are free to move.

**M:** Bend your wrist down, allowing your fingers to straighten at will. Bend your wrist up, being certain that your attendant's hand and fingers do not interfere with your fingers' bending.

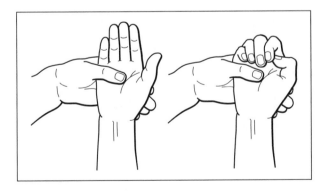

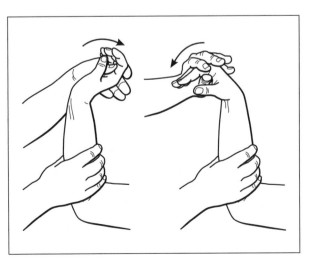

### WRIST DEVIATION

**S:** Keep your wrist in line with your arm, not bent up or down.

## ADAPTIVE DEVICES

Although exercise helps maintain physical function and muscle tone, MS can cause loss of strength, spasticity, and incoordination. Many types of adaptive devices can help you deal with the problems in physical functioning caused by MS. These devices can be thought of as tools to promote safety and maximal function. The best way to determine which device is best for you is to consult a rehabilitation specialist—a physiatrist, occupational therapist, physical therapist, or rehabilitation nurse. A specialist can evaluate your needs and capabilities, and make recommendations that will accommodate fluctuations in your condition.

The following assistive devices are commonly used by people with MS.

### LEG BRACES

If spasticity, which is caused by involuntary muscle contractions, stiffens your knees and hips and pushes down on your feet, you may have trouble stepping high enough for your feet to clear the floor or ground. Climbing stairs or walking uphill becomes especially difficult.

A laminated polyethylene short leg brace can support the dropped foot. This device keeps the toes clear of the ground, thereby reducing the amount of energy needed to walk and lessening the risk of falls. The leg brace fits into a shoe and is not noticeable to others.

### MOBILITY AIDS

If loss of coordination becomes a problem, you can keep your gait within safe limits by using a mobility aid, such as a cane, walker, wheelchair, or electric scooter. Walking aids stabilize locomotion. Different types of aids offer varying degrees of stability, which are determined by the broadness of the walking aid.

Consult with a rehabilitation specialist to find out how much stabilization you require. This specialist can also teach you the best way to walk, go through a doorway, navigate stairs, sit down, get up from a chair, and enter and exit a car while using the aid. Remember that your use of a walking aid must be reevaluated periodically because your body undergoes changes as a result of the MS.

### CANES

If you have only a slight problem with stabilization, a simple cane may be sufficient. Canes are usually used on the side toward which the individual staggers (the weaker side). A quad cane—that is, a cane with four supporting points at the base—offers greater stabilization than a cane with a single tip. Quad canes come with a stable or a swivel-action base, depending on the amount of stability required. (See Figure 6.1.)

To determine the proper height of a cane, stand upright with the cane at your side. The height is correct when your elbow is at a 30-degree angle.

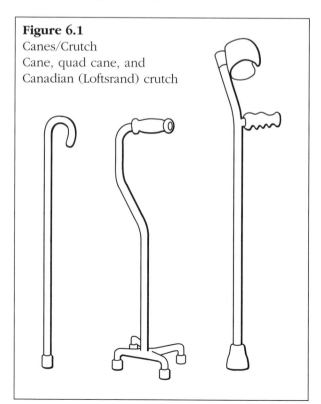

**Figure 6.1**
Canes/Crutch
Cane, quad cane, and
Canadian (Loftsrand) crutch

## WALKERS

Walkers are light aluminum structures with two supporting points on each side. Walkers are lifted and advanced prior to each step. Walkers offer greater stability than canes. The proper height for a walker is the same as for a cane.

Folding walkers are available and are more convenient to transport from one location to another. Occasionally, a wheeled walker or one with a seat might be prescribed. These may come with baskets to carry personal items. Please make sure that your walker, if it has wheels, is fitted with a safe braking apparatus.

Some people resist using a walking aid because of its appearance. However, the price of not using an aid is further restriction of movement. Some people with MS confine themselves because they fear for their safety or feel they will appear to be intoxicated in public. If you need a walking aid, consider the many advantages it will provide. Being able to visit friends, shop, or frequent a park will broaden your horizons and deepen your connection to the world.

## WHEELCHAIRS

It is possible that a person with MS will reach a point in the progression of the disease where walking is no longer possible, despite every effort to restore or maintain it. Although almost everyone fears the prospect of using a wheelchair, those who do so find that even occasional use increases their sense of freedom and conserves their energy. Many people begin using a wheelchair part-time, when they must travel long distances or when walking becomes too tiring.

Not all wheelchairs or wheelchair users are alike. If you still have arm motion, a wheelchair can help you maintain physical fitness because so much energy is required to move the chair. However, if your upper extremities are too weak or uncoordinated

to move the chair, or if you find the process too exhausting, a better option might be a motorized chair or vehicle such as a scooter. Consult a rehabilitation specialist to help you find a wheelchair that is right for your physical capabilities, lifestyle, and body size. Don't buy a wheelchair from someone else because it probably won't be right for you and your insurance won't pay for it. Do not use a wheelchair that has worn or missing brakes. Do not allow anyone else to use or play with your wheelchair, because wheelchairs can and do get broken.

Your safety and comfort come first! The narrower and simpler the wheelchair, the better. A chair with removable armrests will enable you to fit the wheelchair under a desk or table, and to transfer in and out of it more easily. Footrests should swing away to allow for ease in transfer and maneuverability. The seat cushion should align the body properly to prevent skin breakdown, assist with transfers, and promote overall comfort.

For the best fit, sit in the wheelchair and check the following:

- Is there a hand's width space between the seat edge and the back of your knee?
- Is there room for two fingers between your thighs and the wheelchair sides?
- Is the backrest comfortable? The top of the rest should end at about the middle of your shoulder blades.
- Do your arms rest comfortably on the armrests?
- Are your thighs parallel to the floor?

Currently, there are many options for wheeled mobility. These include motorized wheelchairs with adaptations such as "tilt-in-space" to relieve continual pressure on your buttocks; scooters for those of you who are able to walk but not long distances; and motorized units that combine features of wheelchairs and motorized tricarts. These devices are costly and may or may not be covered by insurance. Please check with your carrier and make sure all necessary paperwork is completed before you move forward in what can be a very costly purchase.

Consider getting special training to help you learn how to transfer yourself from the wheelchair to a bed, to another seat, into a shower or bathtub, and into an automobile.

Transfer training will also teach you:

- What supporting surfaces are most effective.
- How to use sliding boards when your arms are weak.

- How to strengthen the muscles required for transferring.
- How to move in the shortest and most direct way.

If you have maintained your range of motion, you can often do transfer maneuvers by yourself, so that your activities are restricted only minimally.

All of these adaptive devices—leg braces, canes, walkers, and wheelchairs—promote maximum independence and minimal risk. They can boost your spirits and raise your quality of life.

# Chapter 7
# Bladder and Bowel Management
Nancy J. Holland, EdD, RN, MSCN and Margie O'Leary, MSN, RN, MSCN

PROBLEMS WITH the passage of urine and stool as the result of multiple sclerosis (MS) can be a source of discomfort as well as great embarrassment and distress. Losing full control over these functions may make you feel like a small child again. Fortunately, there are ways to regain control that will also help you to feel better about yourself.

## BLADDER MANAGEMENT

Proper treatment of urinary dysfunction is probably the greatest factor in increasing the life expectancy of people with MS and in reducing the number of MS-related hospitalizations. In addition to interfering with daily activities, bladder infections and other urinary complications can cause serious illness. The good news is that bladder symptoms can be controlled and complications prevented with proper assessment and treatment.

Understanding how the urinary system works will help you to make sense of the problems you encounter and the ways to address them. The urinary system consists of the kidneys, ureters, bladder, sphincters, and urethra (see Figures 7.1 and 7.2). Urine is produced in the kidneys from waste that is filtered out of the bloodstream and mixed with water. Urine passes out of the kidneys through thin tubes, called *ureters*, into the bladder, where it is stored until about a cupful has accumulated. Under normal circumstances, the urge to urinate (void) is experienced at this time. The external sphincter is voluntarily relaxed, and urine is released down the urethra and out of the body through the meatus. Normal urination involves coordinating the bladder muscle

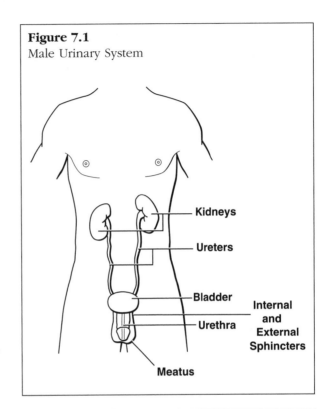

**Figure 7.1**
Male Urinary System

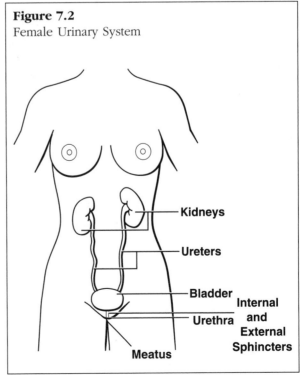

**Figure 7.2**
Female Urinary System

(called the *detrusor*, it has elastic properties like a balloon), which contracts to push the urine out, and the external sphincter, which relaxes to allow free flow of the urine out of the body.

TYPES OF BLADDER DYSFUNCTION

Several types of dysfunction in the urinary system can occur:

*Storage dysfunction.* Storage dysfunction occurs when the bladder signals the urge to urinate even though only a small amount of urine has accumulated. The bladder muscle contracts excessively.

*Emptying dysfunction.* Emptying dysfunction occurs when the bladder does not signal the desire to urinate at the proper time and allows an excessive amount of urine to collect. This stretches the elastic balloon-like detrusor muscle and makes it less able to perform effectively.

*Combined dysfunction.* Combined dysfunction occurs when the bladder signals the urge to urinate when only a small amount of urine has collected and at the same time the sphincter contracts, resulting in incomplete emptying. Because the bladder continues to push urine against a partially closed sphincter, the urine may be forced back up the ureters into the kidneys, causing damage.

SYMPTOMS OF URINARY DYSFUNCTION

Urinary dysfunction in MS is associated with spinal cord disease and is called *neurogenic bladder.* The following symptoms may occur:

*Urgency.* Once the urge to urinate or void is experienced, it cannot be postponed. The person must always be near a toilet.

*Frequency.* Urination occurs more often than every 3 hours.

*Hesitancy.* The urge to urinate is experienced, but the person has difficulty initiating the flow of urine.

*Incontinence.* Urine leaks before the person can reach a toilet.

*Nocturia.* The person awakens during the night to urinate.

*Urinary tract infection (UTI) or cystitis.* This occurs when bacteria in the bladder multiply and cause inflammation. Anyone can develop a bladder infection, but if you have MS, you should suspect neurogenic bladder and check beyond just treating the infection. Incomplete bladder emptying can lead to UTI, because the accumulated urine provides a place for bacteria to multiply. Symptoms of UTI may include any combination of the following:

- Burning or pain during urination (dysuria)
- Frequency
- Urgency
- Incontinence
- Pain in the lower back or abdomen
- Foul-smelling urine
- Fever and chills

ASSESSMENT OF BLADDER DYSFUNCTION

Bladder problems cannot be diagnosed on symptoms alone. Testing is always necessary. The first step is to check for possible bladder infection. Two laboratory tests are used for this purpose: urinalysis and culture and sensitivity.

*Urinalysis.* The urine is tested for the presence of white cells or nitrates, which indicate an infection is present.

*Culture and sensitivity (C&S).* If the urinalysis indicates an infection, a C&S will be done. A few drops of urine are placed on a culture medium in the laboratory, and the bacteria are allowed to grow for 48 hours. The bacteria are then identified and tested against a series of antibiotics to determine the most effective treatment for the infection.

A sterile urine specimen is needed, which is most often obtained using the "clean catch" technique. You will be given a special kit, sealed to ensure sterility, for obtaining a clean catch. Follow these steps with the kit:

1. Clean the urinary opening, using a front-to-back motion, with the towelette provided.
2. Pass a few drops of urine into the toilet to clear the urinary passage.
3. Pass urine into a sterile container without touching the inside of the container or cover.
4. Keep the specimen cool until you deliver it to the laboratory or doctor's office.

If the urinalysis indicates that an infection is present, the physician or healthcare provider will often prescribe an antibiotic for you to take until the C&S results are available. When the results are known, the doctor can determine which antibiotic is best for the particular strain of bacteria growing in your system.

RESIDUAL URINE DETERMINATION

Residual urine determination is measurement of the amount of urine left in the bladder after an attempt to fully empty it. Incomplete emptying can cause any combination of the symptoms described earlier. It also poses a serious risk to your health. Retained urine provides a place for bacteria to multiply, causing recurrent UTIs, and allows mineral deposits to settle and form stones, called calculi. Calculi are contributing causes of UTIs. They also irritate the bladder. Several tests are designed to determine the presence of residual urine.

*Diagnostic catheterization.* After an attempt to fully empty your bladder, the nurse or physician passes a thin hollow tube, called a *catheter*, through the meatus to drain the remaining urine.

*Ultrasound.* Conductive jelly is applied to the lower abdomen, and an instrument that looks like a microphone is moved slowly over the area. This is replacing diagnostic catheterization as the most common method used to check for residual urine.

*Radioisotope renal/residual urine study.* This test looks at kidney (renal) function, as well as at residual urine. A radioisotope is injected into a vein and the abdominal area is scanned to visualize the entire urinary system.

*Intravenous pyelogram (IVP).* This test, which also requires an injection into a vein, visualizes the entire urinary system. However, IVP is an X-ray that requires an empty bowel for the urinary system to become visible. This makes IVP less desirable than other procedures, because laxatives and enemas must be used.

*Urodynamic studies (UDS).* UDS involves measurement of pressure within the bladder and direct assessment of the function of the external sphincter, as well as other factors. The test is performed with the person lying on an examining table, with feet in stirrups. A urinary catheter is put in place for the duration of the procedure, as well as a probe in the rectum. The results of UDS help the urologist determine the nature of the problem and the appropriate treatment(s).

*Cystoscopy.* A thin tube with a light and a magnifier is passed through the meatus and urethra into the bladder, permitting the physician to look directly into the bladder for inflammation, polyps, or other abnormalities.

### TREATMENT OF STORAGE DYSFUNCTION

To control storage dysfunction, the hyperactive bladder must be relaxed by medication, such as imipramine (Tofranil®), oxybutynin (Ditropan or Ditropan XL®), tolterodine actrate (Detrol®) or tropsium chloride (Sanctura®), which may be prescribed for you. These drugs are effective, but you may need to try them all to find which one or which combination at what dosage works best for you. The main side effects are dry mouth and constipation. When nocturia is not relieved by these drugs (or others that have a similar anticholinergic effect), desmopressin acetate (DDAVP) may be helpful. This drug is taken either as a nasal spray or an oral tablet at bedtime.

In addition to the medications, or if you prefer not to take medications, the following nonmedical measures will help.

*Normally, you should drink plenty of fluids.* Water, especially, is necessary to flush wastes, mineral deposits, and bacteria from your urinary system. Try adding fluids slowly if bladder infections have been a problem.

*A paradox: Restrict your fluids.* Beginning about 2 hours prior to an activity where a bathroom is not available, begin restricting your fluid intake. You will have to time yourself to get an accurate personal picture. It is important not to restrict fluids on a continuous basis, however, because the resulting concentrated urine will be an irritant that can worsen the problem. If you are bothered by nighttime frequency, restricting fluids 3 hours before bedtime may be helpful.

Limit fluids that contain caffeine, aspartame (an artificial sweetener), or alcohol. These substances can increase bladder

symptoms. Controlling them will help you control the symptoms associated with storage dysfunction.

*Wear absorbent pads.* Absorbent pads can give you additional security. A variety of products is available. Each contains a powder that turns to a gel when fluid is added.

If you are a man, you may find a condom catheter useful at certain times. A condom catheter is a condom-like sheath attached to a tube leading to a drainage bag that is strapped to the leg.

If these measures do not control your symptoms, especially incontinence, your doctor may prescribe a high dosage of an anticholinergic medication, which may convert your bladder to the emptying dysfunction type. Management of this condition is described below.

### TREATMENT FOR EMPTYING DYSFUNCTION

Intermittent catheterization has had a dramatic effect on management of emptying dysfunction. This eliminates residual urine, which causes UTIs and stones, and contributes significantly to overall health. A catheter is inserted through the meatus into the bladder to allow all the urine in the bladder to empty, usually into the toilet. The process is as follows:

1. Wash hands and urinate.
2. Wash around the urinary opening, perhaps using a towelette.
3. Insert the catheter and allow urine to flow into the toilet.
4. Remove the catheter, wash it with soap and water, dry it, and place it in a plastic bag. The catheter may be reused as long as it remains clear.

This procedure may sound difficult or unpleasant but, with practice, it is easily carried out in just a few minutes.

When intermittent catheterization is not possible, a catheter may have to be left in full-time, or a surgical procedure may be required. Whatever method is used, the critical element is not to have urine stagnate in the bladder. If urine is being retained, it is helpful to promote an acid urine, because bacteria do not thrive in an acid environment. The following measures can help:

- One gram of methenamine mandelate (Mandelamine®) or hippuric acid (Hiprex®) two times per day.
- Limit citrus juices because they produce an alkaline urine despite the presence of ascorbic acid.
- Drink cranberry juice or have cranberry tablets several times daily to aid urinary acidification.
- Limit your intake of red meats, concentrate on "white" meats—chicken, fish, etc.

### TREATMENT FOR COMBINED DYSFUNCTION

Treatment for both storage and emptying dysfunction employs a combination of measures. Taking anticholinergic medication relaxes the hyperactive bladder, and intermittent catheterization removes dangerous residual urine. Complex bladder problems may require a urologic consultation.

### SUMMARY

Bladder symptoms are unpleasant and may be embarrassing. They can greatly interfere with your enjoyment of life and, if the proper interventions are not carried out, bladder problems can pose a serious threat to your health. The good news is that bladder symptoms can be managed and serious complications can be prevented. For this to happen, it is crucial that your urinary function be assessed. Symptoms alone are never sufficient to diagnose the underlying pathology and initiate treatment. Maintain awareness of your urinary function, follow the appropriate management program, and be an active member of your MS care team.

Techniques such as biofeedback and electrical stimulation can be helpful. You can take control of your urinary health!

## BOWEL MANAGEMENT

Most people with MS had little reason to think about their bowel function prior to their diagnosis. Although some people with MS continue to function without difficulty, most experience constipation, a small number have bowel incontinence, and some have both constipation and loose stool. Recommendations for handling both types of problems follow.

### CAUSES OF CONSTIPATION

Constipation is defined as infrequent (less often than every 3 days) or incomplete bowel movement (when the stool is retained in spite of an attempt to have a bowel movement). The digestive process can be traced in Figure 7.3.

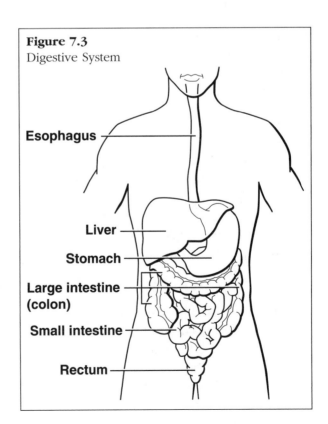

**Figure 7.3**
Digestive System

Esophagus

Liver

Stomach

Large intestine (colon)

Small intestine

Rectum

A number of factors contribute to constipation. For example, the problem may be a result of the following:

- Direct MS involvement of that portion of the nervous system that controls bowel function, producing a sluggish bowel that moves waste slowly through the digestive system.
- The body's absorbing excessive water from the stool, leaving it hard and difficult to eliminate.
- Weakened abdominal muscles, which make "bearing down" less effective.
- A decrease in physical activity, which reduces peristalsis, the process that moves the stool through the lower intestines.
- Urinary problems can also play a role, because attempts to control bladder dysfunction through fluid restriction and medication are likely to contribute to constipation.

### MEASURES FOR GOOD BOWEL FUNCTION

- Drink 1.5 to 2 quarts of fluids per day.
- Eat plenty of fiber every day to stimulate movement of the stool toward the rectum. Fiber can come from cereal, fruits, vegetables, and other sources.
- Engage in regular physical activity and exercise.
- Try to evacuate your bowel at the same time each day; the emptying reflex is strongest within 20 to 30 minutes after a meal or drinking warm fluids.

### WAYS TO MANAGE PERSISTENT CONSTIPATION

Follow all of these measures for good bowel function:

- Take a stool softener daily.
- Take a natural fiber supplement daily.
- Take a mild oral laxative such as milk of magnesia nightly.
- Insert a glycerin suppository 30 minutes prior to a planned bowel evacuation (be

sure to place it against the rectal wall and not in the stool).
- If the glycerin suppository is ineffective, try a mini enema.
- Use bisacodyl suppositories when glycerin suppositories are no longer effective.

### WAYS TO ADDRESS SERIOUS CONSTIPATION IN PERSONS WITH PHYSICAL LIMITATIONS

- Try all of the procedures outlined above.
- Explore possible non-MS causes.
- Stimulate evacuation by inserting a gloved finger into the rectum.
- Remove the stool manually, using latex gloves and lubricant.

Like many conditions imposed by MS, constipation ranges in severity. Patience is needed, because the bowel is highly responsive to repetitive routines. You can find a comfortable routine to relieve constipation.

### BOWEL INCONTINENCE

Episodic loss of bowel control is a very real and extremely distressing manifestation of MS. One cause may be loose stool, because the anal sphincter cannot easily contain liquid stool. A second possible cause is loss of sensation in the rectum, which causes the rectum to fill beyond its usual capacity before the desire to defecate is experienced. An unexpected, involuntary relaxation of the anal sphincter can occur, resulting in bowel incontinence. When non-MS causes, such as the flu or colitis, have been ruled out by your physician, the following interventions can be implemented.

Establish with your healthcare team, then rigorously maintain a regular bowel program. The following are tips for bowel incontinence:

- Follow all of the previous recommendations to control constipation.

- Be alert for signals indicating the need to defecate, especially 20 to 30 minutes after meals.
- Be aware that coffee and other hot liquids may stimulate a sudden urge to have a bowel movement.
- Be aware that anticholinergic medications may relax a hyperactive bowel (see section on treatment of Storage Dysfunction).
- Wear protective undergarments, as needed.
- Consider exploring innovative techniques, such as biofeedback.

## SUMMARY

Constipation and bowel incontinence concern and frustrate many people with MS. Beyond an understanding of the problems and consistent application of proper management techniques, the most important factor is patience. Bowel training can be successful, but it occurs slowly. Trial-and-error will give you the experience you need to develop a firm management plan that works. You can manage bladder and bowel problems successfully!

Chapter 8
# Skin Care
Linda Guiod, RN, BA, BSN

THE SKIN IS the largest and most visible organ, covering the entire body in a four-layer sheath. Like all organs, skin serves specific purposes that contribute to overall physical well-being. Limited ability, for example, to sense potential dangers to the skin or to turn or position oneself, can result in damage to the skin and cause it to break down. Proper skin care is essential to maintain function and prevent breakdown of this vital organ. An understanding of basic anatomy, skin functions, and proper care will allow you to prevent and manage skin problems.

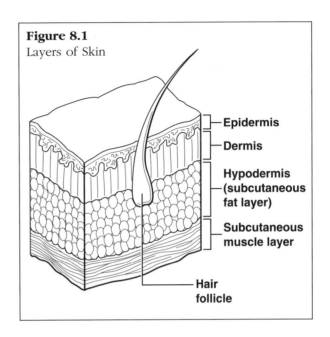

**Figure 8.1**
Layers of Skin

- Epidermis
- Dermis
- Hypodermis (subcutaneous fat layer)
- Subcutaneous muscle layer
- Hair follicle

## WHAT IS SKIN?

Skin is the largest organ in the body. In an average-sized adult, skin covers approximately 20 square feet and weighs from 6 to 8 pounds. The skin's thickness varies depending on the area it covers. For example, the eyelids are covered with 1/50 of an inch of skin, while the palms of the hands and feet are covered with approximately 1/3 of an inch. Moreover, the appearance and quality of skin depend on what body part it covers, the flow of blood to that part, and the amount that is covered with hair. The quality of skin can also tell something about a person's lifestyle. For example, a person with smooth, unblemished skin probably has avoided the sun, while a person with tanned and wrinkled skin probably has spent a fair amount of time in direct sunlight.

Skin may be likened to a four-ply tissue, because it has four layers (see Figure 8.1). The top, outermost layer, or *epidermis*, is the body's defense against infection. This layer constantly sheds through daily wear and tear and is replaced with newer cells from a different part of the epidermis. This layer also contains the cells that determine the pigment or color of your skin.

The *dermis*, located directly beneath the epidermis, provides support and nutrition to the epidermis. The dermis contains blood vessels, nerves, hair follicles, and sweat glands. The supply of blood to the dermis originates in the underlying muscles. Although the skin usually does not require all of its blood supply to function, the muscle and fatty layers beneath it cannot function properly when the blood supply is compromised.

The dermis also contains sensory nerves, which help you determine changes in pressure, temperature, pain, and touch. Some people with MS have areas of demyelination over the nerves that should tell them when to change position, when to regulate the source of heat or cold, or if there is an irritation. People with this condition need to protect themselves by always being aware of what is touching their skin and potentially damaging it.

The *hypodermis*, or subcutaneous tissue, is also referred to as the fat layer. It provides insulation, absorbs shock, and cushions the layers above. It acts as a nutrient reserve when the body is exposed to illness or starvation. The distribution of fat is influenced by age, heredity, and gender.

The muscles, blood vessels, and nerves are covered by *fascia*. It is dense, firm tissue that varies in thickness and strength throughout the body. Fascia's elastic properties facilitate the movement of various parts of the body.

## SKIN FUNCTION

The skin has four major functions, each of which helps the fat, muscles, and bones underneath to perform optimally. These functions include:

- Protection
- Sensory communication
- Temperature and fluid regulation
- Fat and water storage

The most obvious function of the skin is protection. The skin is a barrier to bacteria, dirt, and ultraviolet rays from the sun. Skin should be smooth and resilient. It becomes dry and wrinkled when the body is dehydrated, and taut and shiny when excess fluid is present.

Skin changes color in response to different internal conditions. A red or purple color indicates that blood flow to the area has increased. The skin may feel warm in response to inflammation or infection. A pink or pale color indicates that the blood supply to the area has decreased, and the skin may feel cool to the touch.

When the body's temperature rises, sweat glands produce sweat, a secretion of water and salt, that evaporates from the skin's surface to help maintain normal body temperature. Usually the body is able to distinguish degrees of temperature, touch, and pain on the skin surface. But people with MS may experience sensory symptoms, such as numbness, that prevent adequate sensation. If you lose sensation in your skin, you are at risk for damage from burns. Sometimes you may be unaware that a skin burn has occurred. Some common causes of burns are:

- Hot drink spills
- Hot running water
- Hot water bottles
- Hot stove burners
- Heating pads that are too hot
- Metal parts of a wheelchair exposed to the sun

## CARING FOR THE SKIN

Your skin should be inspected at least once a day—and more frequently if you are less mobile. Areas over a bony prominence should be inspected for redness or deepening in color. Do not massage these areas! Redness or deepening in color indicates increased blood flow, and the chance of damaging tiny blood vessels and tissue beneath is very high. If an area remains red for more than an hour, inform your physician or other healthcare professional. He or she will advise you on how to prevent any progression.

Skin should be cleaned immediately when it is soiled. Urine and stool can irritate the skin and cause skin breakdown. Use warm water and a mild cleansing agent. Some soaps contain harsh perfumes that can be drying and irritating, particularly to people with sensitive skin. Wash your skin with a soft cloth and pat it dry. Avoid rubbing.

Keep your skin well lubricated. This is important because if your skin is too dry, the potential for breakdown is greater. A variety of skin care preparations is available. If you see an opening on your skin, do not attempt to treat it yourself. Notify your physician.

Remember the following key points when caring for your skin:

- Keep your skin clean and dry.
- Do not remain in the same position for more than 1 hour.
- Report persistent skin irritations to your physician.

## MEDICATION-INDUCED INJECTION SITE REACTIONS

Recent studies have shown that disease modifying therapies alter the natural course of MS and slow the progression of disability. These medications are injectable either subcutaneously or intramuscularly. So while it is important to stay on treatment for as long as your health provider recommends it, it is important to take care of your skin. Some people who are using disease modifying therapies such as interferon beta-1b (Betaseron®), interferon beta-1a (Avonex®, Rebif®), and glatiramer acetate (Copaxone®), experience discomfort during the injection or a site reaction after the injection. This reaction may be as mild as redness or as severe as an infection.

The following rules of thumb will help you minimize your discomfort and maintain healthy skin while taking injectable medications:

- *Warm medications to room temperature.* Allow medications that have been refrigerated to reach room temperature for at least 30 minutes prior to injecting. You can also warm the solution closer to your body temperature by holding the syringe in your hand and slowly rotating it.
- *Proper injection technique will ensure correct drug administration and help*

*maintain skin integrity.* If you are just starting a self-injectable medication, ask your health provider for clear instructions and demonstrations on how to administer your injection. If your drug is administered subcutaneously (just under the skin into the fat layer between the skin and the muscle), gently cleanse the injection site and hold the syringe at a 90° angle to inject. For intramuscular injections (into a muscle with a longer needle), stretch the skin taut and also hold the syringe at a 90° angle.

- *Consider using an autoinjector device.* These devices deliver a prescribed amount at a consistent depth and at the correct angle for subcutaneous sites only.
- *Select a different area and side of the body for each injection.* The medication guide that is included with your medicine shows several possible areas of injection. Subcutaneous injections are best administered in the thigh, the outer surface of the upper arm, stomach, and buttocks. These areas are away from joints, nerves, and bones and the skin in these areas is loose and soft. Intramuscular injections are best given in the upper arms and thighs. Each area has several injection sites. Never use the same injection area twice in a row and choose a different injection site from the last injection. Record each injection site on a calendar to better track the areas and sites as you use them. Meticulous injection site rotation greatly lowers the risk of developing a dimpling effect of the fatty layer that makes the skin appear lumpy (lipoatrophy) and the ulcerated skin areas that can occur with frequent subcutaneous injections.
- *Allow at least 1 week to pass before reusing an injection site.*
- *Briefly apply ice to the site for 30 to 60 seconds before injecting* if you experi-

ence pain when the needle enters the skin. You can also try applying Orajel® or LMX cream or other over-the-counter topical creams that help provide a local anesthetic effect.

- Control slight redness, itching, or swelling by applying an over-the-counter 1% hydrocortisone cream.
- Carefully examine the injection site before each treatment.
- Do not inject any area that is irritated, reddened, bruised, tender, hard, or discolored.
- Do not allow the medication to come in contact with your skin. Inject with a "dry" needle tip by leaving a tiny air bubble in the syringe.

If an injection site develops redness that progresses to painful swelling, or if it looks infected, notify your physician immediately. Injection site skin reactions tend to diminish over time, so don't get discouraged. Knowing how to prepare your injection site, practicing good injection techniques, and carefully monitoring your skin for reactions are critical components to maintaining healthy skin while taking disease modifying treatments for MS.

## PRESSURE SORES

A pressure sore—also called a *decubitus ulcer* or *bedsore*—is an injury to the skin and to the underlying layers of tissue. As the name implies, pressure sores are usually caused by unrelieved pressure to a particular area. This continued pressure causes a decrease in blood flow through the vessels that supply the area with oxygen and nutrients. Fragile skin cells then begin to break down. People who are less mobile or remain still for long periods are susceptible to skin breakdown caused by continual pressure on a body part, such as the buttocks or heels. Diminished sensation can

contribute to lack of awareness and the development of pressure sores, thus emphasizing the need for frequent skin checks.

Pressure sores can sometimes be painful, slow to heal, and easily infected. Though they range in severity, pressure sores are always serious and must not be ignored. In most cases, pressure sores are preventable. In addition to practicing all the techniques for good skin care, it is important that you do the following:

- Understand why pressure sores develop.
- Know the most common sites for pressure sores to occur.
- Understand how pressure sores can progress if left untreated.
- Learn ways to prevent and treat pressure sores.
- Learn ways to evaluate your risk for developing pressure sores and to manage your risk factors.

Causes of Pressure Sores

Several factors contribute to the development of pressure sores. These factors include the following:

*Pressure.* Pressure is the amount of force placed on an area. When too much force is placed on the skin, the tiny blood vessels become compressed. If this force is applied long enough, the vessels collapse and stop delivering the oxygen and nutrients that skin cells need to remain healthy. Most people respond to prolonged periods of pressure by changing body position before healthy cells begin to die. However, diminished sensation can reduce the body's normal cues to shift position.

*Shear.* Shear is force that occurs when opposite but parallel motions compress blood vessels. This can happen, for example, when you slide down in a chair. The tissues that are attached to your bones pull down because of your body weight, while the skin and surface tissues either pull up or remain stationary. This type of force can cause obstructed, torn, or stretched blood vessels that decrease blood supply to the area.

*Friction.* Friction occurs when two surfaces rub against one another. Friction injuries to the skin can happen when you move across bed linens or other objects. Such injuries are common among people who have involuntary movements or spasticity, or who wear braces or appliances that rub against the skin.

*Moisture.* Excessive moisture can contribute to the development of pressure sores in two ways. First, continued exposure to moisture—such as sweat, urine, or stool—causes the skin to soften and become water-logged. Once soft, the outer layers of the skin can break down more easily. Second, moisture provides a medium for bacteria to grow. If you have bowel incontinence, the skin is exposed to bacteria from the stool that can add to the risk of infection.

*Infection.* Some evidence suggests that if an area is subjected to pressure, it becomes less resistant to bacterial infection. Pressure decreases the flow of oxygen to an area, which weakens the first line of defense against bacterial invasion.

DETERMINING YOUR RISK: RISK FACTORS FOR DEVELOPING PRESSURE SORES

Anyone can develop a pressure sore if the right forces are present. It takes only about 1 to 2 hours of unrelieved pressure to start the process of skin breakdown. Most able-bodied people can move easily enough to prevent pressure sores, but some people with MS are prone to this complication.

Vulnerability increases with each risk factor and with the seriousness of the factor. Controlling your risk factors is essential—not only to avoid pressure sores, but also because your body's ability to heal depends on your overall state of health. The three most common risk factors for people with MS are immobility, loss of sensation, and bowel or bladder incontinence, but other factors such as nutrition, age, and weight compound the risk.

*Immobility or inactivity.* This is the greatest risk factor for people who have MS. The risk increases for those who use a wheelchair, who have spasticity that keeps them from shifting the position of their limbs, or who are primarily in bed.

*Decreased sensation.* If part of the body does not sense pain, discomfort, or pressure, you may leave it in a pressure position too long even if you are able to move it.

*Bowel or bladder incontinence.* Incontinence creates moisture and exposes the skin to chemical toxins that can irritate. Wet skin is more easily injured than dry skin.

*Nutrition.* A well-balanced diet based on the nutritional pyramid, with adequate proportions of carbohydrates, proteins, and fats, is essential for strong, healthy skin. If the skin is not healthy, pressure sores are more likely to form, wounds will not heal properly, and infections will be more likely to develop.

*Age.* Many changes occur in the skin as you age. For example, sweat glands diminish in number and the fatty layers under the skin, especially in the legs and forearms, become less substantial. As a result, bony prominences become more prominent and less padded. The skin also becomes drier. All of these factors contribute to an older person's risk of developing pressure sores.

*Obesity.* Skin breakdown or irritation occurs more often in overweight people than in people of normal weight. Pressure sores can develop in areas where skin touches skin, causing friction, for example, between the legs and buttocks, in abdominal folds, and under the breasts.

*Underweight.* The likelihood of skin breakdown and infection also increases if you are underweight. This is because underweight people have more bony prominences or protrusions of bones, particularly on the hips, buttocks, and back.

*Dry skin.* Dry skin is more likely than normal skin to lose its integrity when the forces of pressure, shear, and friction are applied.

*Smoking.* Smoking causes tiny blood vessels to constrict, allowing less oxygen and nutrients to reach the skin and its supporting structures.

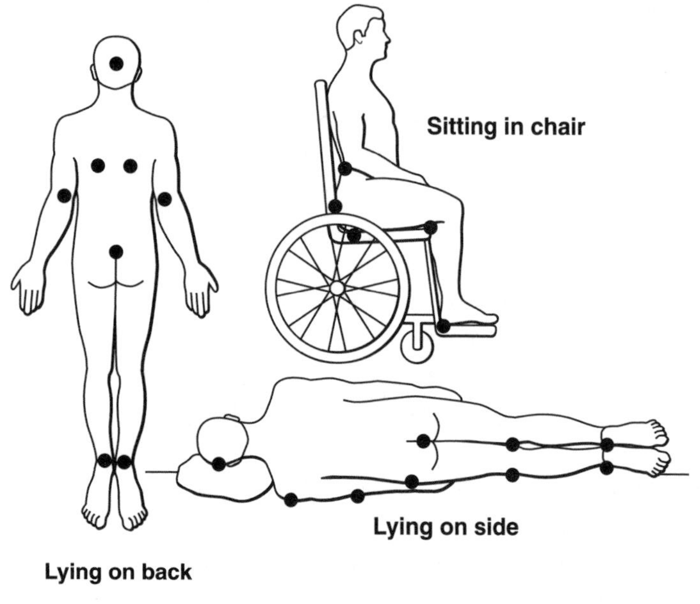

*Medical conditions.* Diabetes, anemia, and cardiovascular disorders increase the risk of skin breakdown.

*Mental confusion.* If you are not aware of what forces are contributing to the formation of pressure sores, you cannot prevent them. Changes in awareness can be brought about by MS, by other health problems, and by medications.

IDENTIFYING YOUR VULNERABLE AREAS: COMMON SITES FOR PRESSURE SORES

Pressure sores usually develop over bony areas, commonly called pressure points, because they bear the weight of the body when it is in a particular position. A pressure point is an area where a bone puts its greatest force on the skin and tissue, thereby reducing the flow of blood to that area. Bony prominences are susceptible to pressure sores because they have the least amount of cushioning. Pressure sores form when these bony parts press against a chair, a mattress, another surface, or other parts of the body. The areas of your body most vulnerable to pressure sores are determined by the positions in which you spend the most time (see Figure 8.2).

If you spend long periods of time in a chair or wheelchair, the spots where pressure sores form will be determined by your sitting position. The most common areas are:

- Shoulder blades
- Elbows
- Tailbone
- Buttocks
- Backs of the knees
- Heels
- Other body parts—such as the back of the head—that create pressure, depending on your wheelchair's design

**Figure 8.2**
Common Pressure Sore Sites

Sitting in chair

Lying on side

Lying on back

If you spend long periods of time lying on your back in bed, the most common areas are:

- Back of the head
- Shoulder blades
- Elbows
- Sacrum
- Heels

If you spend long periods of time lying on your side in bed, the most common areas are:

- Sides of the head
- Ears
- Shoulders
- Upper thigh bones
- Knees
- Ankles

People who are at risk for developing pressure sores are at greater risk when sitting than when lying down. This is because there is more body weight pressing onto a smaller surface area when one sits. When the body is flat in bed, there is a greater surface area over which to spread body pressure.

STAGES OF PRESSURE SORES

You must learn to recognize when pressure sores are starting because sores left untreated can progress rapidly. Although pressure sores do not always progress from one stage to another in an orderly fashion, it is helpful to consider how serious they are based on the amount of tissue that is damaged (see Figure 8.3).

*Stage I.* Pressure sores usually begin with a change in the color of intact skin that remains for about 5 minutes after the pressure is relieved. The skin appears pink, red, or dusky in color and does not become pale when you press on it with your fin-

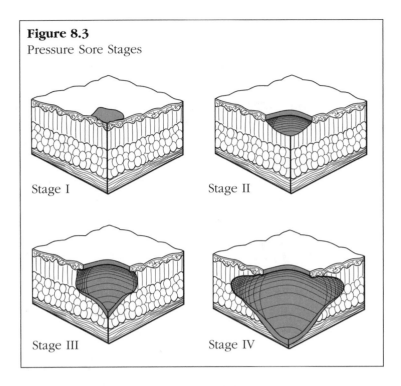

**Figure 8.3**
Pressure Sore Stages

Stage I

Stage II

Stage III

Stage IV

gers. In black-skinned individuals, the skin appears purple. Skin can also feel warm and hard to the touch and appear slightly swollen. This early stage of skin breakdown is reversible if the source of pressure is removed.

*Stage II.* The outer layers of the skin begin to break down. There may be swelling, redness, or blistering, and the area may feel warm to the touch. This stage can take 1 to 2 weeks to heal.

*Stage III.* The ulcerated area extends to the deep skin layers and to the fat and muscle directly under the skin. Live tissue begins to die. The sore looks like a crater or hole and has a foul-smelling drainage. This stage can take months to heal.

*Stage IV.* The sore reaches into deep muscle tissue and bone. Infection can occur and tunnels can develop and extend the size of the sore. This stage requires aggressive medical intervention and takes months to heal.

## What You Can Do to Prevent Pressure Sores

Preventing pressure sores is easier than trying to heal them. Prevention begins when you identify which risk factors apply to you, then incorporate into your daily routine as many of the following measures as you can.

1. Keep moving, or improve your ability to move. When you move and shift your weight, you relieve pressure on vulnerable sites.
2. If you can easily walk and move around, do so. You are probably not at risk for pressure sores as long as you maintain activities that keep you moving.
3. If you use a wheelchair or tend to sit for long periods of time:
   - Shift your weight from one buttock to the other every 15 minutes, if you are able.
   - Change your position at least every hour.
   - If you have enough strength in your arms, try doing wheelchair pushups. Grip the arms of the chair and push down with your hands and arms to raise your body off the seat. You can also use this technique for shifting your weight from one buttock to the other. Hold each new position for about 1 minute.
4. If you are in bed for long periods:
   - Change your position at least every 2 hours. You may need someone to assist you, or you may have a special piece of equipment such as a trapeze attached over your bed to help you move.
   - Place pillows under your legs, from midcalf to ankles, to keep your heels off the bed.

*Practice good skin care.* You are the one closest to your skin and can spot and alleviate problems the earliest.

1. Inspect your skin at least once daily, using a mirror for areas that are hard to see. Pay special attention to common areas of pressure sores and to areas that remain discolored after you have changed position and relieved the pressure.
2. Use warm water and mild soap when bathing.
3. Prevent dry skin by using skin creams or oils. Avoid very cold or dry air.

*Relieve areas of pressure.* Assistive devices and exercise can prevent sores from developing.

1. If you spend most of your time in a chair or wheelchair:
   - Use cushions of foam, gel, or air to relieve pressure. These cushions come in many designs. Ask your doctor to refer you to a healthcare professional or seating clinic that can evaluate your needs both in wheelchair structure and design and in special seating cushions for pressure relief.
   - Do not use donut-shaped cushions because they reduce blood flow, cause tissues to swell, and increase your risk of developing pressure sores.
2. If you are in bed for long periods and cannot move about freely:
   - Use a special mattress that contains foam, air, gel, or water, all of which help to prevent pressure sores. Such mattresses vary in cost and effectiveness, so it's wise to talk to your doctor about which would be best for you.
3. Ask your doctor or nurse about physical rehabilitation and range-of-motion exercises to improve your ability to move and reduce the effects of pressure on tissues.

*Protect your skin from injury.* Avoid movements that increase pressure on vulnerable tissue.

1. Never massage your skin over the bony parts of your body. Massaging the skin damages the tissue under the skin.
2. While sitting or lying down, reduce friction during repositioning by lifting, not dragging, your body.
3. Reduce the risk of damage from friction by applying a thin layer of cornstarch to vulnerable areas.
4. Do not raise the head of the bed more than 30 degrees. Raising the bed higher can force your body to slip down and cause skin damage when you slide over the bed surface.

*Start an incontinence management program.* Wet or soiled skin is more susceptible to breakdown.

1. Ask your physician and nurse to determine if you need a management program for bowel and bladder incontinence.
2. Clean the skin immediately after any incontinence. Use a soft cloth to reduce injury to the skin.
3. If moisture cannot be controlled, use pads or briefs that absorb urine and that have a fast-drying surface that keeps moisture away from the skin.
4. Apply cream or ointment to protect the skin from urine and stool. Your nurse or physician can recommend products for you to use.
5. A number of adult incontinence devices are designed to prevent skin irritation and have no offensive odors. Ask your doctor or nurse which of these devices might be useful for you.

*Develop good eating habits.* You are what you eat—and so is your skin.

1. Eat a balanced diet. The basic nutrients necessary for good health are discussed in Chapter 15, "The Role of Nutrition in MS."
2. Talk to your physician or nurse if you cannot eat a normal, balanced diet. He or she can recommend nutritional supplements or refer you to a nutritionist who can help determine the best way for you to attain the nutrition you need.

WHAT YOU CAN DO IF PRESSURE SORES DEVELOP

Left unattended, pressure sores can lead to serious infection and lengthy healing times. Fortunately, you can prevent pressure sores from worsening. The first step is to learn to recognize the signs of a developing pressure sore. The second step is to work with your healthcare team to devise a treatment plan to heal existing pressure sores and prevent new ones from developing. Remember that you and those close to you are the most critical members of your healthcare team.

Healing a pressure sore involves three main principles. Although the principles of healing are similar to the principles of prevention, they become more important once the skin has begun to break down.

*Relieve the pressure.* Taking pressure off a sore is the first step in healing. Unrelieved pressure will only worsen the sore and slow the healing process. You can relieve pressure by:

- Changing your position often, that is, every hour while sitting in a chair or every 2 hours while lying in bed.
- Using support surfaces to provide support for your body. Several kinds of support surfaces, such as special beds, mattresses, and seat cushions, are available. The one that is best for you will depend upon your general health, your ability to change positions, and the severity of

your pressure sore. Consult your nurse or doctor to help you decide which surface will work best for you.

*Maintain correct body position.* Body position is important in relieving pressure on a sore. Do not lie on a sore. Use pillows to keep knees and ankles from touching each other. Keep the head of the bed raised less than 30 degrees from horizontal. Maintain good posture while sitting. This will help you to move more easily and prevent new sores.

*Report skin problems.* Let your healthcare provider know immediately if your skin begins to break down. Other forms of treatment may be required once an assessment is done by a healthcare professional. These include applying protective dressings to the skin, removing dead tissue, absorbing wound drainage, taking antibiotics, and, in some cases, undergoing surgical procedures.

*In most cases, skin breakdown is preventable.* Become aware of your skin now. Knowing the vital functions of the skin, taking good care of your skin, and understanding how skin breakdown can be prevented and managed are the key steps in maintaining healthy skin. Remember, no one can take better care of your skin than you!

# Chapter 9
# Addressing Cognitive Problems

Nicholas G. LaRocca, PhD and Rosalind C. Kalb, PhD

MULTIPLE SCLEROSIS (MS) is a disease that affects both the body and the mind. It causes damage to tissue in both the brain and the spinal cord. When it affects the brain, MS is highly likely to affect cognition. Cognition includes high-level functions carried out by the human brain, including comprehension and use of speech, visual perception and construction, calculation ability, attention (information processing), memory, and executive functions such as planning, problem-solving, and self-monitoring.

Changes in cognition can occur at any time in the course of the disease. They are not confined to people who have had MS for a long period or who are severely disabled physically. Although about 50 percent of people with MS have some degree of cognitive dysfunction, very few suffer from severe cognitive problems. Most people who are affected have only mild or moderate changes. However, these changes are enough to make daily life a challenge.

## COPING WITH COGNITIVE CHANGES

Having cognitive deficits does not mean that you are stupid. In the context of MS, it means only that some of your cognitive functions do not work as well as they did before the disease affected them. The emphasis is on "some" because MS tends to affect a few areas of functioning while leaving others intact. The following are some of the most frequently cited problems:

- Memory: difficulty remembering names and appointments, keeping track of belongings, or learning new material.

- Abstract reasoning: trouble performing tasks that require complex analysis, such as solving mysteries.
- Slowed information processing: difficulty responding quickly when information comes from several different directions.
- Word-finding problems: problems remembering words or phrases (the tip-of-the-tongue phenomenon, when you just can't come up with the word you want to say).
- Visual and spatial organization: problems finding your way when driving, using maps and diagrams, or understanding assembly instructions.
- Ability to shift between tasks: inability to switch from one task to another without losing track of what you're doing.
- Attention and concentration: trouble screening out distractions or keeping your mind from wandering.
- Organizing and executing complex sequences: difficulty organizing a project, deciding what should be done first, setting up an order for the various steps, and implementing a plan.

## DEVELOPING STRATEGIES

Just a few years ago, people with MS who had cognitive deficits were rarely offered help. Poor memory was regarded as the fate of those with the disease. But many strategies can be adopted that are extremely helpful to those with MS-related cognitive changes. Many of them can be incorporated into your life with little or no money or outside expertise required. But first, you need to acknowledge the problems you are having.

*Admit that you have some cognitive deficits.* Once you have identified the problem, you can begin to accommodate.

*Discuss the situation with your doctor.* Some people who think they are having cognitive loss due to MS may simply be depressed, under a lot of stress, or subject to other factors that affect cognition. Your doctor may refer you to a neuropsychologist who has experience in MS. A good neuropsychological evaluation, which can take more than 6 hours to complete, will provide you with definitive information concerning the nature and severity of any cognitive problems you have. Briefer assessment batteries have been developed that take 2 hours or less. However, the 5- to 10-minute test of mental status that may be part of the routine neurological exam is not sensitive enough to evaluate the types of cognitive changes that occur in MS.

After an in-depth assessment, cognitive rehabilitation may be recommended and a specialized program will be designed to improve your functioning. A trained professional will conduct the program over the course of weeks or months. This professional may be a neuropsychologist, a speech pathologist, or an occupational therapist.

*Find a buddy.* If your cognitive deficits do not warrant professional intervention, find a friend or relative to help you set up a cognitive self-help program. A buddy can help keep your motivation high.

*Adapt.* Let go of the idea that the world will come to an end unless you are able to do everything you used to do as well as you once did and in the same way. Substitution is the key to making cognitive self-help work.

*Be consistent.* Use the strategies you develop—such as a family calendar or an appointment book—to help you cope with cognitive changes. Such strategies will be of little assistance unless they are used consistently.

*Battle fatigue.* Many people with MS find that cognitive functions don't work as well when they are tired. This "cognitive fatigue" is now a scientifically demonstrated phenomenon in MS. If you experience cognitive fatigue, try to schedule tasks so that you tackle the most demanding ones when you are at your best. Plan rest periods so that you can restore energy and alertness and then return to the task at hand. You might also want to consider the measures that are available to manage fatigue, such as regular exercise and certain types of medications.

## GET ORGANIZED

MS makes the mind feel sort of slippery, because information that it used to store now seems to slip away. To counteract this feeling, you need to capture information in such a way that it cannot slip away and is organized for easy reference and retrieval. There are several ways to do this.

*Buy a journal.* One of the simplest and most versatile ways is the familiar organizer book that many people use in their business and personal lives. Such a book can function as a sort of second brain by organizing and storing bits of information that are too numerous and complex to keep in your head.

An outgrowth of the old appointment books, the new books have many sections in addition to the traditional appointment section. The appointment part of the book can be used as a "tickler file" in which you record tasks that you need to do at a certain time in the future, such as having the furnace cleaned in October. Another section may contain lists of things to do. To-do lists can be prioritized so that you know what needs to be done right away and what can be left for another week or month. The organizer can also have a "memory bank" section containing information that you would like to keep with you. For example, you could record the clothing sizes and color preferences of various family members to help you when shopping. The possibilities are unlimited.

*Use a computer.* Electronic organizers come in many forms, ranging from desktop computers to pocket-sized personal digital assistants (PDAs). Computers are wonderful tools for storing all sorts of information.

A special class of software, known as the personal information manager (PIM), can help you use the computer as an organizational tool. PIMs come in many varieties, although this type of software has largely been replaced by the PDAs. PDAs range tremendously in price and complexity. Some are relatively simple, with a calculator, phone list, and one or two other functions. The more expensive models are fully functional computers, with word processing, spreadsheet, database, wireless Web access, a digital camera, etc. Cellular phones are also available that include many of the same functions as PDAs, such as appointment calendars, along with address books.

*Voice-activated organizers.* These use no tapes, but record your voice on a chip instead. Some voice-activated organizers can do many of the same things that paper organizers can, including recording appointments and memos.

*Substitute organization for memory.* In addition to the organizer book, computer, and other gadgets, some simple ideas include:

- Hang a family calendar in the kitchen or other central room to keep track of family members' commitments.
- Establish a single place for frequently misplaced items, such as keys, and always return them to that spot.
- Use a checklist when you are shopping, packing for a vacation, or engaged in any activity that requires you to follow a number of steps or remember various items.

- Avoid putting things off; try to complete tasks while you are thinking of them.

*Jog your memory.* Remembering the names of people you meet or things people tell you in passing can pose one of your greatest challenges. It may not be convenient to whip out your PDA and type in notes at a cocktail party. However, many people compensate for memory loss by carrying a few 3 × 5-inch index cards on which they can make quick notes.

A number of purely mental strategies, such as visualization and association, can also enhance verbal memory. For example, if you meet somebody named Tom Firestone, you might imagine him playing a tom-tom while sitting in front of a burning rock—a "fire stone." To enhance this memory, visualize the stone on fire burning furiously. You might also review Firestone's name with a list of his most striking characteristics, such as hair color, eye color, height, and build.

To sum up, it does not matter whether you are more comfortable with high-tech or low-tech approaches to organization. Many techniques are available to help you substitute effective organization for those slippery-mind functions. Experiment with methods until you find those that work best for you, then use them consistently. The rewards will more than justify the time and effort you invest.

## ENHANCING YOUR ABILITY TO CONCENTRATE

Attention and concentration are like pillars upon which all other cognitive functions stand. When these functions are affected by MS, there can be a ripple effect that touches memory, organization, and other everyday tasks. Attention and concentration can be addressed in a variety of ways, depending on the nature of the difficulty.

- Pinpoint what sorts of things distract you and under what conditions. Then work on removing or avoiding the offending conditions.
- Establish quiet times and places in the home. Tell family members when and where you are going to balance your checkbook, for example, so they get the message, "Please do not disturb!"
- Determine the optimal times for you to work on tasks requiring concentration. Some people are at their best in the morning, while others get a second wind in the early evening.
- Learn energy-conserving and pacing strategies. Getting enough sleep at night or taking naps during the day can help enormously.
- Identify your comfortable attention span and break tasks into chunks of that length. If you begin to drift off after half an hour of sustained attention, for example, try working in 30-minute blocks with a brief break between blocks to refresh yourself.
- Keep your powers of concentration in top form. Working on puzzles, meditating, and reading will all enhance your ability to concentrate.

To a great extent, good powers of concentration are a matter of practice. With the right strategies, consistently applied, you can do much to improve your ability to focus and concentrate.

## PROCESSING INFORMATION

In MS, the processing of information may be slowed. The ability to process information can be particularly problematic when the information is coming from more than one source. In these situations, it's important to alert the people around you that you need them to slow down and that they need to speak in turn, rather than all at once.

Many people with MS report that they can still do all the cognitive tasks they used to do, but that they need more time in which to do them and need to focus on one task at a time.

## HANDLING WORD-FINDING PROBLEMS

Word-finding problems can be the most socially frustrating of the cognitive changes brought about by MS. Feelings of anxiety about finding yourself searching for a particular word can make it worse. The following are the best strategies:

- Give up on the idea that you must think of one specific word. Instead, let it come to you later.
- Try talking at a slower pace. Sometimes you may be talking faster than your brain can process requests for words. By slowing down, you give the brain crucial additional seconds to process.
- Study and expand your vocabulary. When you have trouble thinking of a word, nothing is more useful than having a good synonym at your disposal.

## INVOLVE YOUR FAMILY

Your loved ones may be puzzled by your failing memory and may not connect it with the same demyelinating process that has you walking with a cane and going to the bathroom every half hour. Family members and friends need to be educated concerning the realities of cognitive dysfunction and MS. Without accurate information, those around you may attribute your cognitive changes to stress, depression, age, menopause, stubbornness, laziness, or any of a myriad of other mistaken notions.

In addition, many of the strategies you work out for yourself will require active cooperation on the part of family members, friends, and coworkers. For example, if you establish quiet times and places to do your work, those around you will need to respect those boundaries. If you institute a family calendar and telephone message center, everyone must establish new habits to make the system work. Most important, you need your family and friends to understand your limitations without treating you with condescension. Their expectations for you should be set neither too high nor too low.

Cognitive changes, like other symptoms of MS, can have wide-ranging effects on any number of everyday activities. Fortunately, these cognitive problems generally are not severe and can be countered in a variety of ways. Look for practical solutions. Even simple self-help strategies can help you regain control over your life. Focus on what you can do, then do it well. You may be pleasantly surprised by the results.

# Chapter 10
# Adjusting to Changes in Sexual Function in MS

Frederick W. Foley, PhD and Audrey Sorgen, PhD

NORMAL SEXUAL FUNCTION changes throughout one's lifetime, but having multiple sclerosis (MS) can profoundly affect an individual's sexual experience in a variety of ways. The most frequently reported change in men is diminished capacity to obtain or maintain an erection (impotence), while the most frequent change reported by women is partial or total loss of libido (sexual desire).

Symptoms that can affect sexual activity include:

- Fatigue
- Muscle weakness
- Spasticity
- Hand tremors
- Bladder or bowel dysfunction
- Cognitive dysfunction
- Depression
- Sensory changes (e.g., numbness, tingling, burning sensations)

These (and other) MS symptoms can cause:

- Changes in family roles
- Lowered self-esteem
- Grief and other feelings of distress
- Difficulties in meeting expectations about sexual expression, which can particularly affect those who live with a disability

Certain MS medications can also interfere with sexual functioning. For example, certain antidepressants can cause this difficulty.

## THE BRAIN AND SPINAL CORD AND MS

Sexual response is controlled by emotional responses in concert with the central nervous system: the brain, and the spinal cord.

The brain is involved in many aspects of sexual functioning, including sexual desire, the perception of sexual stimuli and pleasure, movement, sensation, cognition, and attention. Throughout the sexual response cycle, sexual messages are communicated between the brain, spinal cord, and the genitals. Because MS can cause lesions along myelinated pathways, it is not surprising that changes in sexual function are reported so frequently by people with MS.

## SEXUAL RESPONSE CYCLE

Two pioneering researchers, William Masters and Virginia Johnson, identified four stages of sexual response. These stages—excitement, plateau, orgasm, and resolution—are known as the human sexual response cycle. Two basic processes occur during sexual response: vasocongestion and myotonia. Vasocongestion refers to the concentration of blood in the blood vessels and in the tissues of the genitals and breasts. In men, vasocongestion occurs when arterial blood flow to the penis increases and venous outflow decreases. Erection is a result of increased blood flow to the spongy tissue (corpora cavernosa) of the penis, causing these tissues to expand. In women, this inflow of blood causes the clitoris to enlarge, the labia to swell, and the vagina to lubricate. Myotonia, or neuromuscular tension, refers to the increase of energy in nerves and muscles. During sexual activity, myotonia takes place throughout the body, affecting both involuntary and skeletal muscles.

### COMPLICATIONS OF MS

MS can interfere with the excitement and plateau phase of the sexual response cycle.

MS lesions in the brain can interfere with the perception of sexual stimulation so it no longer has an arousing effect. Lesions of the spinal cord can interfere with the transmission of nerve signals to the genitals and prevent vasocongestion, resulting in diminished or absent erections, clitoral swelling, or vaginal lubrication.

In men, orgasm takes place in two phases, emission and ejaculation. In the emission phase, increased tension leads to a series of rhythmic contractions that drives semen into the bulb of the urethra. The second phase, ejaculation, is marked by contractions that force semen out of the urethra.

Some men with MS experience orgasmic contractions without ejaculation (nonejaculatoy orgasms) or ejaculation without orgasm. Some men and women with MS report loss of orgasm, although their excitement and plateau phases are unaffected. More commonly reported are less frequent orgasms, which can stem from direct physical, indirect, or psychosocial causes.

## COPING WITH MS-RELATED CHANGES IN SEXUAL RESPONSE

### COMMUNICATING WITH HEALTHCARE PROVIDERS

Some healthcare providers rarely bring up the subject of sexuality, perhaps because they feel uncomfortable with it, lack professional training in the area, or fear being overly intrusive. Most providers are willing to discuss sexuality, however, if you bring up the subject.

You need to discuss changes in your sexual feelings and ask what treatments are available to enhance your sexuality. Communicate your concerns to your healthcare provider, including your current medications.

### COPING WITH ALTERED GENITAL SENSATIONS

To enhance sexual response, increase stimulation to other responsive areas such as breasts, buttocks, ears, and lips. Conduct a sensory body map exercise by yourself or with your partner to explore the exact locations of pleasant, decreased, or altered sensations. This exercise can enhance intimacy, as well as teach you about changes in your sensual and sexual pleasure zones. As with the treatment of all sexual symptoms in MS, experimentation and communication are the keys to maximizing sexuality.

Increase genital stimulation through oral stimulation or through mechanical vibrators. This can help stimulate erections in men and provide direct clitoral stimulation for women.

Painful or irritating genital or body sensations can sometimes be treated with medications such as amitriptyline, carbamazepine, and phenytoin.

### COPING WITH LOWERED LIBIDO

If you are in an intimate relationship, focus on the sensual aspects. Sensual contact is nongenital; it includes back rubs, gentle stroking of nongenital body zones, and other touching that you find physically and emotionally pleasing. During periods of diminished sex drive, partners often neglect the sensual, nonsexual aspects of their physical relationship.

Make a date for a sensual evening. Partners can enjoy each other physically and engage in sensual exploration of each other's bodies, without the pressure of having to have sexual intercourse.

Restore the special nature of your relationship by showing your partner how important he or she is to you. Loving gestures are often forgotten under the pressure of coping with MS and other stresses. When you treat your partner as a special person, you set the stage for increased intimacy, which can sometimes stimulate libido.

### COPING WITH ERECTILE PROBLEMS

A number of oral medications are available to treat erectile dysfunction. The FDA has approved several medicines called phosphodiesterase-type-5 (PDE-5) inhibitors. PDE-5 inhibitors work by blocking a chemical in the erectile tissues that causes erections to become flaccid. These medicines include sildenafil (Viagra®), vardenafil (Levitra®), and tadalafil (Cialis®). To date, only sildenafil has been completed in clinical trials with men who have MS, although the other medicines are highly similar and can be prescribed for persons with MS. These medicines do not improve libido, but are helpful in maintaining erections when they occur. They are typically taken an hour before anticipated sexual activity. The effects of vardenafil and tadalafil are reported to last somewhat longer than sildenafil, although they have not been directly compared in persons with MS. These medicines cannot be used with some nitrate-based cardiac medicines, since they interact with each other and can lower blood pressure excessively.

In addition to the PDE-5 inhibitors, other oral medicines are in development for erectile dysfunction that work by enhancing or blocking chemical pathways in the brain and spinal cord that are related to sexual function. To date, none of these have been tried in MS.

One noninvasive way to achieve an erection is to use a vacuum assistive device. With this method, a plastic tube is fitted over the flaccid penis, and a pump creates a vacuum that subsequently produces an erection. Then, a latex constriction band is slipped from the base of the tube onto the base of the penis. The band maintains engorgement of the penis for sexual activities, although it cannot be used for more than 30 minutes. If you achieve erections readily, but have trouble maintaining them, you may be able to use the constriction band alone.

Alprostadil is a medicine that can be can injected into the penis, or it can also be used in an urethral suppository. The injections can be easily done with an auto-injector, although it is important to be properly trained in this technique by a urologist or advanced practice nurse. To use the suppository, a small plastic applicator is inserted into the urethra. Through either method, the drug is absorbed into the penile tissues, stimulating a satisfactory erection in most men with erectile dysfunction. However, there is typically some penile discomfort, although the overall satisfaction ratings by men who use these methods are quite high. In rare instances, priapism can occur (prolonged erection).

A more invasive form of treatment for erectile problems is the penile prosthesis. The two types of penile prostheses are: semirigid and inflatable. With the semi-rigid type, a flexible rod is surgically implanted in each of the erection chambers (corpus cavernosa) of the penis. These rods can be bent upward when an erection is desired, and bent downward at other times. Following insertion of the rods, the penis remains somewhat enlarged, with a permanent semi-erection.

With the inflatable type, a fluid reservoir and pump are surgically implanted in the abdomen and scrotum, with inflatable reservoirs inserted into the penis that inflate when an erection is desired. This type of prosthesis is barely noticeable, but the potential risks are significant. Surgical complications, infection, scarring, and difficulty operating the pump can create long-term problems.

Approximately 80 percent of the men who use these types of prostheses find them satisfactory. In general, a penile prosthesis is only recommended when other efforts to manage erectile dysfunction have not been successful.

In coping with erectile dysfunction, it is important to discuss the situation with your partner, particularly if you are in a long-term relationship. Such discussions can enhance feelings of intimacy by allowing partners to learn and explore together. If you are afraid or inhibited about talking openly about these issues, counseling with a mental health professional who is knowledgeable about MS may help.

## COPING WITH VAGINAL DRYNESS AND TIGHTNESS

Similar to the erectile response in men, vaginal lubrication is controlled by multiple pathways in the brain and spinal cord. Psychogenic lubrication originates in the brain and can be enhanced by creating a relaxing, romantic, or stimulating setting for sexual activity; by incorporating relaxing massage into foreplay activities; and by prolonging foreplay. Lubrication can sometimes be increased by manually or orally stimulating the genitals. The simplest way to compensate for vaginal dryness is to apply generous amounts of a water-soluble lubricant. Healthcare professionals advise against using petroleum-based jellies for vaginal lubrication because they can promote bacterial infections and may erode condoms, making them ineffective for birth control or disease prevention.

Although a small trial of sildenafil has been tried in women with MS to enhance sexual response, the results were disappointing. Women with MS seem to have a more complex view of their sexuality than men with MS. It is possible that medicines for MS women with sexual dysfunction may be more effective if they are delivered with counseling that enhances the overall relationship.

## COPING WITH SPASTICITY

Spasticity in the legs can make finding a comfortable position for intercourse difficult. Stretching prior to intercourse can help. Medications such as baclofen or tizanidine, especially when taken about 1 hour before sexual activity, may reduce this problem. Be sure to discuss any medication changes with your physician.

Another approach for coping with spasticity is to explore alternative positions for intercourse. Women with spasticity of the adductor muscles, which draws the thighs together, may be more comfortable lying on their sides, with the partner approaching from behind. Men who have difficulty straightening their legs may be more comfortable sitting upright in an armless chair while the partner mounts the erect penis. However, everyone's body is different, and the key to finding alternative sexual positions is open exploration and communication between partners.

## COPING WITH FATIGUE

You may find it helpful to take fatigue medication about 1 hour before sexual activity. You may also compensate for fatigue by having sex in the morning, when energy levels are higher, and by exploring sexual positions that minimize weight-bearing or tiring movements.

## COPING WITH WEAKNESS

You can compensate for weakness by finding new positions. Reclining may be less tiring, and pillows can improve positioning and reduce muscle strain. Try the new positions before sex to help you determine whether they are comfortable without the anxiety of introducing them during sexual activity. Finally, oral sex requires less movement than intercourse, and hand-held or strap-on vibrators can provide sexual satisfaction without producing fatigue.

## COPING WITH BLADDER DYSFUNCTION

The basic approach to coping with bladder dysfunction is to treat the symptoms when you anticipate sexual activity.

Strategies include the following:

• If you are taking an anticholinergic medication, which is frequently prescribed for bladder storage dysfunction, take it 30 minutes before sexual activity to minimize bladder contractions during sex. Because vaginal dryness is a side effect of these medicines, use a water-soluble lubricant to compensate for this.

- Restrict fluid intake for several hours before sex.
- Empty your bladder or catheterize just before sexual activity.

Men who have small amounts of urine leakage can wear a condom during sex. Women who have indwelling catheters can tape the catheter securely to the abdomen, empty the collecting bag before sexual activity, and put additional tape around the top ring to minimize the chance of leakage. Lying in a spoon position, with the woman in front, will avoid putting pressure on the catheter or the collection bag.

## COPING WITH CHANGES IN ATTENTION AND CONCENTRATION

Changes in attention and concentration may derail your ability to sustain interest in sex. Feelings of confusion, guilt, and rejection may result. Negative feelings can, in turn, increase distractibility or cause you to avoid sex altogether.

Problems with attention and concentration tend to be worse when you are tired, so fatigue must be dealt with. Use a variety of stimulating techniques, such as talking in sexy ways, touching both the sensual and erotic parts of your body, and playing romantic music, to help maintain your focus.

Briefly switching from erotic to nonerotic touching when you lose focus can create an atmosphere of acceptance, and ease both you and your partner back into the right mood.

## COPING WITH EMOTIONAL CHANGES

MS is frequently associated with grief, demoralization, changes in self-esteem and body image, and clinical depression. These emotions can temporarily dampen sexual interest and pleasure. To cope with these changes, obtain a professional assessment of your situation, educate yourself about the disease and possible treatments, and learn strategies for coping.

Temporary changes in self-esteem are often part of the grief process that occurs in response to chronic illness. Normal grieving tends to ebb and flow, as you work to redefine yourself in terms of the MS. You can work through the grieving process by learning about the disease, comparing your experiences with others, discussing disappointments, and exploring new options. Support groups can be particularly helpful and private counseling may also speed the adaptation process.

If you are clinically depressed, that is, if you suffer from long-term depression, medications and psychotherapy can usually offer relief and restore sexual interest. Some antidepressants can cause loss of libido or interfere with orgasm. Talk with your physician or healthcare provider about all potential side effects before you begin antidepressant medication.

## COPING WITH ROLE CHANGES AND LOSS OF INTIMACY

In our society, people believe that sex should be spontaneous and passionate. When these expectations are not met, lovers can be so disappointed that they withdraw from the sexual relationship. They fail to explore other possibilities.

Women, in particular, are susceptible to the effects of negative body image, which MS may worsen. Men with MS may view themselves as failures because they do not live up to their ideal role as breadwinners or as sexual initiators. Sometimes the struggle with role expectations, for both yourself and your partner, results in a gradual loss of sexual feeling. This process may be accelerated if the able-bodied partner provides extensive caregiving to the partner with the disability. If caregiving becomes a large part of a relationship, it is difficult for the caregiver to relax and have fun.

Accompanying these role changes, partners may feel a sense of isolation in the relationship and less compassion for each other's concerns. The diminishing capacity to understand and work through such issues creates greater isolation and misunderstanding. In this atmosphere, resentments may grow.

Solutions to the loss of intimacy that stems are not simple. You may need first to develop a language so you can talk comfortably with your partner about issues concerning sexuality and intimacy. Educational materials can facilitate such discussions. Check what is available through the National Multiple Sclerosis Society (NMSS), Paralyzed Veterans of America (PVA), and United Spinal Association. Many self-help books available from local bookstores and libraries are designed to enhance communication.

The following tips may help you and your partner begin to reestablish a dialogue:

- Read books and watch educational videos with your partner. Set aside time to talk about what you are learning, whether or not it applies to your relationship.
- Talk about sexuality and intimacy.
- Make regular dates, free from the responsibilities of work, caregiving, and childrearing, to rediscover your partner. Try to recreate the feeling of romance that characterized your relationship before it was swept away by the burdens of career, parenthood, and MS.

Because MS brings about so many changes, couples living with the disease need to compare their expectations to reality and to share their feelings about the ways in which their lives have changed. In an atmosphere of caring and support, those shared feelings can rekindle the flame of intimacy.

# Chapter 11
# Understanding Complementary or Alternative Treatments

Patricia Kennedy, RN, CNP, MSCN and Nancy J. Holland, EdD, RN, MSCN

THE TERMS ALTERNATIVE, complementary, or unconventional therapy cover a broad range of healing philosophies and approaches. Some approaches are consistent with the physiological principles of Western medicine, while others constitute independent healing systems. Some alternative therapies are far outside the realm of accepted medical theory and practice, while others fit within the traditional system.

Conventional medicine has been defined as those therapies that are taught in medical schools or are available in hospitals (i.e., medications and surgery).

Alternative treatments include a wide variety of remedies, supplements, and techniques commonly thought to be outside the scope of conventional medicine and used instead of conventional therapies. Today, however, more and more major hospitals are establishing centers for alternative medicine and allowing many alternative treatments to be used in conjunction with traditional medicine. Consequently, the distinction between conventional and alternative medicine is becoming blurred, and complementary and alternative medicine (or CAM) is gaining in popularity.

## KINDS OF ALTERNATIVE TREATMENTS

Because alternative medicine encompasses such a wide range of treatments, it is useful to divide them into categories. The following is the classification from the National Institutes of Health:

- *Biologically based therapies* include vitamins, minerals, herbs, dietary supplements, and other natural substances. This category would include bee venom, homeopathic remedies, and marijuana. Because the course of multiple sclerosis (MS) can vary markedly within any individual, without carefully controlled clinical trials, it is impossible to discern whether the benefits claimed for these natural substances result from the treatment itself, from spontaneous improvement in the disease, or from placebo effects (which can be unusually active in people with MS). Few scientific clinical studies demonstrate the benefit of most of these substances for treating MS, to date, nor have claims of benefits been supported by reliable reports of objective changes in the disease observed by physicians.

- *Special diets* are considered biologically based. Many people with MS have tried the Gerson, McDougall, Swank, and macrobiotic diets. Some of these diets stress lowering the amount of saturated fat eaten, while others emphasize eliminating certain foods such as dairy products, wheat, or corn, which are believed to be related to personal allergies. Some people with MS use such diets in the hope that they will slow the progression of the disease. Others use them to enhance their overall health and sense of well-being.

Following a diet that is low in saturated fats and higher in polyunsaturated fats and that includes foods such as complex carbohydrates, protein, fruits and vegetables, and dairy products (if there are no allergies) is a reasonable and healthy choice. Daily food intake is best consumed throughout the day for optimal benefit.

- *Alternative medical systems* include such therapies as ayurveda and acupuncture. Many of these therapies have their roots in Eastern medicine and have been practiced for centuries. People living with MS report, anecdotally, that they perceive benefit from many of these therapies. Research into acupuncture indicates that it is widely practiced with benefit reported in relief of pain, spasticity, and improvement of general well-being.

- *Mind-body interventions* include prayer, relaxation, meditation, biofeedback, hypnosis, yoga, and t'ai chi. People who practice these therapies believe that the mind and body are connected and that the mind can influence the body. These are practices that many people participate in whether they have MS or not. There are studies that look at some of these methods such as yoga and t'ai chi in people with MS. Anecdotal reports and some studies suggest that these therapies may improve quality of life and may provide symptom relief. Further clinical investigation is needed.

- *Manipulative and body-based methods* are those such as chiropractic, osteopathy, and massage. These have been used for many years for many conditions. People with MS report benefits that include pain relief, spasticity reduction, increased flexibility, and improved quality of life.

- *Energy therapies* include the use of magnets, therapeutic touch, and reiki. Some studies of magnet therapy and electromagnetic therapy have shown some benefit in symptom management such as bladder function, spasticity, and pain. The Food and Drug Administration has not approved any magnets for use in MS. Therapeutic touch and reiki therapy are reported by some who practice them to provide benefit in some symptom management and quality of life.

- *Lifestyle enhancement and disease prevention* may not sound like alternative therapies to most people. These focus not on managing MS, but on prevention of other conditions. Included are exercise, adequate rest, regular visits with a healthcare professional, not smoking, eating well, wearing seat belts, seeking help for psychological issues, managing stress, and participating in leisure activities. Incorporating these into the lifestyle of a person living with MS will help improve the quality of life and will help lessen the impact of having a chronic disease.

## THE APPEAL OF ALTERNATIVE TREATMENTS

Recent surveys have shown that over 50 percent of people with MS utilize some form of alternative medicine in addition to the conventional medicine recommended by their physicians. The reasons given were to improve quality of life and to enhance overall health and sense of well-being. These patients were not looking for a cure. Respondents report both positive and negative experiences with alternative treatments. But because MS is a disease in which symptoms commonly go into remission spontaneously, it is difficult to determine whether any treatment, traditional or alternative, is responsible for a remission.

## SAFETY AND TOXICITY

Many users of alternative treatments do so because they believe that such treatments are natural and, therefore, will have fewer toxic side effects than traditional treatments. Although this is sometimes the case, it is not true of all alternative treatments. Even over-the-counter and natural substances have side effects, especially when taken in large doses or in combination with certain traditional medications. Some people with MS expressed fear of the possible side effects and toxicity of traditional treatments. This should be discussed with a healthcare provider who can help weigh the risks and benefits.

Alternative treatments offer hope. Many people with MS have not been able to find relief for their symptoms through traditional treatments. They are, therefore, willing to give alternative treatments a try. But even though no treatment has been shown, through clinical trials, to cure MS, some alternative treatment proponents make this claim. Such claims, which have no basis in scientific evidence or solid medical research, offer people a hope that traditional medicine simply cannot offer.

Most of the time, such claims are based on anecdotal evidence, that is, on stories of individuals who claim to have been helped or cured by a treatment. Because such individuals were not studied under the controlled conditions necessary to determine if a treatment is effective, it is not possible to tell if improvements were related to the treatment or caused by a remission that would have occurred anyway.

## BE A WISE CONSUMER

Although many people have reported positive experiences with alternative treatments, you need to be a wise consumer. When choosing an alternative therapy, ask these questions:

- Is there any evidence that it is harmful?
- Is there any evidence that it is helpful?
- Is it too expensive for my budget?
- Is it too difficult to access?
- Is there a potential negative interaction with any of my current medications?

In addition, the following guidelines can be helpful:

- *Beware of alternative therapies that make "hard to believe" claims or are supported by pages of testimonials from users.* The old adage, "If it sounds too good to be true, it generally is" holds true here. As Ellen Burstein MacFarlane pointed out, all human beings, no matter how strong and independent they normally are, become vulnerable to manipulation or fraud when they are faced with a crisis such as a diagnosis of MS or a worsening condition. At those times when people want to believe something, they are more vulnerable and, therefore, need to be skeptical.

- *Conduct research.* When choosing an alternative therapy practitioner, investigate the person's background, training, credentials, and specific area of expertise. Think of your doctor or other practitioner not as an authority figure, but as someone you want to have on your team.

- *Ask questions.* Find someone with whom you feel comfortable asking whatever questions are on your mind and who takes the time to give you truthful and thorough answers. If you are considering an alternative practitioner, ask how this person feels about combining alternative and traditional treatments. Be suspicious if his or her advice is to abandon traditional treatments. Choose a physician who is comfortable with your use of CAM and who will work with you in your choices.

- *Interview several potential practitioners before making your decision.* Be wary of practitioners who tell you not to listen to people who report negative experiences, or who make you feel as if you have a negative attitude if you ask questions. Asking questions is a sign that you are in charge of your life. You have a right to be fully informed!

- *Get information from as many sources as possible.* Don't rely solely on the practitioner whose treatment you are seeking or on the clients he or she tells you to call. If possible, seek out on your own people who have undergone treatment with this particular practitioner. Speak with people who have had positive experiences, as well as people who have had negative experiences. In this way, you can get a balanced view of the advantages and disadvantages of the treatment and a particular practitioner.

- *Talk with family members and friends.* In addition to discussing alternative treatments with your doctor, talk to family members or trusted friends. Get their opinions concerning the treatments and the practitioners—both traditional and alternative—that you are considering.

- *Remember that you have choices.* If any doctor or health practitioner claims that he or she is the only one who can help you, run in the other direction!

Although there is no cure for MS, there are many safe and effective ways to improve the quality of your life and enhance your overall wellness.

For additional resources, please see Appendix A.

# Chapter 12
# General Health Issues
June Halper, MSCN, ANP, FAAN

SOME HEALTH ISSUES affect all women and men, whether or not they have multiple sclerosis (MS), but are of particular concern when they may add to the symptoms or functional impairment brought about by a disabling condition. Therefore, health maintenance is extremely important in MS. Be aware that not all symptoms are related to MS.

General healthcare should include regular general checkups by your primary care physician, with assessments appropriate for your age and current symptoms and concerns. Assessment of current symptoms and problems, blood pressure assessment, Pap smears, prostate examination, and tests and examinations appropriate for the person's age are indicated. Table 12.1 summarizes the National Multiple Sclerosis Society's preventive care recommendations for adults with MS.

Examples of screening for all people include:

- Fasting cholesterol every 5 years starting at age 20.
- Fecal blood annually over age 50.
- Sigmoidoscopy every 5 years or colonoscopy every 10 years over age 50.
- Clinical breast examination annually over age 40 in women.
- Mammography every 1 to 2 years over age 40 in women.
- Vision exam annually over age 65.
- Hearing exam every 5 years over age 50.

## CANCER

### GENERAL CONCERNS

*Breast cancer.* Breast cancer strikes one in nine women in the United States, and 1,300 men a year. Cancer is actually a number of diseases, including leukemia and Hodgkin's disease, caused by the abnormal growth of cells. Often, the cells grow out of control and form masses known as tumors. Malignant or cancerous tumors not only invade normal tissue, but also travel to other parts of the body to form more malignant tumors. This spreading is called metastasis.

Breast cancer most often begins as a painless lump or thickening in the upper outer portion of the breast, but it can occur anywhere, including the nipple (see Figure 12.1). Breast cancers may spread to the lymph nodes in the arm pit and then throughout the body. Because the cause of breast cancer is unknown, there is no way to prevent it.

Risk factors for developing breast cancer include:

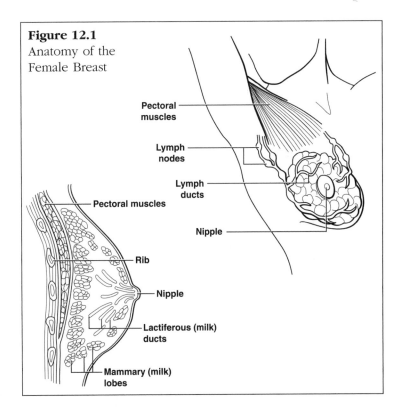

**Figure 12.1**
Anatomy of the Female Breast

Pectoral muscles

Lymph nodes

Lymph ducts

Pectoral muscles

Nipple

Rib

Nipple

Lactiferous (milk) ducts

Mammary (milk) lobes

**Table 12.1**   Preventive Care Recommendations for Adults with MS

| Medical Tests: | Recommendations: | Note dates of last & next test |
|---|---|---|
| Blood Pressure & Pulse | Yearly if normal. | |
| Height & Weight (Technically not a test, but important to track) | Test at initiation of interferon therapy, repeat in 1 month, then every 3 months thereafter. | |
| Thyroid | Consider for anyone with symptoms of fatigue. | |
| Urinalysis | Yearly and following the completion of treatment for a urinary tract infection, as per physician recommendation. | |
| Chest X-Ray | Discuss with healthcare provider. | |
| Electrocardiogram (EKG/ECG) | Discuss with healthcare provider. | |
| Total Skin Exam | Discuss with healthcare provider. Sun avoidance and sunscreen use are recommended. | |
| Dental Cleaning and Examination | Every 6 months. (Note: If daily tooth care becomes difficult, discuss with healthcare provider and consider electric appliances.) | |
| **Over age 20** | | |
| Fasting Cholesterol (with HDL, LDL, and triglycerides) | Every 5 years starting at age 20. | |
| Fasting Blood Sugar | Every 5 years starting at age 20. | |
| **Over age 40** | | |
| Thyroid | Consider for women age 40 and older and for anyone with symptoms of fatigue. | |
| Vision/Glaucoma | Every 2–4 years for ages 40–65, then yearly. | |
| **Over age 50** | | |
| Stool for Occult Blood | Yearly (three stool guaiac cards) starting at age 50. | |

*(continued on next page)*

**Table 12.1**  Preventive Care Recommendations for Adults with MS *(continued)*

| Medical Tests: | Recommendations: | Note dates of last & next test |
|---|---|---|
| Sigmoidoscopy/Colonoscopy | Every 5 years starting at age 50 for sigmoidscopy or every 10 years for colonoscopy. Begin screening high-risk individuals earlier. Consult with physician about frequency. (Reference: American Cancer Society.) | |
| Hearing | Every 5 years over age 50. | |
| **For those with risk factors** | | |
| Bone Density Test | Once, for everyone with risk factors including prolonged use of steroids or anticonvulsants, a family history of osteoporosis, and a sedentary lifestyle. Retest periodically, especially women near onset of menopause. | |
| PPD (purified protein derivative) | Every 1–2 years if at high risk for tuberculosis (including healthcare workers, persons with HIV, persons living in areas where TB is prevalent). | |
| Fasting Blood Sugar | More frequently than every 5 years for those with risk factors such as obesity or family history of type II diabetes. | |
| **Women Only** | | |
| Pap Smear | At least every 1–3 years for women who are or have been sexually active and have a cervix. The American Cancer Society recommends initiation no later than age 21. Other organizations recommend age 18 because of the high prevalence of sexual activity. | |
| Clinical Breast Exam (by healthcare provider) | Yearly. | |

*(continued on next page)*

**Table 12.1**  Preventive Care Recommendations for Adults with MS *(continued)*

| Medical Tests: | Recommendations: | Note dates of last & next test |
|---|---|---|
| Self Breast Exam | Monthly. | |
| Mammogram | Every 1–2 years starting at age 40. (The American College of Obstetricians and Gynecologists recommends every 1–2 years from age 40–49 and annually over 50 years. The American Cancer Society recommends annually starting at age 40.) If there is a family history of breast cancer, consult with a physician about appropriate beginning age. | |
| **Men Only** | | |
| Prostate Exam (digital rectal exam) | Yearly starting at age 50, except for African-Americans or those who have a family history of prostate cancer, then start at age 40. | |
| PSA (prostate-specific antigen) Test | Yearly starting at age 50, except for African-Americans or those who have a family history of prostate cancer, then start at age 40. | |
| Clinical Testicular Exam (by healthcare provider) | Yearly. | |
| Testicular Self Exam | Monthly. The American Academy of Pediatrics recommends starting at age 18. | |

| Vaccines: | Recommendations: | Note dates |
|---|---|---|
| **Immunizations** | | |
| Tetanus-Diphtheria | Boosters every 10 years. | |
| Rubella (German measles) | Women of child-bearing age. | |
| Varicella (chicken pox) | Women of child-bearing age who have not had chicken pox. | |

*(continued on next page)*

**Table 12.1**  Preventive Care Recommendations for Adults with MS *(continued)*

| Vaccines: | Recommendations: | Note dates |
|---|---|---|
| Flu Vaccine | Yearly for those who are susceptible to the flu, likely to be exposed, or have respiratory problems or certain chronic disorders. Pregnant women who will be in second or third trimester during flu season should also receive a flu shot. | |
| Hepatitis B Vaccine | Healthcare or public safety workers who have exposure to blood at workplace. Household contacts and sex partners of those infected with hepatitis. Sexually active men and women with more than one partner in last 6 months or with recently acquired sexually transmitted diseases. Intravenous drug abusers. | |
| Pneumococcal Pneumonia Vaccine | Once at age 65 or older. If received before age 65, need booster after 5 years. | |
| Other Immunizations | Supplemental immunizations (Hepatitis A, for example) may be needed in special circumstances such as overseas travel. | |

*Acknowledgments:* Thank you to the National Multiple Sclerosis Society's National Council of Clinical Advisory Committee Chairs for professional reviews, and to the Southern California Chapter for initiating this project.

To reach the nearest Society office: 1-800-FIGHT-MS

Web site: nationalmssociety.org

## General Health and Safety Recommendations

- *Stop smoking (or don't start)* to reduce your risk of cancer and heart disease. It's not too late to join a smoking cessation group and/or consider medication to help decrease the desire to smoke.

- *Exercise regularly.* Check with your doctor before starting on a new exercise program.

- *Eat a well-balanced diet.* Limit fat and cholesterol. Emphasize fruits, grains, and vegetables to reduce risk of heart disease, control constipation, and maintain a healthy weight.

- *Drink fluids.* Drink plenty of fluids every day to maintain general health and health of the urinary system, and to lessen constipation.

- *Maintain a healthy weight.* If you are overweight, lose weight to reduce your risk of developing heart disease, hypertension, diabetes, and other diseases.

- *Consume adequate calcium.* Adults between ages 19–50 should consume 1,200 mg daily. Women aged 51 and older and men aged 65 and older should consume 1,200–1,500 mg daily.

- Women of childbearing age should be consuming 0.4–0.8 mg of *folic acid every day* to prevent common birth defects (neural tube defects or spina bifida). Folic acid (or folate) is a vitamin that is contained in many multivitamin supplements.

- *Alcohol* can affect balance, coordination, and thinking. It depresses the nervous system and may interact with your medications. Check with your doctor about whether alcohol is safe for you, and if so, how much and how often.

- *Protect yourself against sexually transmitted diseases* by using condoms whenever appropriate, and by using your best judgment with sexual partners.

- *Wear lap and shoulder belts* while driving or riding in vehicles.

- Install and maintain *smoke detectors.*

---

- Having close relatives, such as a mother, sister, aunt, or grandmother, with breast cancer.
- Giving birth to a first child after age 30, or not giving birth at all.
- Having an abortion during first pregnancy.
- Being obese.
- Having early onset of menstruation, before age 12.
- Experiencing late menopause.
- Smoking cigarettes.
- Eating a diet that is high in fat.
- Consuming alcohol.

Women with neurologic disease are at no greater risk for breast cancer than the general population, although inactivity may lead to weight gain and altered mobility, which can in themselves increase the risk of developing breast cancer. Access to regular medical care may thus be affected. Men too, have a risk (less than women) of breast cancer. Reduced hand function and sensation may interfere with monthly breast self-examinations, which are recommended for all women. If you use a wheelchair, you may find it challenging to get into the proper position for a mammogram.

To reduce your risk for breast cancer, follow these guidelines:

- Maintain a healthy weight and reduce your fat intake.
- Eat foods that are high in fiber.
- Include plenty of deep green vegetables in your diet.
- Limit salt-cured, smoked, or nitrite-cured foods, such as ham, hot dogs, bacon, and sausage.
- If you have fluid-filled sacs or small cysts in your breasts (called *fibrocystic breasts*), decrease or eliminate caffeine.
- Maintain moderate use of alcohol.
- Stop smoking.

In addition, the American Cancer Society recommends the following:

- Examine your own breasts monthly, so you can detect changes early.
- See your health professional at least every 3 years until age 40, and annually thereafter, for a clinical breast examination.
- Obtain a baseline mammogram by age 40 and annual mammograms after age 50.
- Request a biopsy of all suspicious lumps.

---

**Figure 12.2**
Breast Self-Exam (BSE)

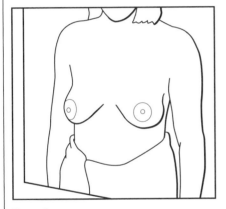 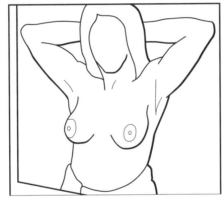 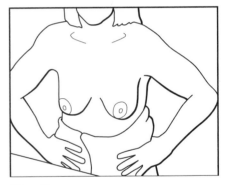

**Step 1**
Here's what you should do to check for changes in your breasts. Stand or sit before a mirror (above). Check each breast for anything unusual, such as any discharge from the nipples, puckering, dimpling, or scaling of the skin. Each time you examine your breasts you will become more familiar with how they appear and feel, making it easier to notice any changes that may occur. Notice the normal size and shape of each breast (it is not unusual for one breast to be larger than the other) and the normal position of the nipple.

**Step 2**
Clasp your hands behind your head and press them forward. You should feel your chest muscles tighten. Look in the mirror at the shape and contour of your breasts. Take your time; again, look for any changes in the size and shape of each breast and look for any swelling, dimpling, rash, discoloration, or other unusual changes in the skin.

**Step 3**
Next, press your hands firmly on your hips and bend slightly toward your mirror as you pull your shoulders and elbows forward. Once again, you should feel your chest muscles tighten. Look for any change in the shape or contour of your breasts.

**Step 4**
Gently squeeze each nipple and look for a discharge. If present, see your doctor. In fact, if you have a discharge at *any* time you should check it out with your doctor.

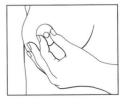

Monthly self-examinations involve inspecting the breasts in a mirror to look for lumps, changes in breast shape, or discharge from the nipple. Use your fingers to evaluate your breasts for lumps or pain. Feel your breasts in overlapping areas about the size of a dime. Remember to also check the underarm and upper chest areas (see Figure 12.2).

If MS interferes with your ability to perform a self-examination, you can teach your husband, care partner, or care provider to assist you. Ideally, this examination should be done four to seven days after your menstrual period (if you are still menstruating) or on a regularly scheduled basis (if you have gone through menopause).

Self-care to identify changes in breast tissue is very important. If breast cancer is treated at its earliest, noninvasive stage, the survival rate is almost 100 percent.

*Ovarian and cervical cancer.* Ovarian and cervical cancer are also life-threatening problems if they go unrecognized and, therefore, untreated. Every woman should have an annual pelvic examination with a Pap smear performed by a gynecologist or by a trained nurse practitioner. If you practice birth control, evaluate its effectiveness

---

**Figure 12.2**
Breast Self-Exam (BSE)

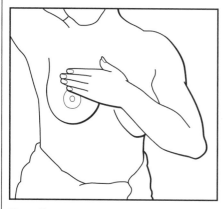
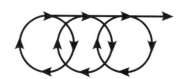
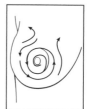
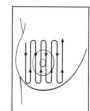
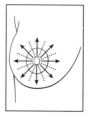

**Step 5**
The next step is done standing or sitting straight up. Raise your left arm. Use the pads of your fingers of your right hand to check your left breast and the surrounding area—firmly, carefully, and thoroughly. Some women like to use lotion or powder to help their fingers glide easily over the skin. Feel for any unusual lump or mass under the skin. A lump is unusual if it has not been felt during earlier breast exams and it now stands out against the normal feel of your breast.

Use the pads of your fingers.

Feel your breast in overlapping areas.

Some research suggests that many women do breast self-examinations more thoroughhly when they use a pattern of up-and-down lines or strips. Other women feel more comfortable with another pattern. The important thing is to cover the entire breast and to pay special attention to the area between the breast and the underarm, including the underarm itself. Check the area above the breast, up to the collarbone and all the way over to your shoulder.

Feel the tissue by pressing your fingers in small, overlapping areas about the size of a dime. To make sure that you cover your entire breast, *take your time* and follow a definite pattern; circles, lines, or wedges (see above).

**Figure 12.2**
Breast Self-Exam (BSE)

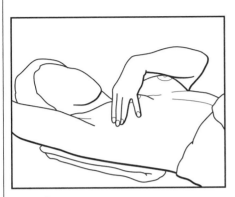

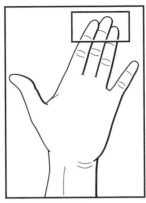

**Step 6**

Repeat step 5 lying down. Lie flat on your back, with your left arm over your head and a pillow or folded towel placed under your left shoulder. This position flattens the breast and makes it easier to examine. Check the left breast and the area around it very carefully, using one of the patterns described in step 5. Repeat the exam on the right breast.

If your breasts are large, you may need to hold the side of each one steady with your other hand while you are performing the examination.

**Step 7**

Some women repeat step 5 in the shower. Your fingers will glide easily over soapy skin, so you can concentrate on feeling for changes underneath.

*hypertrophy* (enlargement) is one of the most common conditions affecting middle-aged and older men. Enlargement can interfere with the flow of urine, because the prostate surrounds the urethra, the tube that carries urine out of the bladder. This enlargement is identified through a rectal examination and a blood test called prostate-specific antigen (PSA). Prostatic hypertrophy can be treated with medication to reduce the swelling or with surgery performed by a urologist.

Prostate cancer is now the most common form of cancer in men. About 100,000 men are diagnosed with prostate cancer each year. Most men do not die from the disease. Treatment for prostate cancer may consist of surgery, radiation therapy, chemotherapy, or a combination of regimens.

The most important element in the treatment of prostate cancer is diagnosis. If you are over age 50, you should visit your physician annually for a checkup. African-Americans or men with a family history of prostate cancer should start at age 40. The prostate gland should be examined for enlargement, hardness, or lumps.

*Testicular cancer.* The testes are walnut-shaped glands that reside in a protective

regularly with your physician. If you are approaching menopause, discuss your options for hormone replacement therapy (HRT). Menopausal symptoms, your potential for developing osteoporosis, and your risk for developing cardiovascular disease should be part of this discussion.

## MEN'S CONCERNS

*Conditions of the prostate gland.* The prostate gland straddles the urethra and is the size of a chestnut. It is shaped like a doughnut and is gray to red in color. It contains and secretes fluid involved in the ejaculation of seminal fluid. *Benign prostatic*

sac called the scrotum (see Figure 12.3). The primary functions of the testes are to produce sperm and hormones, called androgens, that become testosterone. As sperm are manufactured, they travel through a tube called the epididymis, into another tube, the vas deferens, where they are stored. The testes of a young adult male produce about 120 million sperm each day. During intercourse, fluids from the prostate and seminal vesicles and sperm from the vas deferens are pumped into the upper part of the urethra, where they mix. This mixture comes out of the urethra during intercourse.

Testicular cancer, while not as common as prostate cancer, can occur throughout a man's lifetime. It is most common among men between the ages of 20 and 35. Two groups are particularly susceptible: men whose testicles descended into the scrotum after age 6, and men whose testicles never descended. Men who were born with low birth weight are also at higher risk. If the disease is diagnosed early, survival from testicular cancer is better than 90 percent.

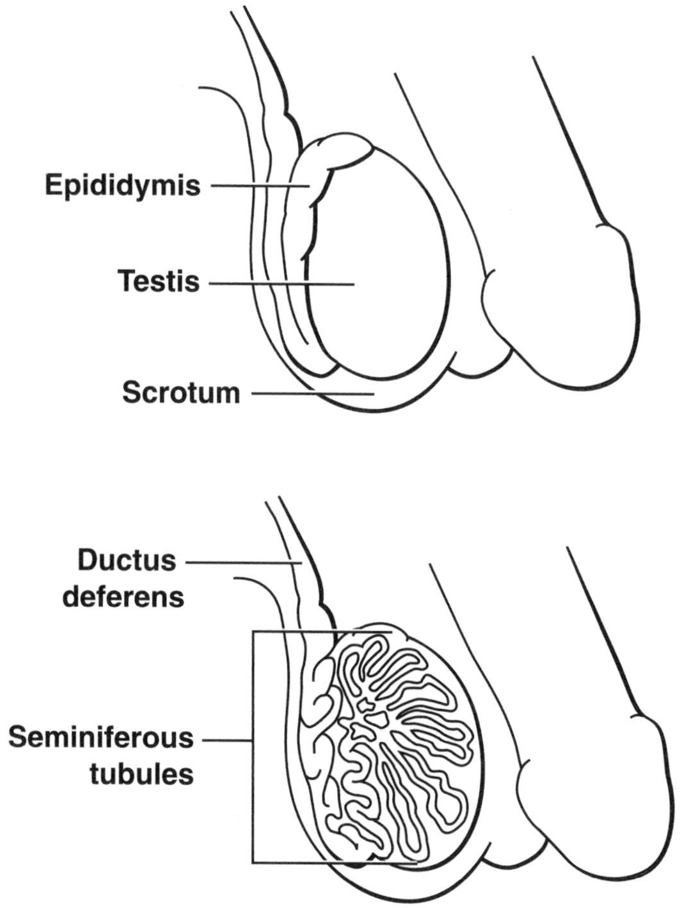

It is extremely important for a man to perform testicular self-examination on a monthly basis (see Figure 12.4). You need to become familiar with the usual size, shape, and consistency of your testicles. They should be smooth, egg-shaped, and firm. Also note the color of your scrotum, the sac of skin that holds your testicles. Do not be alarmed if one testicle is larger than the other. This is normal. You may also feel a cordlike structure on the top and back of each testicle. This is the epididymis. Try to perform your self-examination after a warm bath or shower because the scrotal skin is looser at the time. Visually inspect for changes of color and appearance. Examine each testicle with both hands by placing the index and middle fingers under the testicle and the thumbs on top. Gently roll, feeling for changes. The first sign of testicular cancer is usually a hard, painless lump the size of a pea. Also examine the penis for lumps, sores, ulcers, or changes in color.

*Epididymitis.* Other problems, such as *epididymitis* (inflammation of the epididymis), may go unrecognized without self-examination or visual inspection. Men with MS may have diminished hand function or sensation. Examination by a spouse or care provider will be a key factor in the early identification of changes and potential problems. Lumps, redness, swelling, pain, or discharge should signal the need for contact with a physician and prompt medical attention.

**Figure 12.3**
Male Reproductive Anatomy

Epididymis

Testis

Scrotum

Ductus deferens

Seminiferous tubules

**Figure 12.4**
Testicular Self-Exam (TSE)

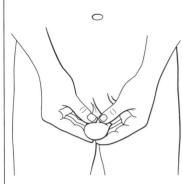

**When and how to do a testicular self-exam**

Try to perform TSE after a warm bath or shower. The scrotal skin will be loose and the testes easier to examine. Follow these steps:

1. Visually inspect the scrotum for changes in color—reddening, for example—or appearance, such as darkening.

2. Examine each testicle with both hands by placing the index and middle fingers under the testicle and the thumbs on top. Gently roll the testicle between the thumbs and fingers, feeling for any changes—whether it's more or less firm  or whether there are lumps, swelling, or painful spots. The first sign of testicular cancer is usually a hard, painless lump about the size of a pea.

3. Follow the same procedure on the other testicle.

Also examine the penis for lumps, sore, ulcers, or a change in color.

**What to expect if you find something abnormal**

If you find a lump—or any other abnormality—make an appointment with your doctor right away. The doctor will want to see you to rule out less serious causes. Inflammation, for instance, can be caused by viral or bacterial infection. Swelling may be the result of swollen veins within the scrotum, a collection of fluid, or a cyst.

If the doctor suspects cancer, he or she will refer you to a surgeon who will need to remove the testicle for direct examination. There's no other way to confirm the diagnosis. If cancer is confirmed and it's in an early stage, the removal of the testicle may have been enough to cure the disease.

The surgeon will also order a CT or ultrasound scan and lab tests to see if cancer may have spread to other parts of the body. Even if there's no sign of spread, the surgeon may suggest radiation therapy to the remaining testicle and lymph glands as a precaution. If the disease has spread, chemotherapy is likely.

Although removal of a testis for diagnosis reduces sperm count, it doesn't interfere with sexual function or preclude reproduction. Dealing with the loss of a testicle may well be difficult for you, but you can take comfort in knowing that by doing TSE, you've maximized your chances of surviving this disease.

ADDITIONAL INFORMATION

For additional information about cancer, self-examination, or other issues see Appendix A, Resources.

## VISION

Although some vision problems may be due to MS, do not assume that all visual effects are a result of the disease; all of the common visual problems seen in other people occur in people with MS. Regular checks of vision should be made and those that can be corrected with lenses should be managed normally. MS-related visual problems cannot be corrected by lenses, but the need for reading glasses by the age of 40, and the incidence of glaucoma, uveitis, cataract, and other disorders are the same as for everyone else.

## HORMONALLY MEDIATED EVENTS

Many women with MS notice changes in their symptoms related to the menstrual cycle, such as a return of previously experienced problems. This "relapse" usually improves as the flow begins. If this is a significant problem, controlling the menstrual cycle with a birth control pill may alleviate these symptoms; you should consult your gynecologist.

Women who are in their childbearing years and have MS should be in contact with their gynecologist when considering pregnancy. Prenatal and postnatal counseling and support are important to guarantee adequate rest, avoidance of infection, and management of stress. First-time parents need a lot of education and advice, and the experienced mother needs additional support, as her other children have their own needs and household responsibilities continue.

Menopause may cause uncomfortable symptoms in many women and can be controlled to a great extent by HRT. Some of these symptoms, "hot flashes," fatigue, and bone thinning (leading to osteoporosis) can intensify symptoms and problems related to MS. Osteoporosis has been linked to the treatment of MS with steroids, and this condition may worsen during the perimenopausal or menopausal state of life.

Unfortunately, there is some controversy in the medical community about the benefit/risk ratio of HRT and women should consult their personal physician and gynecologist to discuss the pros and cons of these medications. There are other reasons your physician might suggest HRT for a person with MS, as they can reduce postmenopausal complications that include osteoporosis, weight gain, fatigue, vaginal dryness, diminished libido, increased cardiovascular disorders, and decreased exercise tolerance.

## PSEUDORELAPSES

### HEAT AND HUMIDITY

Symptoms of MS may be aggravated by heat in approximately 80 percent of patients.

When this occurs in a hot room, in a hot bath, or on a hot muggy day, it may mistakenly be identified as an MS attack, even though the symptoms often disappear as soon as you move to a cooler place. People with MS often note that they may become so weak after a hot bath that they must lie down to rest and may even have trouble getting out of the bath. On a hot muggy day, you may be so affected by heat that you feel dizzy, weak, and very ill. Such episodes are not attacks, and you must be advised about avoiding heat, taking cold drinks and cool showers, and using air conditioning.

### EXERCISE

Exercise is important for people with neurologic problems, but some will note worsening symptoms and weakness when their body heat increases. Most people do well with exercises in a swimming pool because the water cools the body during exercise, thus increasing exercise tolerance. An individualized conditioning program, designed to be reasonable about a balance between the benefits of exercise and the fatigue that it may cause may be the best option.

### INFECTION

Infections can increase symptoms by increasing body temperature, but they last longer because an infection may go on for many days. Because infections may precede an acute attack, the situation may have to be assessed carefully to see if this is a transient episode related to the temperature and symptoms of the infection or a longer lasting problem requiring immediate medical attention.

### INTERFERON THERAPY

Pseudorelapses also may occur when a person first begins interferon therapy, as there may be a period during which the side effects, which may be accompanied by some aggravation of spasticity, can feel like an acute attack. In such cases, a reduction of the dose, slowly increasing as the person adjusts to the drug (see Chapter 3, "Disease Management"), usually will manage this situation; if the side effects remain intolerable, the person might be switched to glatiramer acetate (Copaxone®).

## INFECTIONS

People with MS are not more prone to infection than other people are, except when they develop bladder involvement or when inactivity or being confined mainly to bed makes them less resistant to respiratory tract infections.

Viral infections can be a problem because they not only make the person weaker, but also may precipitate an attack of MS. Because they do not respond to antibiotics, prevention is the best plan. Vaccinations to prevent influenza are helpful for MS patients, as they, to a significant extent, prevent the major anticipated influenzas for that season. They have been shown to be relatively safe for MS patients.

An interesting coincidence is that *amantadine*, an antiviral agent that can treat influenza, may also be helpful in treating the fatigue that is so common in MS patients.

Good general management of infections with fluids, acetaminophen, nonsteroidal anti-inflammatory drugs (NSAIDs), and rest can make the person comfortable until the infection has passed.

## COMPLICATIONS OF TREATMENT

Many of the treatments for MS may result in drug side effects and complications. It is a good principle for physicians to outline the common or expected side effects and possible complications to patients, and for patients to be sure that they understand the drugs they take. Interferons may aggravate some symptoms when initiated, and these drugs as well as glatiramer acetate may cause allergic responses.

- Steroids may cause *Cushingoid* features (facial fullness, acne, easy bruising, and risk for osteoporosis) if used for weeks or more, which is not recommended.
- An occasional patient who has had repeated courses of steroids may develop aseptic necrosis of the hip. The pain and increased difficulty in walking is often attributed to progression of the MS, and may result in an inappropriate course of steroids.
- Osteoporosis, as discussed earlier, is a common problem in older women and is increased in MS because of inactivity and the use of steroids. Recognizing the risks and identifying the problem is important, as this can further disable MS patients, and treatment and prevention can be helpful.

Perhaps the easiest discussion is the list of diseases that are associated with MS. One might think that there would be an association with other immunologic diseases because MS has an immunologic aspect. In fact, there is little evidence for such an association, aside from anecdotal reports that might be expected just by the expected incidence of these disorders in the general population. Because there may be 400,000 people with MS in the United States alone, a large number of diseases would be expected to occur due to the natural incidence of these conditions. There is no more cancer, rheumatoid arthritis, or other common illness in people with MS than in any other group of people.

## OTHER DISEASES

Other illnesses in people with MS can occur unrelated to MS or be complications related to MS.

Illnesses that can occur in anyone else can occur in people with MS, but may be difficult to identify, especially if the symptoms are similar to those produced by the disease.

- Hypothyroidism can cause slowing down, fatigue, weight gain, slowing of thinking, and even neurologic symptoms.
- Hypertension is common in our society, and this important risk factor must be assessed in MS patients, like anyone else, and treated if blood pressure remains elevated.
- The aches and pains of arthritis and fibromyalgia are often ascribed to MS. Because nonspecific pain occurs in approximately half of all MS patients, it needs careful assessment to determine how to manage it best.
- Insomnia is another common problem in the MS population and can make dealing with other symptoms difficult, especially fatigue.

## COMMON COMPLICATIONS RELATED TO MS

- Bladder infection is a common complication of the neurologic involvement of the bladder and must be recognized and treated. Adequate fluids, cranberry tablets, and good perineal hygiene are important in preventing infections, and prophylactic antibiotics may be necessary.
- Decubiti, or pressure sores, can be prevented by good skin care, shifting weight frequently while sitting, and turning the entire body while in bed, with attention to mattresses, pillows, and chair seats.
- Pressure palsies can occur as the result of pressure on a peripheral nerve, and the sensory loss or weakness that results

may mistakenly be blamed on MS.
- Trigeminal neuralgia occurs in a small number of patients with MS and responds to the usual therapies, including carbamazepine, baclofen, or local neurosurgical procedures.
- Epilepsy (seizure disorder) is not common in MS, but does occur in 5 percent of patients; it also responds to the usual treatments for seizures.

## HEALTH ISSUES FOR CAREGIVERS

The health of family members who often provide extensive home care services (caregivers) is extremely important, but often neglected in the discussion of MS needs and supports. It may be neglected by the person with MS, who sees all others as healthy, in comparison; it may be neglected by the physician, who concentrates on the more obvious needs of the person with MS and, more importantly, it is often neglected by the caregivers themselves, as they believe their problems and needs are minor compared with those of their loved one with MS.

Many studies have shown that caregivers neglect their own health. They do not get regular checkups, do not have their blood pressure taken regularly, and are not being treated for important problems and risk factors when they are present. It is interesting that this is different for women and men in many cases, as women more naturally move into the caregiver role and pay less attention to themselves in view of the new responsibilities, whereas men assume the role in a more organized manner and often include their own health issues as part of the overall project. Thus, women are more likely than men to neglect their health, their personal lives, and their exercise as part of caregiving.

Caregiving is a natural part of a relationship, and when both members are healthy, the caregiving is balanced and equal. When one becomes ill, the balance shifts, and as the disease progresses, the weight of caregiving falls mostly on the shoulders of the "healthy" partner. The number of tasks performed by the caregiver often increases over time, and the caregiver and the healthcare professionals must recognize that it is in the interest of the patient as well as the caregiver to make sure that the caregiver's health is a priority.

All of the aforementioned recommendations about general healthcare apply to the caregiver as well. Caregivers should also recognize that the National MS Society has useful information on the nature and role of caregivers, and can also advise about respite programs and self-help groups aimed at more successful and healthy caregiving.

## SEEKING WELLNESS

When confronted with the challenge of neurologic conditions with no cure and complex treatments, the patient and family must assume ongoing responsibility for healthcare and self-monitoring. The *wellness model* is a collaboration between the person with MS and the healthcare team, a positive striving toward self-awareness and self-responsibility. Wellness is a positive striving, unique to the individual, in which a person can have a disease and still be well, with a deep appreciation for the joy of living and with a life purpose. General guidelines include weight control, keeping cholesterol and other blood fats within normal limits, eating a well-balanced diet, managing stress, and getting adequate rest. In addition, balancing work with fun, incorporating hobbies and other life-fulfilling activities, and interacting with a supportive social and family network, are all wellness activities that have been shown to result in better health. It is important to put one's life and life's challenges into perspective and to deal with each day as a new opportunity for fulfillment and satisfaction.

# Chapter 13
# Exercise Options and Wellness Programs
Brian Hutchinson, PhD and Richard W. Hicks, PhD

EXERCISE IS OFTEN the focal point of a comprehensive wellness program. Recent research projects have examined the effects of exercise and broader based wellness programs on people with multiple sclerosis (MS). Prior to this research, it was thought that exercise and wellness programs were either inappropriate or futile. It was thought that exercise may actually increase the disease process of MS. Wellness programs were thought to be either complementary or alternative and therefore not relevant to a person with a chronic disease such as MS. Now we are learning the importance of exercise and wellness programs in improving or maintaining overall physical and psychological health.

Many problems are associated with decreased activity, a sedentary lifestyle, poor nutrition, and increased emotional stress, as follows:

- Decreased activity leads to decreased endurance.
- A sedentary lifestyle means that fewer calories are expended during the course of a day, making weight gain much more likely.
- Obesity, secondary to decreased activity or poor dietary habits, is a risk factor for heart disease and stroke, two of the top three killers in our society.
- Poor dietary habits are also related to increased blood lipid levels, another risk factor for heart disease.
- Inactivity is associated with feelings of depression and anxiety.

Exercise programs have been shown to improve strength, flexibility, and endurance and promote a greater sense of well-being.

Increased activity has been positively correlated to decreases in the risk for heart disease. Exercise has not been shown to affect the disease process either positively or adversely, but it has been shown to decrease the complications that arise from a sedentary lifestyle. These benefits can improve overall mobility. Wellness or health promotion programs focus on areas that empower program participants to take charge of their health. These programs generally complement existing treatment.

## PHYSICAL FITNESS, PHYSICAL ACTIVITY, AND EXERCISE

Physical fitness is the outcomes or traits that relate to the ability to perform physical activity. Physical activity is any bodily movement produced by skeletal muscle that results in caloric expenditure. Exercise is a subcategory of physical activity—physical activity that is planned, structured, and repetitive. Exercise has been shown to be effective in improving physical fitness and quality of life. The purpose of an exercise or physical activity program is to improve overall health. In part, physical activity determines physical fitness, but many other factors have a role in physical fitness and these will be covered in the section on wellness programs.

Exercise can be broken down into three main categories: aerobic or cardio-respiratory exercise, strength training, and stretching and flexibility activities. Most people can benefit from a comprehensive program that includes all of these areas, but some people choose to emphasize one area over another, based on individual needs and preferences.

## AEROBIC/CARDIORESPIRATORY EXERCISE

Aerobic exercise consists of rhythmic, large-muscle movements at moderate to high intensity. Activities such as walking, bicycling, swimming, cross country skiing, and stair stepping are considered aerobic exercise. Regular aerobic exercise reduces the risk of myocardial infarction, high blood pressure, excess body fat, resting heart rate, and lung function. In addition, aerobic exercise has been positively correlated with improvements in emotion and mood.

A cardiorespiratory exercise "prescription" generally consists of four areas: *Frequency*, *Intensity*, *Time* or Duration, and Mode or *Type* of Activity, often referred to as the *FITT* principle. Recommendations in these different areas are dependent upon the goals of your exercise program. The following recommendations, suggested by the American College of Sports Medicine, are geared toward: 1) enhancing physical fitness, 2) reducing risk for future development or recurrence of cardiovascular disease, and 3) ensuring safety during participation in exercise.

- *Frequency*—3 to 5 times per week
- *Intensity*—55 to 90 percent of maximal heart rate
- *Time*—15 to 60 minutes
- *Type*—Any activity that uses large muscle groups, can be maintained for prolonged periods, and is rhythmic

These are good guidelines to keep in mind when beginning an exercise program; however, sometimes they are merely guidelines. Multiple sclerosis can add some different challenges when recommending aerobic exercise. For instance, some people with MS demonstrate blunted heart rate responses to exercise—a condition in which the heart rate does not increase with exercise intensity—and may find it hard to achieve the "tar-

**Table 13.1** Rate of perceived exertion (RPE) scale

| | |
|------|------------------|
| 0 | Nothing at all |
| 0.5 | Extremely light |
| 1 | Very light |
| 2 | Light |
| 3 | Moderate |
| 4 | Somewhat heavy |
| 5 | Heavy |
| 6 | |
| 7 | Very heavy |
| 8 | |
| 9 | Extremely heavy |
| 10 | Maximal |

get" heart rate. Therefore, it may be more effective to think about the *FITT* principle in the following manner.

- *Frequency*—Don't miss more than 2 days in a row. Try to move every day, but don't worry if you miss a day. Be kind to yourself as you slowly develop this "therapeutic ritual."
- *Intensity*—Utilize a rate of perceived exertion (RPE) scale (see Table 13.1). The RPE scale is a numerical scale that will help you define the proper level of exertion for an exercise session. The most effective way to determine the proper RPE is through a graded exercise test with your healthcare specialist. This will be particularly helpful to those with the blunted heart rate response described earlier.
- *Time*—Start a time that is comfortable for you and progress from there. Progression should be approximately 10 percent per week. Don't try to increase the time too much or too quickly.

- *Type*—Pick something you enjoy and that is available. You may need to look at ways to modify the activity (e.g., specialized bike pedals), but if you enjoy something, you are more likely to stick with it.

Starting an aerobic exercise program takes commitment! It is important to set realistic goals and utilize your healthcare team in identifying an appropriate exercise prescription. Some tips to keep in mind when beginning your program include:

- Approach your exercise as a "therapeutic ritual." Schedule your exercise on certain days and do your best to stick with it. There will be times when it is not possible, but to "build the habit," it is important to incorporate it into your life.
- Five-minute rule—Because exercise is a therapeutic ritual, begin your activity on the days you have set. If after 5 minutes of the activity you feel "increased fatigue," then stop the activity and schedule it on another day. If you feel better, which is often the case, then complete your activity for that day.
- Two-hour rule—If 2 hours after you have finished exercising, you don't feel as well as you did before you started, then you probably exercised too hard. (This usually manifests as an increase in fatigue.)
- It is OK to break up your exercise throughout the day. If you experience increased fatigue with 20 minutes of continuous exercise, try two separate 10-minute sessions. Think in terms of cumulative increases in exercise, not necessarily what you do in one session. It is what you do every day that counts, not what you do on a single day.
- Drink plenty of fluids to stay hydrated and cool.

- Pick an appropriate time of day to exercise to avoid overheating and increased fatigue.
- Consider exercising with a group of people. This will increase socialization and commitment to the exercise program.

## STRENGTH TRAINING

Many people with MS experience a decrease in muscle strength, power, and endurance. Research has demonstrated that people with MS, as a group, have less strength than people without MS. The loss in strength is often secondary to decreased nerve signals to the muscle, resulting in neurological weakness. However, other studies have shown that people with MS can improve their muscle strength with a regular exercise program.

In addition, muscle spasticity will often affect the strength of the opposite muscle group. For example, spasticity in the biceps, which help flex or bend the elbow, may accentuate or increase weakness of the triceps, which help extend or straighten the elbow. It may be difficult for the triceps to generate enough force to overcome the spasticity of the biceps.

Muscle weakness can also be caused or accentuated by deconditioning secondary to disuse. Loss of muscle strength can increase problems with balance, mobility, endurance, and fatigue. Strength training exercises are designed to correct muscle weakness caused by deconditioning. Strengthening exercises seek to improve muscle power and endurance, both of which are necessary for you to perform your daily activities.

A physician or physical therapist should assess your need for a strength training program and identify the muscles or muscle groups most in need of attention. In addition, they can help identify the source of weakness and design an appropriate program to gain the greatest results. Muscle strengthening is best accomplished through "progressive resistance." Resistance can be in the form of weights, resistive tubing or bands, manual resistance, your own body weight, or gravity. Consult your physical therapist, occupational therapist, exercise physiologist, or exercise specialist to help you determine the type and amount of resistance you need and the number of sets and repetitions you should perform for optimal benefit.

Strength training for a person with MS requires the expertise and experience of a therapist who works with neurological conditions. Strength training principles for a person with MS are different from those for orthopedic conditions such as fractures, sprains, or muscle strains. The primary difference is the separation of neurological weakness from deconditioning. Overexercising a neurologically weak muscle can increase the muscle's weakness, and generally leads to frustration and discontinuation of the strength program.

*Closed chain exercises* are exercises in which the extremity is fixed and there is motion on both sides of the joint. Examples of closed chain exercises are squats, stair stepping, and push-ups. *Open chain exercises* are exercises in which the extremity is free to move. Examples of open chain exercises are knee extensions, leg curls, and biceps curls. Both types of exercises have advantages. Closed chain exercises often add an element of balance, which is often appropriate for the person with MS, while open chain exercises are generally safer for people with significant balance difficulties. Because many daily activities incorporate both closed and open chain activities, you need to incorporate both into your strength training program.

Design of a strength training program requires two primary considerations, safety and balance. Some strengthening exercises are best performed in a standing position. But be aware that balance difficulties can result in injury. Muscle fatigue, incorrect performance of an exercise, and inappropriate equipment also can increase your risk of injury. You do not need to work your muscles to the point of fatigue, and you may require some modifications to the equipment to optimize muscle function. Finally, be sure to perform strengthening exercises through a full range of motion, both to strengthen the muscle throughout the range and to avoid abnormal muscle shortening.

## STRETCHING AND FLEXIBILITY

A regular stretching program is important to maintain optimal length of muscles and other soft tissue structures (e.g., tendons, fascia, and connective tissue). If you have tightness in any areas, you increase your risk of injury or possible contractures secondary to abnormal shortening of the muscles or other soft tissue structures. Ultimately, such tightness reduces mobility, because of the decrease in range of motion, and makes you more prone to sprains and strains. Finally, a stretching program reduces muscle tension and increases relaxation.

Many people with MS experience spasticity. Increased spasticity will often increase muscle stiffness and tightness. If untreated, spasticity can result in pain, reduced range of motion, and even contractures. Studies have shown that a combination of antispasticity medication and stretching is the most effective means of treating mild to moderate spasticity.

Stretching is best performed slowly and statically. Slow, static stretching—stretching that does not include bouncing—prevents the stretch reflex from being activated. Any time muscles are stretched too far (or too quickly), a nerve signal is sent to the muscle to contract. Therefore, if you stretch too far, either by bouncing or overstretching, the muscle will contract to keep from being injured and eliminate positive effects of the stretch.

Stretching should be relaxing and feel comfortable. To promote good muscle length, you should hold mild tension in the muscles or other soft tissue structures for 20 to 60 seconds. You should perform each stretch three to five times. Your program may be designed for you to be in a sitting, lying, or standing position. It may be beneficial to perform your stretching program either with an assistant or with assistive aids such as belts, towels, or other everyday items.

Generally, stretching programs are performed once per day, but in certain cases, they may be recommended more often. Consult with your healthcare professionals to assess your degree of tightness—and spasticity—to determine how often you need to perform your stretching exercises. They will also be able to help you with the appropriate types of stretching exercises to maximize benefit and minimize fatigue.

There are books on stretching which provide information and illustrations on different types of stretching. Many of these books are available through the National Multiple Sclerosis Society.

## OTHER TYPES OF EXERCISE

*Balance.* Some exercises can improve balance. For example, you can use balance boards, Swiss balls, and variable surfaces to assist in balance training. However, balance problems are individual, and a balance training program should be designed by your healthcare professional to address your specific needs and maximize safety. A study evaluating a structured Awareness through Movement program to improve balance demonstrated improvements in balance, balance confidence, and self-efficacy.

*Yoga.* Yoga has become a very popular activity for many people. Yoga for people with MS can be beneficial in improving overall flexibility and body awareness. In addition, yoga is performed at the level of the participant, so fatigue and balance problems can be minimized. Yoga can be performed through organized classes or by using video tapes to guide you through the different poses. When researching yoga classes, discuss with the instructor any limitations you may have and how they will be accommodated during the class. Many MS clinics and local chapters of the National Multiple Sclerosis Society offer yoga classes specifically for people with MS.

*Pilates.* The Pilates method has become a very popular form of physical activity. The Pilates method consists of specific body movements in which the individual is focused on the muscles being used. Pilates proponents claim increased benefits with strength and flexibility. Individuals with MS have reported that the Pilates method is helpful and allows them to participate in activity without increasing fatigue or core body temperature. An individual should receive training from a trained instructor before continuing on a home program.

*Hydrotherapy.* Hydrotherapy and water exercise can be an excellent form of activity for people with MS. In the buoyancy of water, you can perform many activities you may not be able to perform on land, and in the coolness of water, you usually will not become overheated. It is important to be aware of water temperature when choosing a pool for a hydrotherapy program. A temperature of approximately 80 to 84 degrees Farenheit is most often recommended. However, you may find that a slightly higher or cooler temperature works best for you. Aquatic exercises can include stretching, strengthening, aerobic, balance, and relaxation. Hydrotherapy includes specific techniques, usually facilitated by a trained aquatics instructor, which incorporate a variety of functional activities.

*T'ai chi.* T'ai chi is another popular activity, which consists of slow, rhythmic body movements. Research has shown that tai chi does increase strength and flexibility and may also improve fatigue. T'ai chi is often performed as part of a group, which may provide significant benefits with socialization. Many people with MS feel that t'ai chi is effective in improving balance and mobility and reducing stiffness. It may be an effective form of activity for people with MS, but individuals should receive training from an individual trained in working with people with disabilities.

*Therapeutic horseback riding or hippotherapy.* Hippotherapy and therapeutic horseback riding are activities often used along with physical therapy. Hippotherapy and therapeutic horseback riding are very popular techniques for the pediatric population, but have become more popular with adult neurological populations, such as those with MS. Hippotherapy is felt to be beneficial for reducing spasticity and improving balance, and other movement dysfunctions. Individuals with MS report significant physical and psychological benefit with hippotherapy and therapeutic horseback riding. The majority of the studies have been done with children with cerebral palsy, but many of the same benefits may be seen for people with MS.

## WELLNESS PROGRAMS

Wellness programs or wellness interventions are variable, but all include education in health-promoting behaviors. Characteristics of wellness programs are that they are participant-centered and multidisciplinary, with a focus on self-care in the areas of physical, psychological, or spiritual health. The aims of health promotion/wellness programs are to reduce secondary conditions (e.g., obesity, hypertension, pressure sores), maintain functional independence, provide an opportunity for leisure and enjoyment, and enhance the overall quality of life by reducing environmental barriers to good health. This may incorporate, as stated earlier, starting an exercise program, practicing stress management techniques, and/or incorporating dietary changes to improve blood lipid profiles.

A review of the literature on wellness interventions showed positive benefits for those who participate. The review also suggested that this type of intervention reduces health service usage. Another study supported the positive effects of a wellness intervention which included lifestyle-change classes and telephone follow-up, in improving health behaviors and quality of life. The study also reported that goal setting and goal attainment were important mechanisms to promote behavior change. Goal setting is an important step in behavior change and the Stuifbergen study identified that the goals should address continuing behaviors and not one-time behaviors. For example, the goals should center around activities such as consistently participating in an exercise program or practicing relaxation strategies and not on getting a flu shot or mammogram.

Wellness programs have become very popular for the MS population. This is in part due to disease-modifying agents slowing the progression of disability and decreasing exacerbations in relapsing forms of MS. Wellness programs are offered by MS clinics, MS Society chapters, and other organizations that specialize in wellness programs for people with MS like the Heuga Center. The Heuga Center has been providing health promotion programs and supporting research into the effects of exercise on people with MS.

More research is needed into the effects of wellness programs on people living with MS and their family members. Those who participate in these programs report improvements in overall health and quality of life, an important factor in adjusting to life with MS.

# Chapter 14
# Your Lungs and Heart
Linda Lehman, MSN, RNCS, FNP and June Halper, MSCN, ANP, FAAN

MULTIPLE SCLEROSIS (MS), a disease of the central nervous system, may be affected by other diseases or conditions. Therefore, it is important to take steps to remain well. Your heart and lungs (cardiopulmonary system) are vital organs and must be protected by wellness activities.

## RESPIRATORY SYSTEM

The respiratory system consists of the windpipe (trachea); bronchi (respiratory tree), which connects to the lungs; diaphragm (the main muscle of breathing); and the intercostal muscles (the muscles between the ribs that are used for coughing and deep breathing) (see Figure 14.1).

Protected by the breastbone, ribs, and spine, the lungs function primarily in breathing and filtering air. Air, which consists of nitrogen, oxygen, water, carbon dioxide, and other particles, enters through the nose and mouth; travels through the larynx (voice box); and proceeds down the trachea (windpipe), through the bronchi, and into the lungs. The lungs consist of millions of alveoli (air sacs) in which there are meshworks of capillaries where the exchange of oxygen and carbon dioxide takes place.

The act of breathing is controlled by the brain, normally about 10 to 20 times per minute, although you can consciously regulate the rate. Messages are sent from the respiratory center of the brain to the diaphragm and to certain rib muscles, which contract. This contraction pulls the lower surfaces of the lungs downward and air is inhaled. Stretch receptors in the lungs then send signals back to the brain, making the diaphragm and rib muscles relax, causing an upward movement and exhalation of air.

The respiratory muscles in the chest assist in breathing and ventilation by compressing and distending the lungs, causing an expansion and contraction of the alveoli. The lungs, which are elastic in nature, facilitate ventilation (or breathing), as does the presence of *surfactant*, a material found in the lungs of healthy individuals. This surfactant acts like a detergent and facilitates gas exchange.

The function of respiration is under the neurologic control of the medulla and pons, areas of the brain with nerves that affect functions such as chewing and swallowing. For this reason, people who have MS lesions in the medulla may not only have difficulty with breathing but with swallowing (dysphagia), which may predispose them to aspiration (drawing of foods and liquids into the lungs). Your respiratory rate or breathing rate can increase with fever, increased blood pressure, exercise, or anything that produces more carbon dioxide in your body. The rate decreases during sleep or periods of rest, or with a decrease in

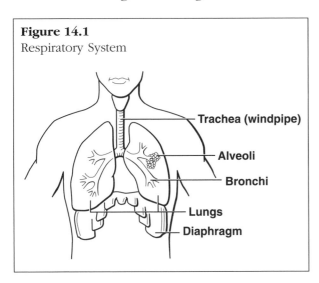

**Figure 14.1**
Respiratory System

Trachea (windpipe)

Alveoli

Bronchi

Lungs

Diaphragm

body temperature, blood pressure, or oxygen in the body.

Each lung is covered by a *pleura*, a lining that protects the lung and helps it expand and contract inside the chest. Lungs are spongy in consistency, light in weight, and can float in water. Normally, the lungs can avoid infection because the nose and respiratory system filter the air, and the trachea and bronchi produce mucus, which assists in trapping and carrying away contaminants. *Cilia*, small hairs that cover the entire respiratory tract, move the mucus and contaminants along by rapidly beating back and forth, in some areas at a rate of up to 1,000 times per minute.

Infections can cause your MS to feel worse, with intensified symptoms and increased weakness. Therefore, it is important to understand what types of infections can occur and how they can affect your ability to function. There are noninvasive devices that are helpful to people who are experiencing breathing difficulties on a continuous basis due to MS. BiPap™ machines and portable volume ventilators can help inflate the chest cavity when muscles are too weak to sufficiently contract. These devices can be used either throughout the night or on an as-needed basis. You should inform your healthcare provider if you feel you need mechanical assistance for breathing or clearing secretions in your throat.

### ASTHMA

Asthma is usually a chronic, inflammatory condition that can cause attacks of wheezing, dry coughing, or breathing difficulties. These attacks can be provoked by emotions, irritants, exercise, respiratory infections, fatigue, or allergies. When a person is exposed to a provoking agent, the overly sensitive bronchi respond by going into spasms and narrowing. The result is an asthma attack. People with asthma usually have little or no trouble breathing in (inspiring), but may have problems breathing out (expiring).

### BRONCHITIS, PNEUMONIA, AND INFLUENZA

The human body has natural defenses to prevent infection, such as the cilia that trap mucus and other contaminants. However, in people with underlying weakness and impaired ability to clear secretions, there may be a greater predisposition to react to infections, which can lead to bronchitis (inflammation of the bronchi) or pneumonia (inflammation of the lungs with accumulation of secretions).

Bronchitis, influenza, and pneumonia are lung-related conditions that occur more frequently in people with MS who are inactive and do not breathe in and out deeply. These illnesses can occur in individuals who are minimally disabled as well. They are frequently caused by infectious organisms, such as bacteria or viruses, or by exposure to irritants, such as chemicals. People with MS and other disabling diseases should talk to their physicians about obtaining a flu shot, which is given annually, and a pneumonia vaccine, which is needed less frequently. These injections may help prevent or reduce the occurrence of influenza and pneumonia.

### CIGARETTE SMOKING

Cigarette smoking is known to damage the respiratory system, blood vessels, heart, and other organs. Men who smoke have a 70 percent higher death rate from diseases of the heart and respiratory system than men who do not. Smoking interferes with the lungs' natural ability to rid themselves of pollutants. Smoking is associated with increased coughing, breathing problems, respiratory infections, pneumonia, stroke, hardening of the arteries (arteriosclerosis), gastrointestinal ulcers, and cancer of the mouth, throat, esophagus, lungs, kidneys, bladder, and pancreas. Smoking during pregnancy increases the risk of miscarriage and fetal death. Secondhand smoke has been reported to increase the risk of respiratory and middle-ear infections in children and to cause about 3,000 deaths from lung cancer and about 36,000 deaths from heart disease each year.

SELF-CARE STRATEGIES FOR RESPIRATORY HEALTH

- Limit or stop smoking. Avoid passive smoking by discouraging friends and family members from smoking in your presence.
- Treat upper respiratory infections promptly with fluids and decongestants. Contact your healthcare professional if a fever develops or if a cold or sore throat does not go away within a week.
- If your mobility is decreased, remember to take deep breaths throughout the day to aerate your lungs. Breathe in as deeply as you can, count to three, and push all the air out. Do this 5 to 10 times each session.
- Try to avoid known pollutants such as dust, mold, fumes, and dangerous chemicals. They can damage or destroy the cilia that protect your lungs.

## CIRCULATORY SYSTEM

The circulatory system consists of the heart, blood, blood vessels, and lymphatic vessels. Its purpose is to deliver oxygen and nutrients to all parts of the body and to pick up waste materials and poisons that the body eliminates. The various types of blood vessels are: arteries, arterioles (smaller arteries), veins, venules (smaller veins), and capillaries. These vessels are part of what is generally considered to be two systems: the *systemic* circulatory system, which carries oxygen-rich blood from the heart to the organs and tissues, and the *pulmonary* circulatory system, which carries oxygen-poor blood and other

materials to the lungs where carbon dioxide is released and oxygen is picked up. The blood then returns to the heart to be pumped out to the body (see Figure 14.2).

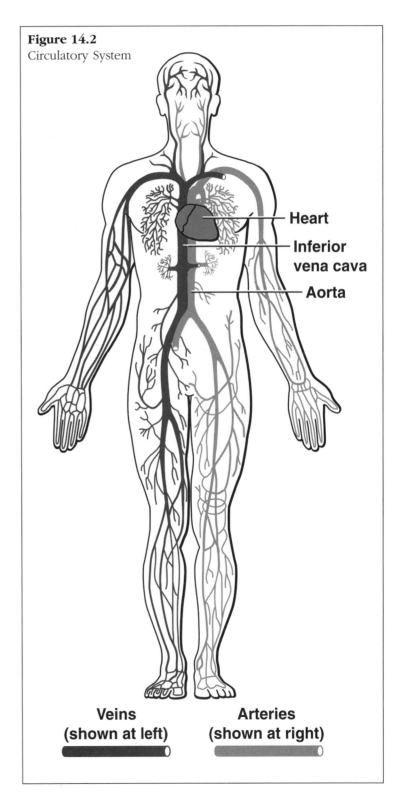

**Figure 14.2**
Circulatory System

Heart

Inferior vena cava

Aorta

**Veins (shown at left)**

**Arteries (shown at right)**

Blood transports oxygen and waste products, keeps the body's temperature stable, promotes defense against infection, and facilitates hearing. Blood is channeled through the arteries, which are thick walled and carry blood with a high concentration of oxygen. The largest artery is the aorta, which rises directly from the heart. The coronary arteries rise directly from the beginning of the aorta and feed blood directly back to the heart. Arteries can be narrowed by deposits of fatty substances within the vessels (atherosclerosis), or they can become brittle and stiff (arteriosclerosis). These changes can occur because of age, obesity, or poor dietary habits, which might include a high intake of fats.

Veins are thin-walled vessels that carry blood with a lower concentration of oxygen. One exception is the pulmonary veins, which carry blood that is full of oxygen from the lungs to the heart.

Your heart is composed of muscles that work together as a pump. The heart has four compartments: two *atria*, or upper chambers, and two *ventricles*, or lower chambers. Blood is returned from the body to the heart by two large veins—the superior and inferior vena cava on the right side of the heart—and from the lungs by the pulmonary veins to the left side of the heart.

Your heartbeat is sustained by a part of the heart that functions as a pacemaker. A healthy heart has a regular beat of 60 to 100 beats per minute. Heart rate varies with age, sex, physical activity, and emotions. During checkups, your physician listens to your heart with a stethoscope, measures your blood pressure, and checks your pulse. Blood pressure is a measure of the force with which your blood goes through your veins. It is regulated by how well your heart pumps blood and how much tension is in your arteries. A wide range of blood pressures is considered normal. A stable blood pressure is one that remains within a consistent range. Your personal physician is in the best position to determine what blood pressure is normal for you. In general, 140/90 is often considered borderline for high blood pressure and should be further investigated by a visit to your doctor.

The nervous system controls the diameter of the blood vessels, adjusting it to body position and level of activity. When you move from sitting to standing or from standing to lying down, the diameter changes to accommodate blood flow. Some people with MS develop swelling (edema) in the legs. This may be associated with changes of color (mottling) of the skin and with changes of skin temperature (frequently cool to very cold). Edema can be reduced by wearing compression or support hose, maintaining the regular range of motion of the legs, and elevating the legs frequently during the day.

To determine the health of your circulatory system, your physician may order a range of tests, such as electrocardiograms, echocardiograms, stress tests, and blood counts. As with most tests, none of these is 100 percent accurate in determining heart disease, although each can provide your doctor with valuable information about your body's ability to function.

SELF-CARE STRATEGIES FOR CARDIAC HEALTH

- Reduce your intake of dietary fats and increase your intake of complex carbohydrates, such as grains, oats, rice, pasta, and barley; fresh fruits and vegetables; and lean meats, fish, chicken, and turkey.
- Maintain your body weight to within 5 pounds of the ideal.
- Keep your alcohol consumption moderate.
- Avoid cigar and cigarette smoke.
- Exercise to the best of your ability.
- Monitor your cholesterol level regularly.
- Check your blood pressure regularly.

An additional resource is the American Heart Association, which provides information on the prevention and treatment of heart disease. Call the Consumer Nutrition Hotline, which is run by the American Dietetic Association, at (800) 366-1655 for information about diet and nutrition.

Chapter 15
# The Role of Nutrition in Multiple Sclerosis
Susan Goodman, MA, RD, CDN, CDE

ADEQUATE NUTRITION traditionally has been recognized as a key factor in maintaining health—both for people already in good health and for those with a chronic illness such as multiple sclerosis (MS). Healthcare professionals as well as people affected by MS have investigated the role of nutrition in the course of MS for more than 50 years. Attention has been given to many eating plans—including the Swank diet, the gluten-free diet, and other elimination diets—and to various dietary supplements such as vitamins, oil of evening primrose, and food additives. To date, no dietary regimen subjected to scientifically controlled trial has been shown to be of significant therapeutic merit in the treatment of MS. Therefore, the recommendations for good nutrition for people affected by MS are the same as those for the general population.

Many people affected by MS may feel overwhelmed and not know where to start. They may eat whatever is easy to grab—a candy bar here, a burger there, ice cream, cookies, chocolates, chips—all washed down by copious amounts of soda. These may taste good, but they don't provide the nutrition necessary to help you be at your best. With a little planning and a little practice, you will be able to put together simple, appealing, tasty meals and snacks that provide pleasure as well as provide the many nutrients needed for good health. Let's take a moment to review some principles of good nutrition and then see how we can apply these recommendations to people with MS and to you in particular.

## EAT A WIDE VARIETY OF FOODS

Use the food guide pyramid as your daily guide to good eating. Try to include foods from all the categories of the pyramid every day: grains, fruits, vegetables, lean meats and meat alternatives, and low fat dairy products. Varying your choices within each group from day to day will keep meals and snacks interesting and help promote a good appetite.

- Select 6 to 11 servings of bread, grains, and other starches daily. One serving equals one slice of bread or 1/2 cup cooked cereal, pasta, or rice. Select whole grains, such as oatmeal, grits, or corn flakes; wheat, rye, or multigrain breads and crackers; and brown rice, whole grain pasta, bulgur, kasha, or barley. Select crackers and baked goods made with liquid oils, not partially hydrogenated fats, which contain unhealthy trans-fatty acids. Whole and enriched grains are good sources of B vitamins; whole grains also contain fiber.
- Select 2 to 4 servings of fruit every day. One serving equals 1/2 cup cooked or one piece of fresh fruit that fits in your hand. Limit fruit juice to one 3/4 cup serving per day. Choose fresh fruits in season; frozen, dried, or canned fruit can be good alternatives, but be aware that some of these may contain added sugar. These foods contain vitamins, minerals, and fiber.
- Select 3 to 5 servings of vegetables per day. One serving equals 1/2 cup cooked or 1 cup raw or 3/4 cup vegetable juice. Choose fresh vegetables in season;

canned vegetables or frozen vegetables prepared without sauces are good alternatives. These foods contain vitamins, minerals, and fiber.

- Select 2 to 3 servings of lean meat or meat alternatives daily. One serving equals 2-3 ounces. Lean meats and poultry, eggs, nuts, nut butters, lentils, dried peas and beans, and tofu are good sources of protein. Choose fish such as tuna or salmon at least two times a week. Trim excess fat from meats and discard poultry skin. Bake, broil, roast, steam, or poach more often than frying.

- Select 2 to 3 servings of low fat dairy products each day. One serving equals 8 ounces of milk or yogurt, or 1-1/2 ounces of cheese. These foods provide calcium as well as protein.

- Choose something from each category for each meal; eat balanced meals. Mom was right!

- Choose healthy snacks: Snack on the pyramid.

- Choose small portions of sweets such as cakes, cookies, and sweet beverages, in addition to, not in place of, the food pyramid foods.

- Include alcohol only if it is permitted by your doctor. Some medications, such as amantadine and baclofen, which are often prescribed for people who have MS, do not mix well with alcohol.

- Choose small amounts of healthy fats, such as olive or canola oil for cooking. Avoid saturated fats like the fat in whole milk, cheese, butter, ice cream, whipped cream, cream cheese, chicken skin, and meat. These are not healthy for your heart or arteries.

## MAINTAIN A HEALTHY WEIGHT

Achieving a healthy weight means eating the right amount of food for you.

- Your current weight is the result of life-long eating habits, heredity, and level of physical activity.

- Changing your weight is a matter of energy balance. Food energy is measured in calories. Carbohydrates, protein, fat, and alcohol are the sources of energy in foods. Fat is the most concentrated source of calories. If you are eating more calories than your body needs, regardless of the source, you will gain weight. If you are not getting enough calories, you will lose weight.

- If you are not as active as you once were, you may need fewer calories to maintain your weight. It may be important to choose more carefully.

- If your dexterity and ability to prepare food have decreased, you may be eating less and losing weight.

- If you have a poor appetite or are too fatigued, you may be eating less and losing weight.

- A healthy weight is important for maximizing your ability to ambulate, as well as helping to control blood pressure, blood cholesterol, and blood sugar.

- To determine if your current weight is healthy for you, find your body mass index (BMI) at www.nhlbi.nih.gov/guidelines/obesity/bmi_tbl.htm. Locate your height and weight on the chart and find the number where they intersect. A healthy BMI is between 19 and 24. A person with a BMI of 25 to 29 is considered overweight. A person with a BMI of 30 or above is considered to be obese. A person with a BMI less than 19 is considered underweight.

## CHOOSE THE AMOUNT OF FOOD THAT IS RIGHT FOR YOU

- If you are underweight, and have little appetite, try eating small frequent meals; eat six times a day.

- Rest before you eat.
- Eat your sandwich or meat, potato, and vegetable first, when you do eat; eat the salad or soup after, if you still have room.
- Save your beverage for after the meal.
- Snack on nutritious foods such as yogurt, pudding, nuts, and fruit; make every bite count.
- Eat foods you enjoy.

- If you are overweight, try to prevent your weight from going any higher.
- If your BMI is over 30, try to lose a small amount of weight and do it gradually. See if you can lose just the amount of weight necessary to lower your BMI by two points (5–10 pounds). This can make a big difference in your overall health and well-being, while still enabling you to include your favorite foods. When you have accomplished this, try for another two points. Gradually changing your weight will help you develop new habits to help you maintain a lower weight. Be realistic in your expectations.
  - Look at what you eat, how it is prepared, and how much you eat. When you eat away from home or get take out, it is difficult to know what and how much you are eating. Many times, there is more fat added in the preparation than you would add at home.
  - Look at your current portion sizes. Estimate how many servings your current portions include. For example, a bagel bakery bagel contains 4 to 5 servings of bread! Try to make your portions a little smaller so you can gradually reach the recommended sizes.
  - What do you snack on? Aim to snack on foods found on the pyramid: fruits, vegetable soup, a sandwich, yogurt, and milk. Make snacks count.
  - What do you drink when you are thirsty? What you drink does make a difference. One 12-ounce can of soda contains 12 packages of sugar; one 16-ounce bottle of Snapple contains 16 packages of sugar! Choose water often; plain tea, coffee, and diet beverages are also good choices. Drink less soda, sweetened iced tea, juice, and juice drinks.

## COMPARE AND EVALUATE

Any diet can help you lose weight as long as you stick with it, but for most people, diets have a beginning and an end. Many people are looking for a quick fix. New solutions are being offered all the time; many diet books become best sellers. How can you evaluate the offerings? If it sounds too good to be true, it probably is! A sound program leads to a moderate weight loss of 1/2 to 1 pound per week. It includes foods from all the categories and allows for individual preferences. It should provide a long-term strategy. It should recommend physical activity for weight maintenance.

Two diets currently in vogue include the Atkins diet and the South Beach diet. How do they stack up? What about Weight Watchers?

- The Atkins diet is essentially high in protein and fat and low in carbohydrate. Depending on individual choices, unhealthy saturated fats may abound. Fruits and vegetables are limited. It is not balanced, and it is not a healthy long-term plan.
- The South Beach diet is similar to the Atkins diet, but it recommends healthy fats and provides more variety. It may be more helpful for long-term weight management. However, it does not address the role of physical activity.

- Weight Watchers provides a balanced diet. There is room for personal preferences. The program teaches how to create a healthy lifestyle over time and how to maintain a healthy weight.

## BE AS ACTIVE AS POSSIBLE

Can you increase your physical activity a little? Physical activity includes walking, gardening, dancing, vacuuming, etc., not just "exercise"; people with limited mobility can do exercises while seated in a chair. Not only will physical activity help you maintain a healthy weight, but it will also help you to have a more positive attitude and actually increase your energy level. A physical therapist can recommend exercises that will be best for you.

## GET ENOUGH CALCIUM

Many people with MS are at risk for osteoporosis. If you are taking corticosteroids or are less mobile (using a wheelchair or confined to bed), you are more at risk for this condition that usually occurs later in life. Be sure to talk to your healthcare provider about having your bone density checked and taking prescription medicines for preventing or treating osteoporosis if necessary. You can decrease the risk by limiting alcohol intake, quitting smoking, doing weight-bearing exercise (like walking, dancing, or stair climbing), and taking in an adequate amount of calcium. Depending on your age, the recommended daily intake of calcium is between 1,000 and 1,300 mg per day, the amount in three to four 8-ounce glasses of low fat milk per day or the equivalent, so be sure to include milk, yogurt, and cheese often. If you are lactose intolerant, you can choose lactose-free dairy products or try Lactaid pills. Calcium-fortified soy milk is another alternative. If you don't like milk:

- Whip up a shake with fruit and milk or fruit and yogurt.
- Add grated cheese to your pasta, soups, and vegetables.
- Include a toasted cheese sandwich or a slice of pizza as one of your meals or snacks.
- Have fruit and cheese and crackers for a meal or snack.
- Cook your oatmeal with milk in place of water.
- Cook canned cream soup with milk instead of water.
- Choose pudding or ice cream for dessert or a snack.
- Choose dark green, leafy vegetables like kale, collards, broccoli, or turnip greens often.
- Eat the bones in *canned* salmon or sardines. (Never eat the bones in fresh or frozen fish!)
- Choose calcium-fortified juices—drink a glass every day.

While food is the best source of calcium, if you do not include the recommended number of servings on most days, speak with your healthcare provider about taking a calcium supplement to supply the difference.

- Take no more than 500 to 600 mg of elemental calcium at one time. This is the amount your body can use at one time.
- If you choose a supplement of calcium carbonate, such as Tums® or Caltrate®, it will be best used if taken with a meal, but not with a high fiber meal. Calcium should not be taken at the same time as iron or with any medication to be taken on an empty stomach.
- If you choose a supplement of calcium citrate, such as Citracal®, it can be taken any time without regard to food, medications, or supplements.

- Be sure to get enough vitamin D with your calcium, but not too much—a total of 400 to 800 IU for the day.

## GET ENOUGH FLUID

Drinking too little fluid can make you feel tired and can contribute to urinary tract infections and constipation, both of which are common problems for people with MS. However, many people affected by MS restrict their fluid intake. Therefore, it is very important to drink enough fluids or liquids. The recommendation is for eight glasses a day. There is no need to drink it all at once. In fact, it is better to divide it up and have some in the morning, some midmorning, some midday, some in the afternoon, some in the evening, some late evening, and some if you are up at night. Water is the best choice. It has no calories and will not put on weight; diet soda, seltzer, plain tea, and black coffee are other calorie-free sources of fluid. Sweet drinks like soda, sweetened iced teas, juices, and juice drinks will add calories. Milk, milk shakes, puddings, gelatin-based desserts, soups, sorbets, and ice cream also count as fluids.

## GET ENOUGH FIBER

Constipation is no fun! Many people with MS suffer from constipation. Limited physical activity and inadequate fluid intake can make the problem worse. In addition, some of the medicines frequently prescribed for people with MS can cause constipation as a side effect. Amantadine and baclofen are two examples. Although only about 2 to 6 percent will experience constipation, it is helpful to be alert to this possibility. So, get enough fluids, include physical activity, and get enough fiber. Like everyone else, you should aim to include 25 to 30 grams of fiber a day. Include a variety of sources such as whole grain breads and rolls; whole

grain cereals such as oatmeal, wheatena, cornflakes, or raisin bran; brown rice and whole wheat pasta; dried peas, beans or lentils; nuts; fruits; and vegetables. Have a salad every day, and include vegetables with each meal. Snack on fruit. If you are going to increase your fiber intake, do it gradually so that your body can get used to the change. Be sure to drink enough water. If increasing your fiber intake through food does not give you relief, speak to your healthcare provider about including a fiber supplement. How much fiber is in your current intake? Use the following guidelines to estimate your current intake:

- Bran cereal
  1 cup                          10–13 grams
- Rye or wheat bread
  1 slice                        2 grams
- Fruit with peel
  1 medium                       4 grams
- Fruit without peel
  1 medium                       2 grams
- Berries
  1 cup                          4 grams
- Baked potato with skin
                                 5 grams
- Vegetables
  1 cup cooked                   2 grams
- Beans
  1 cup                          4 grams

## KEEP YOUR TEETH AND GUMS HEALTHY

Some medicines that are often prescribed for people with MS can cause dry mouth, which can cause increased risk of dental problems. Amantadine is one example. Baclofen also can cause dry mouth. Drink sips of water or calorie-free beverages to moisten the mouth or try sucking on sugar-free candy or chewing sugar-free gum. (Be aware that sweeteners, such as sorbitol, found in sugar-free gum and candies, can cause diarrhea!) Besides eating a healthy diet, the following things can help keep your gums and teeth healthy:

- Brush your teeth twice a day with a fluoride toothpaste; ask someone to help if you cannot do this yourself.
- Floss daily to remove plaque and food particles between the teeth and under the gum line; again, you may need assistance.
- Change your toothbrush about every three months so it can do the best job.
- Visit your dentist regularly. Some dentists make house calls. Ask your doctor or nurse for the name of a dentist who makes house calls if this would be a better option for you.

## IF YOU TIRE EASILY

The following are tips if you tire easily:

- Plan ahead for cooking and food shopping.
- Make a menu for the week. Include six small meals or three meals and three snacks each day.
- Make a list of items to purchase so you can buy everything in one trip and make fewer trips.
- Budget your energy. Eating and drinking throughout the day will help you keep up your energy level during the day.
- Do the more tiring tasks when you have the most energy.
- Rest often throughout the day.
- Take advantage of convenience: use prepackaged cut vegetables and salads; use the salad bar for cut up fresh fruits and vegetables as well as salads.
- Get home delivered meals.
- Take advantage of delivery services from restaurants and supermarkets.
- Purchase prepared foods.
- Engage a home care attendant to help with meal preparation.

- When you do cook, prepare enough for at least one more meal.
- Prepare your own frozen dinners: for example, meatloaf with gravy, mashed potatoes, cut green beans, in covered microwavable pyrex containers.
- Let family members help; children may feel proud to take an active role in preparing and serving meals.

## IF YOU HAVE SWALLOWING PROBLEMS

About half of all persons affected by MS experience *dysphagia* or difficulty in swallowing. Dysphagia can be a serious problem. It can result in choking, aspiration, malnutrition, dehydration or pneumonia. Coughing when drinking water, choking when eating, and/or, having a hoarse, wet sounding voice are indications that you may have a swallowing problem. If you suspect a swallowing problem, you may benefit from a consultation with a speech-language pathologist. Once a specific problem has been identified, the speech-language pathologist can recommend foods, beverages, textures, and techniques to improve the quality, enjoyment, and safety of your eating.

## IF YOU HAVE TREMORS OR WEAKNESS

If you have tremors or weakness, assistive devices such as weighted or enlarged utensils, elongated straws, and lipped plates and cups can be helpful. An occupational therapist can fit you for these special aids.

## FOOD AND DRUG INTERACTIONS

While the prescription medicines you take are doing their jobs, they can sometimes cause unpleasant side effects. Some can affect your appetite and your sense of taste. Some can cause nausea and vomiting. Some can cause constipation. Others can cause diarrhea. Alcohol should be avoided when taking some medicines. Supplements, over-the-counter products, and herbs also can interact with medicines. Always consult with your healthcare provider when considering taking anything in addition to those medicines that are specifically prescribed for you. If more than one provider has prescribed medicine for you, be sure that they are all aware of the medicines the others have prescribed.

## HOW WELL ARE YOU EATING?

Now, let's see how well you are eating. Write down everything you eat and drink today. Note the times; for example, cheese sandwich at 9:00 a.m. Now answer the following questions.

- Did you have a whole grain bread, cereal, rice, or pasta today?
- Did you have any fruit today?
- Did you have any vegetables or salad today?
- Did you have any meat, fish, poultry, beans, or tofu today?
- Did you have any milk, cheese, or yogurt today?
- Did you drink any water today?
- Are you eating throughout the day?
- Are you drinking liquids throughout the day?
- Are your portions right for you? You can use your hand to estimate portions that are right for you. Here's how:
  - A portion of grain products is the size of your fist.
  - A portion of fruit fits in the palm of your hand.
  - A portion of cooked vegetable is the size of your fist.
  - A portion of salad fits in two palms.
  - A portion of meat, fish, or chicken is the size of your palm.

  - A portion of cheese is the size of your two thumbs.
  - A portion of butter or oil is the size of your thumbnail.
  - A portion of cream cheese is the size of your thumb.

### WHAT LITTLE CHANGES CAN YOU MAKE TO IMPROVE THE QUALITY OF YOUR INTAKE?

Here are some simple suggestions that you can use. Which ones will you choose?

- Add a whole grain roll or have a sandwich on whole grain bread.
- Add a whole grain cereal like oatmeal, cornflakes, or raisin bran.
- Add a piece of fruit.
- Add a vegetable.
- Add a salad.
- Add meat, fish or chicken, or rice and beans.
- Add a glass of milk.
- Add a yogurt.
- Drink more water.
- Drink water in place of juice or soda.
- Eat more frequently.

A month from now, write down everything you eat and drink in one day. Answer the same questions. Are there any differences? Keeping track of little changes will show you how they add up over time. By next year, you may be pleasantly surprised to see the changes you have made. Share your progress with your healthcare team.

### WHAT MIGHT BE GETTING IN YOUR WAY?
- Not enough money for food?
- Too tired to eat?
- Feeling down?
- Need help cooking, shopping, or planning meals?
- Hate to cook?
- Need new menu ideas? Bored with eating the same old thing?

| **Breakfast** | **Snack** | **Lunch** |
| --- | --- | --- |
| Oatmeal | Yogurt | Black Bean Soup |
| Milk | Wheat Crackers | Toasted Cheese |
| Sandwich | Water | Cherry Tomatoes |
| Dried Cranberries | | Sliced Pear |
| Coffee | | Iced Tea |
| **Snack** | **Dinner** | **Snack** |
| Tapioca Pudding | Meatloaf | Chocolate Chip Cookie |
| Water | Mashed Potatoes | Milk |
| | Green Beans | |
| | Tangerine | |
| | Lemonade | |

Your healthcare provider can help. Be sure to discuss any concerns at your next visit. A registered dietitian can help you create a personal meal plan tailored to your health needs, functional level, likes, dislikes, budget, and cultural and religious preferences.

## LET'S MAKE A PLAN

Putting together healthy meals and snacks is easy. Make a list of your favorite foods from each of the food groups: grains, fruits, vegetables, lean meats and substitutes, and low fat dairy products. Pick one choice from each group and you have a meal! Be sure it is colorful. Close your eyes now and imagine how it will look and taste. What will you prepare at home and what will you purchase already prepared? Keep it simple and delicious. Continue making your menu until you have meals for three days. Now go back to day one and repeat the three days. Add one day and now you have a menu for a week. Use your menu to plan your market order. Include planned leftovers so you don't have to cook or prepare as often. For example, Monday's meat loaf can become a sliced meat loaf sandwich for Tuesday's lunch. Wednesday's grilled chicken cutlet can become Thursday's sliced chicken on a tossed salad.

Rest before you eat so you will have the energy to enjoy your meal. Be sure your room is a comfortable temperature. Turn on your favorite soothing music. Put everything you need for the meal on the table. Pull up a chair. Relax and enjoy. Bon appetit!

Below is a menu for one day to get you started.

## CONCLUSION

Should you follow a special diet for MS? When you evaluate the claims for "dietary" cures, be aware that the course of MS is somewhat unpredictable. Responses to particular foods and diets may be coincidental. Testimonials by individuals do not substitute for scientific research. Before adopting any diet plan, especially one that eliminates whole categories of food, consult your healthcare provider. See if there is any evidence to back the claim and be sure that the change you are considering will not be harmful.

What about the Swank diet, the macrobiotic diet, and the gluten-free diet? The Swank diet is essentially a low fat, low saturated fat diet. It contains foods from all the categories and seems to be a healthy eating plan, but it is not a cure.

On the other hand, the macrobiotic diet, which attempts to balance the "yin" and "yang" characteristics of foods, is essentially a vegetarian diet with several stages. As one progresses through the stages, the food choices become more limited. At the highest stage, only brown rice is eaten. This diet is not balanced, and is nutritionally inadequate. People have actually died when they have tried to exist at the brown rice only level.

The gluten free diet, which eliminates wheat, rye, and barley (and sometimes oats) in all their forms, is helpful in the treatment of celiac disease. It is not helpful in the treatment of MS.

Now you know the basics of good nutrition and how to create a personalized eating plan to meet your nutritional needs. Being well nourished can help maintain the integrity of your skin, protect your bones, decrease the frequency of urinary tract infections, help prevent constipation, maintain a healthy weight, and maximize your energy level. Take good care of you. You're worth it!

# Chapter 16
# Coping and Stress Management
Rosalind C. Kalb, PhD and Nicholas G. LaRocca, PhD

ALTHOUGH STRESS IS often thought to be a product of an overcharged modern society, it has been a constant companion since time immemorial. Primitive humans did not have to deal with rush-hour traffic, but they did have to worry about where their next meal would come from and whether a predator was lurking behind a nearby bush. Stress is so basic that the human body has developed an elaborate physiological mechanism to deal with it. The "fight or flight" reaction is the body's primitive but adaptive response to stress. As society has developed, the causes of stress have multiplied exponentially, but human physiology has remained basically the same. As a result, the instinctive response to stress may be inappropriate for the complex pressures of modern life. In effect, cave people are now masquerading in modern dress, still primed for fight or flight.

## STRESS: DEMON OF THE MODERN AGE

Many people believe that stress plays an important role either in precipitating the onset of multiple sclerosis (MS) or in triggering exacerbations. Anecdotes abound of people who had their first attack right after a major emotional trauma. Many studies have investigated this possible link, with mixed results. It is therefore unclear whether stress plays a major role in MS disease activity.

Immune dysregulation seems to be the major culprit in MS. There is plenty of evidence, mainly from disorders other than MS, that stress influences the immune system. However, it is not known how this complex relationship plays out in MS or what its sig-nificance may be. Studies in disorders other than MS have indicated that stress, especially severe stress, can promote inflammation. This raises the possibility that stress may be linked to MS by triggering some aspect of the inflammatory process associated with exacerbations. However, much more research will be needed to clarify whether stress plays a significant role in MS and what exactly that role might be.

Unfortunately, belief in the negative effects of stress has caused many productive people with MS to cut short their careers unnecessarily to avoid occupational stress. In addition, many family members harbor unnecessary guilt concerning their role in causing the stress that made a loved one's MS worse. Hopefully, the true significance of stress in MS will be understood some day.

### CAN STRESS BE AVOIDED?

People with MS are often told to reduce or avoid stress in their lives. Avoiding stress is easier said than done, however, because avoiding stress often means avoiding life. Life is full of stress, and the fuller your life, the more likely you are to be exposed to stress. Instead of avoiding stress, you need to learn how to deal with it.

Dealing constructively and creatively with stress will be more satisfying than a futile attempt to escape from stress. For example, if you quit your job to avoid occupational stress, you may encounter the stresses of isolation, loss of self-esteem, and a lower standard of living. Remember, the human body is biologically programmed for fight or flight. Although flight may have worked well in the past, when people were confronted by saber-toothed tigers, it doesn't work well now, when sources of stress can relentlessly pursue you where tigers could never go.

### What Is Coping?

In modern times, a third option has been added to the legacy of fight or flight: coping. The concept of coping is not really new; it is simply a refinement of the fight part of our heritage. Instead of flight from occupational stress, you might decide to stick it out and fight—that is, to try your best to cope with stress in all its myriad manifestations. The best way to understand the nature of coping is to compare it to stress. Stress involves anything that demands a response from you, particularly if the demand is for change. Coping can be thought of as the ability to respond comfortably to stress.

But what does *comfortably* mean in the context of coping? That's a question on which social scientists have disagreed for decades. To some, you are coping comfortably if you are not anxious and depressed. However, in some situations, feeling anxious and depressed may indicate that you are in healthy touch with reality and are processing feelings that you will inevitably have to confront. To others, you are coping well if you forge ahead through life, viewing each stress as a challenge to be mastered through clever problem-solving strategies. Still others believe that it is optimal if a person has a wide variety of coping strategies to draw upon, with the choice of method contingent upon the unique demands of the situation.

Each of these ideas of what constitutes good coping strategies can teach a valuable lesson. If you go through life perpetually depressed and anxious, it's time to take stock of your coping strategies to see if something is lacking. Coping with a chronic disabling disease like MS inevitably demands a lot of concrete problem solv-

ing—for example, how to surmount a curb. Life has a dizzying variety of stressors, and what works in one situation may not work in another.

## COPING AND STRESS MANAGEMENT

Coping is a broad term that encompasses several strategies, including stress management, counseling, psychotherapy, and use of psychotropic medication. Successful coping involves using whatever resources are at your disposal.

The need for professional help may be indicated by a number of situations. For example, if your efforts to manage stress are foundering and you are feeling overwhelmed in spite of your best efforts, you probably need to consult a therapist. Likewise, if you are so depressed or anxious that it seriously interferes with your everyday activities, self-help may not be enough. If you find yourself having recurrent thoughts of death or of hurting yourself or having fantasies that you would be better off dead, you need professional help.

Many determined souls put off seeking professional help, feeling that to do so is to admit failure. Nothing could be further from the truth. Participating in counseling is a form of self-help, and your self-help program should incorporate the notion that, at some point, you may need professional help to get you on track so that you can effectively use other self-help strategies. Championship athletes get to be good through hard work and determination, but few can do so without coaches, trainers, and teammates.

### Managing Stress

In learning how to manage stress successfully, the first step is to take stock of yourself and your life. Although many people know that they feel stressed, they have a surprisingly sketchy idea of why. Keeping a stress record book can help you get in touch with the sources of your stress.

Use your stress record book as a diary to record situations that you find stressful in daily life. Along with entries concerning the who, what, when, and where of each stressful event, record how you reacted to each event in four domains:

- What were your thoughts during and after the situation?
- What were you feeling?
- What did you do?
- What sorts of physical reactions did you have?

For example, if the stressful event was filling out your taxes, it might go like this:

- Thoughts: "This is impossible; I'm never going to get this done."
- Feelings: anxiety, frustration, and hopelessness.
- Actions: organized the necessary papers, read the instructions, and made up a checklist to get it done.
- Physical reactions: headache, indigestion, sweaty palms, and/or rapid heartbeat.

Monitoring stress is not an academic exercise. It helps you to identify and understand where stress is coming from. More importantly, it provides real insights into how you are coping with stress. The stress record book will help you to notice when you are underutilizing certain strategies or overemphasizing others. This may be the first step toward developing a more varied and increasingly successful stress management program.

## INTERPRETATIONS OF STRESS

Taking stock of stress and your reactions to it can help you understand your interpretation of stress, because how you interpret or appraise stress affects how well you cope with it. For example, if you perceive stress as an uncontrollable, overwhelming enemy, you are unlikely to do as well as someone who views it as a challenge to be dealt with creatively. Therefore, a powerful stress management technique is to understand and, if necessary, work to alter your appraisal of stress. Altering your appraisal of stress can make the difference between feeling demoralized and defeated and feeling triumphant.

## STRESS MANAGEMENT TECHNIQUES

In some instances, the emotional response to stress, including the tension and agitation that it produces, precludes any sort of rational appraisal. At such times, it may be helpful to use a technique to foster calmness and tranquillity. Once disruptive emotions are under control, it's a lot easier to confront stress rationally.

*Meditation.* For many, meditation is a useful tool for achieving the requisite state of peace and tranquillity. Although meditation may strike some as a mysterious, almost mystical experience, it is a simple and effective way to achieve a slightly altered state of consciousness that helps to manage stress while promoting a feeling of well-being.

There are many approaches to meditation. The classic technique involves two or three 15- or 20-minute sessions per day. The directions are simple:

- Pick a quiet place, free of noise and interruptions.
- Loosen clothing, close your eyes, and breathe deeply.
- Clear your mind of all extraneous thoughts and focus on and repeat a one-syllable word that has a calming effect.

In some forms of meditation, this one-syllable word is called a mantra. It can be gently chanted (aloud or in your mind) in a slow, rhythmic pace while you breathe deeply. At the end of your session, have a good, slow stretch and return to your normal activities feeling refreshed and renewed.

*Relaxation techniques.* Another classic stress management technique is known as progressive deep muscle relaxation. This technique involves alternately tensing and relaxing a number of major muscle groups such as hands and arms, forehead, stomach, and thighs. The procedure takes about 15 minutes and can be done several times during the day.

Some people with MS find that tensing certain muscles can start a spasm. For this reason, progressive deep muscle relaxation should be used with caution. If you run into the spasticity problem, you may want to consult a professional to help you adapt the technique to your needs.

*Yoga.* In recent years, yoga has become a popular activity for many people with MS. Yoga combines stretching, especially the back, with breathing exercises. But, like progressive deep muscle relaxation, certain yoga exercises and positions may be problematic for people with MS.

In many locales, yoga classes specifically tailored for individuals with MS are offered. A good yoga teacher who is familiar with MS can help you work out a program to suit your special needs. In addition, books, videotapes, and television programs on yoga are readily available.

*T'ai chi.* Like yoga, t'ai chi is an ancient art that can be successfully practiced by young and old alike, regardless of physical disability. The slow, rhythmic movements of t'ai chi are, in many ways, ideally suited to the person who has some weakness caused by neurologic disease. Also like yoga, t'ai chi has more than physical benefits. It tends to facilitate global feelings of well-being that help to neutralize the effects of stress. T'ai chi has gained great popularity in recent years, and many MS t'ai chi groups are available across the country.

*Aerobic exercise.* Stress-reducing exercise does not have to be of the ancient Eastern variety. Many people find that aerobic exercise like swimming, walking, or bicycling have the same benefits as yoga or t'ai chi (see Chapter 13, "Exercise Options and Wellness Programs").

However, when taking part in any exercise program, don't overdo it. Exercising to the point that you feel disabling fatigue and find yourself unable to function the next day will induce stress, rather than reduce it.

*Visualization.* Visualization employs vivid mental images in which you take an active role. You imagine a pleasant and appealing scene in which you are doing things and experiencing the scene through a variety of your senses—sight, smell, hearing, and touch. Many people find it relaxing to imagine themselves on a sunny beach listening to waves gently breaking on the shore. They imagine the smell of salt air, the gentle warmth of the sun, and the soft, refreshing coolness of wet sand. Visualization can be used in conjunction with other techniques, such as deep breathing or relaxation.

Visualization has gotten a bad name in some quarters from unwarranted claims for its ability to alter the physical condition of the body. For example, if you find it relaxing to imagine myelin regenerating itself on nerve fibers damaged by MS, by all means, do so. There is, however, no scientific evidence that visualizing biological events can make them happen any more than your imagining a scene at the beach could give you a sunburn.

*Having fun.* While you're busy imagining going to the beach or the mountains or wherever, why not plan on making your fantasy a reality? One of the most reliable ways to reduce feelings of stress is to have fun.

People with MS often abandon enjoyable activities because they have limited ability to engage in them. The person who used to love museums may stop going because he or she can't handle all the walking. Why not use a wheelchair or scooter and start enjoying life again? Perhaps it's because of the stress of appearing in public in a wheelchair. That goes back to the appraisal of stress—that is, how we interpret stressful situations. When people with MS dust off and reactivate abandoned activities, it can feel like a rebirth.

### COMMUNICATING WITH OTHERS

Stress comes in many varieties, but one of the greatest sources of stress in our lives is other people. Ironically, in many instances, the people we love the most can be the greatest sources of stress.

The ultimate stress reducer for sources of social stress is good communication. What constitutes good communication? Like good coping, there is no universal definition of good communication.

If other people are sources of stress in your life, you need to talk with them about it. You're probably a source of stress for them as well. Maybe an understanding or a change in behavior can take place, leading to greater comfort for all involved. But if communication proves fruitless or seems to make things worse, try to get professional help.

Sometimes talking about stress can help you sort it out and, at the same time, relieve the tension. You can accomplish this by talking to a therapist, but sometimes a friend or family member can be helpful. For many, support groups are indispensable for talking through the stressors found in everyday life.

The important thing to keep in mind is that bringing the causes of stress out in the open and discussing them can be a powerful tool for relief.

### REDUCING UNNECESSARY STRESS

Although trying to avoid stress completely is futile, there are things that everyone can do to reduce unnecessary stress. For example, sometimes stress results from the ways in which you do or do not do things. The key is to learn how to cope with situations that are beyond your control, while trying to modify situations you can control.

Here are a few tips:

- *Give yourself enough time to complete tasks.* A major source of stress for many is feeling rushed because not enough time has been allocated for the tasks at hand.
- *Don't just accept help, ask for it.* Many people feel overwhelmed because they think they have to do everything themselves. Work on that foolish pride that stands in the way of your enlisting the aid of others.
- *Cultivate flexibility, especially concerning time and schedules.* If you find that you don't have time for something you wanted to get done today, relax and reschedule it for tomorrow.
- *Stop being a perfectionist.* Relaxing your standards even a little will relieve you of a major source of stress.
- *Learn to conserve your energy.* People with MS often feel stressed because fatigue interferes with their ability to accomplish things they would like to do. Instead, get to know your energy limits and plan around them. Avoid doing so much in one day that it takes you a day or two to recover.
- *Get organized.* A major source of stress for many is chaos. Disorganization man-

ifests itself in piles of papers, things you can't find, phone numbers scattered all over the house, and schedules you can't keep track of. Get a book on personal organization and follow the suggestions. For example, you can set up a family calendar, create a home filing system, establish bill-paying routines, and use telephone message pads. Staying organized is one of the most effective stress-reducing things you can do for yourself.

- *Think twice every time you find yourself saying something like, "I should...."* Those "shoulds" are really guilt and stress inducers. If you encounter something that you think you should do, ask yourself why you should do it. Do you really have to do it? Can someone else do it? Is it something that can be left undone until tomorrow, next week, next year, or perhaps, forever? If it is something that you really do need or want to do, avoid procrastinating. Putting things off tends to lead to a stress-inducing backlog of tasks, just the thought of which can be overwhelming.

- *Learn to respect the coping strategies of others,* as you pursue what is most comfortable for yourself. There is no one right way to cope. What's best for you may not be best for someone else.

If you repeatedly find yourself in a stress-provoking situation, sit down and try to sort out how and why it's so stressful. Think about how you are handling the situation and whether a different approach to the task or situation might make it less stressful. Talk about the situation with someone whose opinion you trust, and experiment with new approaches.

Stress is an integral part of life. Everyone must deal with stress, but a chronic, disabling disease like MS tends to give you an extra dose. There are a host of ways to deal with stress, many of them simple and inexpensive, and you can become expert in how to use them. Then, if you apply them consistently, you will find yourself feeling that you have mastered stress, rather than being at its mercy.

# Chapter 17
# Work, Family, and Community Participation

Nancy T. Law, BA and Beverly Noyes, PhD, LPC

MOST PEOPLE WITH MS have marketable skills and work experience. Many continue to work after their diagnosis and keep their jobs for a long time, often until the normal age of retirement. Some people with MS, however, have serious difficulties keeping their jobs or are advised by their doctors or employers that quitting work would be the best choice. In fact, within 10 to 15 years after diagnosis, only 25 percent of people with MS still work. This is disturbing because many people with MS do not experience chronic debilitating symptoms. And many who leave work regret doing so, especially when decades of unnecessary unemployment follow.

With MS, continuing to work can be a challenge. You may become frustrated if your symptoms interfere with your job duties. Also frustrating are obstacles in the work place, such as inaccessible offices, lack of social support, or discrimination by employers or coworkers. You can overcome whatever job barriers you face if you commit yourself to the task of overcoming them, are creative in identifying your options, and communicate openly with your employer.

## DECIDING WHETHER TO WORK

Often, one of the first decisions made by people after diagnosis is whether to continue working or to quit. Many people, often in the midst of an exacerbation, decide to quit working without sufficient knowledge or careful consideration of all the factors. It is easy to be influenced by family members, friends, coworkers, and physicians, who, though well-meaning, may have limited information about how people with MS continue to work and the problems they may face.

## DECIDING ABOUT DISCLOSURE

If you want to work, you must address the issue of disclosure. Your symptoms may be invisible, and you may wonder whether it is in your best interest to tell your employer and coworkers that you have MS. This is an individual decision. Many people decide not to disclose, at least at first. However, each person should consider a variety of factors to determine what is in his or her best interest.

Here are some reasons why you may not wish to disclose:

- You believe your condition is no one's business but your own.
- You believe that open communication about personal matters will have negative consequences.
- You believe that disclosing will jeopardize your position or adversely affect your work relationships.

On the other hand, you may feel that disclosure is best. Here are some reasons why you may wish to disclose:

- You have visible symptoms and feel some explanation would help other people cope with changes in you.
- You want your boss and coworkers to know what you are experiencing.
- You anticipate that your condition may affect your ability to do your job.
- You need reasonable accommodations now.
- You want to reduce your level of stress at work.
- You believe that disclosure will put you in a better position of control.

## COMPENSATING FOR CHALLENGES

Another issue in your decision-making process is the extent to which your symptoms interfere with your job duties. Do not assume that, because your symptoms interfere with your job performance, you will have to quit working. There are ways to compensate for many of the challenges MS may present.

Many people with MS, even those with severe symptoms, have continued to work for years. Here are some things you can do to make that possible:

- Talk with your doctor or other health-care provider about the demands of your job. Find out how you can manage your symptoms in light of those demands.
- Organize your workload, set priorities, and pace yourself, especially if fatigue is a problem.
- Arrange your work environment so that you conserve energy and minimize physical demands. The solution may be simple, such as keeping your work tools nearby, or requesting workspace closer to the toilets.
- Make an ongoing effort to assess your work performance.
- Communicate your needs and concerns to your employer.
- Request accommodations if you're having difficulties.
- Use support systems. Let your coworkers or supervisor know when you need help.

Examples abound of people who have successfully kept their jobs in spite of significant barriers. Melissa, a clothing salesperson, is one such person.

Melissa began having difficulty with her job when weakness in her legs made it hard to walk around the store and fatigue caused her energy level to drop in the after-

noons. To keep working, she needed some accommodations.

Melissa approached her employer to discuss the difficulties she was having, and her employer was receptive to making changes. Melissa was given different work hours, which enabled her to cope better with her fatigue. She was also given additional paperwork duties in exchange for one of her coworkers committing more time to floor management.

Melissa also went to her neurologist and described the problems she was experiencing. The doctor prescribed an occupational therapy evaluation of Melissa's workplace. This evaluation helped Melissa organize her work environment, conserve her energy, and become more efficient.

## REMAINING PRODUCTIVE

Though many people with MS want and can continue to work, others find that they must reevaluate and decide how employment fits into their lives. Some, like Laura, a practicing attorney, decide that leaving the workforce is the best choice.

When frequent and severe exacerbations of MS forced Laura to retire, she offered her services to the National Multiple Sclerosis Society (NMSS). Very quickly, Laura became a vital "unpaid staff member" for the organization—as a speaker at chapter programs, a columnist for the magazine *Inside MS*, and an advisor on legal issues and independent living. Although Laura is unable to work at times because of MS, she says her status as a volunteer gives her the flexibility to attend to her healthcare needs and the freedom to decide which projects deserve her energy. Laura says that the lack of salary for her work does not diminish the value of her accomplishments and that pursuing her interest in legal issues for people with disabilities is essential to her self-esteem.

After she was diagnosed with MS, Linda, a registered nurse, opted to quit her job in a hospital to take a less demanding position in a physician's office. But, though her job performance was fine, Linda felt torn between the demands of her career and her two young children. Because of MS-related fatigue, she was exhausted at the end of each work day. After examining her values and priorities and discussing them with her family, Linda decided to quit her job to become a full-time homemaker. She now volunteers at her children's school and is a scout leader. She says her life is full and rich.

Fred retired from teaching high school math because of increasing difficulty with mobility and fatigue. Now he uses his skills to tutor. Fred takes a nap on his tutoring days so that he has energy for this late-afternoon activity. Students are grateful for Fred's services, and Fred enjoys continuing to make a contribution to others.

Laura, Linda, and Fred found alternatives to employment that they find personally rewarding and that support their feelings of self-worth. They all made choices based on their values and interests that focused their energy and maximized their productivity.

## DEVELOPING A LIFE PLAN

If you find that employment is not viable, you can still maintain a healthy quality of life. Development of a life plan is recommended if you are leaving the workforce. A life plan is a contract you make with yourself to take care of your financial, physical, emotional, intellectual, and spiritual needs.

- *Financial plan*. Know how you will support yourself. Do you have a budget? Can you supplement Social Security or other disability income with part-time income? Do you understand your company's long-term disability or retirement package? Will it make a difference in your benefits if you continue to work a few more months? Will your medical expenses be covered by health insurance? The NMSS offers a workbook on financial planning for people with MS that can help you through this process.

- *Physical health*. Pay close attention to your health. Consumption of food, tobacco, and alcohol often increases after retirement. Even a small weight gain can affect your mobility, and the health problems associated with habit-forming substances are well known. Do you have an exercise routine? This is an excellent time to see a recreational or occupational therapist to find the right regimen for you. Establish an exercise routine and stick with it! (See chapter 13, "Exercise Options and Wellness Programs.")

- *Emotional support*. Examine your system of social support. Are you withdrawing from friends and colleagues? Are you isolated by lack of transportation? Explore what your community has to offer and make a plan to access transportation. Are you keeping the lines of communication open in the family, as everyone adjusts to changes in the routine? How is the transition affecting you and members of your family? Is there a cause you are interested in? Volunteer! Are you feeling sad much of the time? It is often helpful to seek counseling during this and other life transitions.

- *Intellectual stimulation*. Develop your interests, even if you must approach some things differently. Learn something new. Practice a hobby. Cable TV stations offer courses on a variety of subjects. This can be fun, but be cautious. Do not let television become your companion; too much TV is intellectually debilitating. Make a daily and weekly schedule and a to-do list, just as when you were working, and follow it. Get up at a regular time, and get dressed even if you are not going out. Rest when you need to, but beware of the mental state of I've Got All Day (IGAD), where hours drift by meaninglessly until bedtime and you find that you have not addressed any daily tasks. IGAD is a common ailment for individuals who are used to having their days programmed in the workplace and must now become self-starters.

- *Spiritual fulfillment.* Develop your spiritual being by becoming involved with a religious or philosophic group, by reaching out to others through volunteer work, or by meditating or undertaking spiritual study. You may have to devote special attention to your self-esteem and self-understanding as you go through this time of change.

In the human hierarchy of needs, as described by psychologist Abraham Maslow, the need to love and be loved and the need to work are secondary only to the need to survive. As you adapt to the changes that MS brings to your life, consider the importance of productivity. Actively address all your needs, whether through continued employment or postemployment activities.

## AMERICANS WITH DISABILITIES ACT

The Americans with Disabilities Act (ADA) was passed by Congress in 1990 to ensure that people with disabilities are treated equitably. ADA contains numerous provisions designed to protect all people with disabilities, including those with a chronic illness such as MS. The most important employment provisions include the following:

- If you are qualified for a particular position, you cannot be discriminated against in any way because of a disability. If, for example, you apply for a posi-

tion for which you are qualified, an employer cannot ask any questions related to your disability. Also, if you are employed and your work performance has been satisfactory, your employer cannot take any action—such as a change in job duties—that discriminates against you because of your disability.

- If you are a qualified individual with a disability, your employer has a responsibility to ensure that you have full and equal access to all aspects of the employment situation, including training opportunities, promotions, compensation, and other privileges of employment.

- Employers must make reasonable accommodations for known physical or mental limitations of qualified applicants or employees with a disability, unless the employer can show that the accommodation would cause an undue hardship on the operation of the business. Therefore, if you are having difficulties with some part of your job because of your disability, you may request a reasonable accommodation that will enable you to perform the task, and your employer is required to consider your request and provide it unless it creates an undue hardship on the employer.

- Employers cannot make medical inquiries or require medical examinations, either of applicants prior to a job offer or of employees, unless there is evidence of a job performance or safety issue.

The Americans with Disabilities Act has been valuable in helping people with disabilities secure and maintain employment. Become familiar with the provisions of this law so that you can understand and exercise your rights. You may need to contact a disability rights attorney for assistance. See Appendix A for resources.

## NATIONAL MULTIPLE SCLEROSIS SOCIETY

The National Multiple Sclerosis Society (NMSS) is a membership organization devoted to education, research, quality healthcare, and advocacy for people with MS. For the past 20 years, NMSS has sponsored employment initiatives. These include job placement programs, employment retention programs, and services to help employers understand MS and make changes in the workplace that will assist employees with MS and other disabilities. Many chapters can provide referral to a disability rights attorney as well. Contact your local NMSS chapter for further information.

# Chapter 18
# Driving and Other Transportation Issues

Frances Tromp van Holst, OTR/L, CDRS and Teresa Valois, OTR/L, ATP, CDRS

MAINTAINING YOUR independence in mobility and transportation is a basic element to your quality of life. Your ability to walk and drive may change as a result of multiple sclerosis (MS). These changes often require use of a personal modified vehicle, or you may choose to use alternative public or private transportation. Depending on your environment, public transportation may be available for access into your community. Public accessibility for travel options, including plane and train travel, is becoming easier for persons with disabilities.

A key to continued independence is recognizing and accepting loss of function. At some point, you must make responsible decisions about changes in your needs and abilities. To do that, you will need to know what options are available to you. Don't wait until you accidentally miss the brake pedal and run into something before deciding to seek help. Anticipate changes in your condition and plan what types of vehicle, equipment, and transportation modes will provide you with safety, security, and freedom.

Research in the area of driver's rehabilitation has focused on self-report, comparative motor vehicle records of crashes, and driving behaviors. Maria T. Schultheis, PhD, from the Neuropsychology and Neuroscience Laboratory, Kessler Medical Rehabilitation Research and Education Corporation, reports that there is a significantly higher number of motor vehicle crashes among drivers with MS than among control subjects. The presence of cognitive impairment in drivers with multiple sclerosis can result in increased risk of motor vehicle crash involvement. Given the high value attributed to driving independence, self-reported information may not include minor crashes or documented reporting to the motor vehicle agencies. Some individuals with MS may strategically limit their driving exposure and rely upon others for transportation; these behaviors represent good judgment and deliberate self-regulation of driving behavior.

## EVALUATING YOUR DRIVING SKILLS

A self-appraisal is necessary whenever your medical status changes. It is vitally important that you recognize when fatigue is overwhelming your abilities and acknowledge if it is no longer safe for you to drive. Ask your family and friends if they see a change in your abilities relative to your decision making and ability to respond to traffic, or if they are concerned about your safety when you drive. You may think that the next step is to go to your state licensing agency, but be aware that state examiners may not have sufficient medical knowledge to evaluate your abilities objectively or to suggest options that may enable you to continue driving safely.

The role of driver's assessment has become an advanced skill of occupational therapists and certified driver rehabilitation specialist (CDRS). "All occupational therapists possess the basic skill set necessary to help clients achieve and maintain community mobility, instrumental activities of daily living (IADL) that includes driving. Driving requires readiness, skill, ability, and competence—activity demands that are addressed across practice areas," says Elin Schold Davis, OTR/L, CDRS, coordinator of the American Occupational Therapy Association (AOTA) Special Interest Section Driving Network Listserv.

You can obtain a comprehensive assessment from a rehabilitation professional that has special skills in driver evaluation and training. The Association for Driver Rehabilitation Specialists and the National Mobility Equipment Dealers Association have established model practices for driver's rehabilitation. These practices define the credentials of the rehabilitation professional and the services of:

- Driver evaluation
- Driver training
- Vehicle consultation
- Vehicle modification recommendations
- Vehicle inspection
- Functional inspection with the consumer

Major rehabilitation medical centers and Department of Veterans Affairs hospitals can refer you to an evaluation center. You may also find a resource person through your local American Automobile Association or through the organizations listed in Appendix A, Resources.

A formal evaluation of driving skills typically includes the following:

- Motor skills tests, especially reaction time, sense of position, balance, endurance, coordination, strength, spasticity, range of motion, fine motor ability, and sensation.
- Visual tests, including acuity, tracking, field of vision, depth perception, color vision, spatial orientation, night vision, glare, double vision, and figure–ground perception.
- Cognitive skills tests, to determine the speed of decision making, the ability to focus simultaneously on multiple tasks, distractibility, and the ability to see the "big picture" while maintaining attention and emotional control.

The assessment usually starts with a clinical screening of the three areas listed above, then moves to a passenger car or modified van in a safe, nontraffic area. The evaluation vehicle may be equipped with a dual-control braking system or other assistive technology.

After completing the evaluation, you should have a clear idea of your driving ability and have recommendations that may include vehicle options, assistive technology, and training with adaptive driving equipment. Your rehabilitation professional may be able to train you to use new equipment; your family members and local driving schools may also be able to help you. Your rehabilitation professional can make referrals and recommendations for training and advise whether your state agency requires you to demonstrate competence with the new equipment through relicensing.

If driving independence is not safe or financially feasible, then your focus may shift to other means of mobility and transportation. Critical to your sense of safety and freedom is the ability to participate in your mobility plan. The communication process between you, your family, and healthcare professionals must be facilitated to meet your goals. When using power mobility such as a scooter or wheelchair, your vehicle transportation needs must be reviewed.

## WHEN TO CONTACT YOUR STATE LICENSING AGENCY AND INSURANCE COMPANY

Each person is responsible for informing the state licensing agency of changes in his or her medical condition. Some states require that you obtain a medical form for your physician to complete. Often this process is initiated when a person with MS who uses a cane enters the office to renew a driver's license. The state licensing agency personnel may use some prescreening observation criteria of your functional limitations. The examiner may ask if you have had any changes in your abilities that could affect your control of a vehicle. Your physician may be asked to report on your current medications and neurological status and to justify the selection of assistive technology. License renewal may be based on periodic review by your physician and on re-examination of your driving skills and knowledge.

It is important that you inform your insurance company of all changes in your condition and of your use of special equipment. In particular, the company needs to know about any pieces of assistive technology that have been installed in your vehicle so that they can be covered by your policy. Your policy rates will be based on both your driving record and the replacement value of your vehicle and special equipment. Make sure that you can afford the insurance premiums before you change vehicles or add pieces of assistive technology.

## SELECTING VEHICLE AND CONTROL MODIFICATIONS FOR DRIVERS

Your rehabilitation professional can help you determine your personal mobility needs and your vehicle's suitability. But, because of the expense of making vehicle modifications, be sure to consider both your current and future needs before you make any costly decisions. The driver rehabilitation specialist should complete a report with recommendations of the modifications to meet your individual needs. This "prescription" usually includes an expiration date not to exceed 1 year. You, your rehabilitation professional, and the company modifying your vehicle must work closely together to ensure you get the most up-to-date and cost-effective equipment that meets your needs and the federal motor vehicle safety standards. Some combination of the following items may help you compensate for your disability.

*Fine motor condition impairments.* Some people use key extensions, dashboard switch modifications, turn signal crossover for operation with the right hand, gear shift extensions for leverage or for the left side, steering knobs, quad grip steering devices, grab bars, and hand-held remote controls.

*Lower extremity weakness, spasticity, loss of sensation, and paralysis.* Options may include a left-foot gas pedal, hand controls, reduced effort braking system, and manual or powered parking brakes.

*Upper extremity weakness, lack of active range of motion, and difficulties with coordination.* As changes occur in upper body weakness, some people use reduced-effort and/or horizontal power steering systems; steering column extensions; electronic steering controls; and seats equipped with support for trunk stability.

*Impaired vision, fatigue, and sensitivity to glare.* You may benefit from custom or wide-angle rearview mirrors, tinted windows, air conditioning, or photosensitive glasses.

*Mobility impairments.* There are transfer seat bases for ease in movement to and from the seat and positioning while in the driver's seat, electric cartop carriers for loading a folded wheelchair, and car and truck lifts for manual wheelchairs and scooters. If you can no longer use a car, you may opt for a minivan that has been modified with powered doors, powered ramps, and lowered flooring; or a full-sized van with a raised roof, wheelchair platform lift, or an under-vehicle lift. In addition, the driver compartment in some vans can be modified with a lowered floor to accept a wheelchair as the driver's seat, with customized seat belts and docking-type wheelchair restraint systems.

If you are no longer able to drive safely, you may need some combination of personal mobility devices, the adaptive technologies listed above, and a driver who is trained in the proper use of such equipment. You may also wish to investigate whether public transportation is a viable alternative, particularly if you live in an urban area. When you use public transportation (accessible bus), for your safety, you will want to use an occupant restraint belt and a wheelchair tie-down.

## SELECTING A VEHICLE

As you begin to integrate mobility devices, vehicles, and driving equipment into your life, consider the following:

- Where will you park?
- Will your new vehicle fit into your garage?
- Do you need a four-wheel-drive vehicle to navigate safely in snow and rain?

Not all vehicle modifications affect other members of your family. For example, a left-foot gas pedal allows a person with right-sided weakness to use the left foot to operate the gas and brake, but another driver can simply fold down the added accelerator and use the conventional pedals.

Consider what investments in technology will meet both your current and long-term needs and serve you at home, at work, and in the community. For example, if you have trouble walking from a scooter lift-mounted on the rear of your car to the driver door, you may be better accommodated by using a traditional four-wheeled power chair and a modified van. The wheelchair could be used as seating in the driver compartment of the van and at your desk at work, thus eliminating additional transfers, increasing safety, and minimizing fatigue.

Finally, make sure you have an up-to-date disabled person parking permit, which you can obtain from your state vehicle licensing agency. To obtain this permit, you must have your physician fill out a special application form verifying your disability.

## ESTIMATING COSTS AND GETTING FINANCIAL HELP

A professional evaluation of your driving skills ranges in cost from $300 to $700. The estimated cost for adaptive driving equipment ranges from $950 for installation of hand controls to $40,000 for a new minivan equipped with a power ramp entry system. Some vehicle manufacturers give up to a $1,000 rebate to purchasers of new vehicles to assist with the cost of add-on vehicle modifications. In addition to evaluation and modification costs, driver's training may be indicated. Training costs are usually based on an hourly rate and may include assistance for obtaining a driver's license.

After the installation of adaptive equipment, it is recommended that the vehicle be inspected. The purpose is to ensure the user has the functional ability to operate all the equipment, and it is consistent with the driver's rehabilitation prescription and meets federal standards.

Your rehabilitation professional can direct you to reputable equipment installers. To find out about the installers' differences and manufacturers' offerings of equipment, obtain competitive quotes from three installers and get the best deal.

## FUNDING RESOURCES

Your state department of vocational rehabilitation may provide funding for evaluation, training, and vehicle modifications. Technology services and devices may be considered as a provision of the 1992 reauthorization of the Rehabilitation Act of 1973.

This legislation authorizes your state to administer assistive technology services under vocational rehabilitation. To establish eligibility, you must outline your vocational objectives and the services necessary to achieve them in an individual written rehabilitation plan (IWRP).

The Social Security Administration (SSA) has programs available for individuals enrolled within the Supplemental Security Income Program, such as a Plan for Achieving Self-Sufficiency (PASS), that assist in purchasing equipment that will help you achieve a vocational objective.

The Department of Veterans Affairs provides assistive technology equipment and related professional services to individuals who have a service-connected disability.

Public sources for funding can come from federal, state, or local levels. Direct inquiries to the National Council on Disability, 1331 F Street, N.W., Suite 3850, Washington, DC 20004; or call (202) 272-2004.

Church congregations and other community service groups can help you with personal fundraising.

## LOOKING TO THE FUTURE

To maintain a level of safety and independence in your driving, periodic reevaluations may be necessary. The exacerbations and remissions associated with MS may affect both the physical and cognitive abilities necessary for safe driving. Changes in medications can also influence your short- and long-term driving abilities.

Advances in technology have enabled people to drive using various ways to access primary (gas/brake) and secondary (signals, cruise control, high low beams, etc.) controls. Although the costs and the risks involved in using such technologies must be examined, people with disabilities have extensive resources and options to facilitate and prolong their ability to drive.

## OTHER TRANSPORTATION ISSUES

An individual with MS looking for alternative transportation might want to consider the following:

- Personal safety
- Sense of security
- Weather conditions and exposure to extreme heat
- Lighting
- Physical stamina for the distance and length of time of travel
- Required transfer and access to public restrooms
- Planning and executing a route
- Need for a companion or care giver
- Knowing the accessibility of the environment at your destination
- Exposure to danger such as pedestrian/traffic collisions and safety around strangers

Community accessible transportation might include:

- Public/paratransit systems:
  - Taxi programs
  - Greyhound and Trailways buses
  - Regional reduced fare permits
  - Special qualifications and fare criteria
- Special services such as when the driver is responsible to be with you at all times
  - Priority seating
  - Early reservations for accessible seating or wheelchair space
- Cars and vans:
  - Car rental agencies can provide fully equipped automobiles with a prior reservation
  - Wheelchair accessible van rentals
  - Cabulance
- Airplanes—The Air Carrier Access Act prevents airlines from discriminating directly or through a contractual arrangement against people with disabil-

ities; this affects all domestic air carriers and all airport facilities:
- Special boarding chairs
- Advance notice requirements
- Seating assignments
- Airline liability for equipment
- Boarding assistance
- Transfer and lifting
- Equipment and storage
- Accommodations for use of the lavatories
- Trains
  - Lifts and platforms for boarding and detraining
  - Bridging ramps and level boarding for the gap of space
  - Accessible seating
  - Accessible restrooms
- Ferries:
  - Access to decks via ramps
  - Elevators
  - Overhead loading ramps
  - Accessible bathrooms
  - Disability travel permits with reduced fares

Depending on your own personal circumstances and need to travel within or outside your community, there are a variety of accessible transportation options. Many of the resources for finding accessible services are available on the Internet and may only take a call or two for you to get details in assisting you to plan your trip.

The following are a few resources to consider:

- Amtrak:
  - www.amtrak.com/plan/tips.html
- Airlines:
  - www.emerginghorizons.com
  - www.gimponthego.com
  - www.access-able.com
- Greyhound:
  - www.greyhound.com
- Accessible vans:
  - www.accessiblevan.com

# Chapter 19
# Fitness and Recreation
James H. Rimmer, PhD

THERE IS A BELIEF among many experts in fitness and recreation that participating in physical activity is a close second in terms of its importance to eating and breathing. What would your life be like if you weren't able to participate in all sorts of leisure, fitness, and recreational activities? In a society filled with many stressful events, the need to "release" by moving in any way, shape, or form that is comfortable and enjoyable to you is critical for maintaining overall balance in your daily life. For some people, yoga, meditation, and relaxation exercises fit the bill. Others must hop on a stationary bike or go for a jog to feel "invigorated." No matter what type of multiple sclerosis (MS) you have or how much you're able to move, exercise, recreation, and physical activity can be adapted to meet your needs. Don't ever underestimate what you're capable of doing. Many experts in engineering, technology, and exercise have found ways to adapt all kinds of physical activity to meet your needs.

Recreation, fitness, and leisure are extremely important for maintaining both physical and psychological health. Lately, I have been using the phrase, the *5 M's to Good Health*, which stands for *Moving More Means More Mobility*. Life requires a balance of movement and nonmovement (i.e., rest such as sleep, meditation, and relaxation), and for each of us, that will depend on how we feel on any given day. First and foremost, you must listen to your body and balance the amount of *movement* and *nonmovement* based on the amount of fatigue you experience, what your body will allow you to do, and your overall health. Because your condition and how you're feeling will vary at certain times of your life, make sure you understand *what* amount of physical activity works best for you, and continue making adjustments to fit your needs and comfort level. Let's begin by dividing physical activity into two types: physical fitness-enhancing activity and recreational/leisure activity. Both should be an integral part of your life.

## PHYSICAL FITNESS

Physical fitness includes activities that will improve your strength, endurance, flexibility, and balance. It is divided into the following components: cardiorespiratory endurance, which is the ability of your heart and lungs to transport oxygen through your body and is commonly referred to as *aerobics*; muscular strength and endurance, which is the ability of your muscles to lift objects such as weights or groceries, and also helps you maintain good sitting posture if you use a wheelchair or better standing balance; flexibility, which is the ability of your muscles and tendons to move your joints through various angles and ranges; and balance, which involves your ability to maintain your center of gravity in a position that does not risk a fall. Depending on your condition, each of these components will require a greater or lesser amount of your attention. For example, someone with poor balance will have to spend more time performing exercises that will help maintain or improve balance. Individuals with poor strength should begin a weight training program to improve their strength.

Physical fitness is a vital part of improving your health, so make sure you focus on several of these areas in your exercise program. Examples of what you can do in each area of fitness are described below.

### Improving Endurance (Aerobics)

Endurance-type physical activity refers to activity that involves large muscle groups and is sustained for a few minutes at a time to 30 minutes or longer. Examples of endurance activity include cycling, swimming, walking, and lifestyle activities such as gardening and yard work that incorporate large muscle groups. The key to performing endurance activity is to make sure you don't experience too much fatigue immediately after the activity or a day or two later. It is important to balance the *amount* of activity with how you feel. Some days will be better than others, so adjust the amount of endurance activity depending on how much energy you have that day. Don't hesitate to adjust your daily routine from a few minutes a day when you are tired or fatigued, to 30 to 60 minutes a day when your energy level is good. Any amount of exercise is good, and moving a few minutes a day is better than doing nothing.

### Strengthening Activities

Strength activities increase your muscle strength and help you perform more easily various activities such as climbing stairs or carrying various items like groceries, luggage, or handbags. You can improve your strength in a number of ways, such as using weight machines, elastic bands, or lifting 1-gallon milk containers filled with water (one full container weighs 8 lbs.). The amount of resistance and number of repetitions you should perform will depend on your current level of strength. In general, one to three sets of 10 to 12 repetitions are recommended for improving or maintaining your strength. As your strength increases, the amount of weight that you lift should also increase. Ideally, strength training should not be performed on consecutive days, in order to allow the muscle groups being used to recover between sessions.

While both upper and lower body muscles should be included in a strengthening program, this will depend on how much use you have in each set of muscle groups in your upper and lower body. Muscles in the lower body (ankles, hips, and legs) are particularly important for mobility, and muscles in the arms are important for performing transfers, getting up from the floor, and lifting and carrying various objects. And remember to strengthen the muscles in your stomach and back area. They are important for maintaining good postural alignment.

### Flexibility Activities

Flexibility activities will help you maintain or increase your range of motion around various joints in your body. It is a good idea to get into a routine of daily stretches, especially if you have a lot of tightness in various parts of your body such as your hips or legs. Some people like to stretch for a few minutes a day before going to work or getting out of bed. They find that it helps "loosen up" tight or spastic muscles. Flexibility activities can be incorporated into your daily routine at work or home, or may be done as part of an exercise class during the warm up and/or cool down phases of the class.

Stretching should include both static and/or dynamic exercises. In *dynamic stretching*, the muscle moves through the full range of motion of a joint, such as when you perform arm circles. A *static stretch* is when the muscle is lengthened or stretched to the point where there is some discomfort or tension, but it is not painful, and you are able to hold this stretch for around 15 to 45 seconds. Static and dynamic flexibility are both very important for keeping your joints moving through their full range of motion.

### Balance Activities

There are two types of balance: static balance and dynamic balance. Just as the name implies, *static balance* is performed by moving into various positions and holding them for a certain amount of time (a few seconds up to a minute). *Dynamic balance* is the ability to maintain your balance while moving. Static balance activities are commonly used in various types of yoga positions, which is an excellent way to maintain and improve your static balance. Yoga can be performed in a chair, lying on a mat, or standing.

Dynamic balance can be improved by decreasing your base of support while walking, such as walking between two narrow lines, walking on a straight line, or walking heel-to-toe or on your toes or heels. If you are having trouble with your balance, try static balance activities holding onto a chair, and dynamic balance activities sliding your hand along the wall as you move across the room. Try not to get frustrated. Some days your balance will be better than on other days. Balance is also affected by the type of medication you're taking. If you have a change in medication, you might notice that your balance has changed. On days when your balance is not so good, try doing sitting balance exercises from a chair or on the floor. It is important that you make balance exercises a regular part of your daily routine. The National Center on Physical Activity and Disability (NCPAD) can provide you with a variety of balance activities that will keep your balance program both interesting and challenging (see Appendix A, Resources).

ADAPTIVE FITNESS EQUIPMENT

There are special types of adaptive fitness equipment that can help with your exercise or recreation program. These are too numerous to list here, but include such things as adaptive gloves and straps that will keep your hand(s) connected to an exercise machine or piece of equipment, and various types of exercise equipment made specifically for people with limited use of their arms and legs. A list of these adaptations and equipment can be found on the NCPAD website at www.ncpad.org or by calling its toll-free number at 800-900-8086. See Resource Appendix for additional places to obtain assistance.

RECREATION AND LEISURE

Recreation and leisure activities are usually not done as regularly as fitness activities. Examples include taking a weekend ski trip, hiking, going for an occasional bike ride or walk, bowling, boating, and sleigh riding, among many others. Highlighted below are some enjoyable recreational activities that can be performed by individuals who have various levels of ability. Note that some recreational activities, such as swimming, if done regularly, can improve your fitness level and will most certainly improve your general well being.

AQUATICS

Aquatic exercise is an excellent low-impact activity for individuals of all abilities and can be performed in either indoor or outdoor pool facilities. There are many different kinds of aquatics activities, from structured classes that improve all aspects of fitness, to swimming laps. If you swim outdoors, be sure to stay out of the sun as much as possible. Also, make sure the pool temperature is at your comfort level. Pools that are too warm can increase your fatigue, and pools that are too cold can increase stiffness in your muscles and tendons. Everyone has a slightly different preference regarding pool temperature, so experiment with what temperature is most comfortable for you. In general, the pool temperature should be less than 85 degrees Fahrenheit. If you have difficulty getting in and out of the pool or the pool does not contain a lift, contact NCPAD and they will explain what options are available for making the pool accessible.

### T'AI CHI

T'ai chi is an ancient Chinese activity and philosophical exercise aimed at harmonizing the mind and body. These series of movements are performed at a moderate intensity and steady rhythm. The exercise builds strength, balance, and endurance. Its smooth, relaxed movements make t'ai chi suitable for individuals with varying levels of MS. T'ai chi can be practiced outdoors or indoors, and does not require any equipment. If necessary, the ways in which the movements are performed can be easily adapted to your specific needs. T'ai chi classes are available at fitness or wellness centers, as well as at park districts or your local YMCA. If you prefer to practice tai chi at home, a number of instructional videos are commercially available. NCPAD contains a library of these videos and can be contacted at 800-900-8086 for more information.

### YOGA

Yoga is an ancient Indian discipline designed to integrate the body and mind. The word yoga literally means "to yoke" or "union." The basic components of yoga include breathing techniques (*pranayama*), relaxation, and performing the different postures or movements called *asanas*. Movements can be performed while seated, standing, or in a reclined position, and at a slower pace if you have trouble performing certain movements. The benefits of yoga include increased flexibility, balance, muscle strength, and endurance. There are many different styles of yoga, so find the appropriate style that matches your needs.

### HANDCYCLING

Handcycling has become a very popular activity for many individuals who do not have good balance or cannot use their lower legs to propel a bike. Handcycles are just like bicycles, except that the exercise is performed with your arms instead of your legs. The other difference is that you are in a recumbent (seated) position with a supportive backrest. The seats are very comfortable and many people with lower extremity disabilities enjoy taking their bike out to the park and handcycling for a couple of hours on the weekend.

### EXERSTRIDING

Exerstriding is a type of walking activity that involves holding a set of poles (similar to ski poles). The poles were originally developed for injured athletes who were not able to run or jog, but are extremely beneficial to anyone who has difficulty with their balance. They can even be used by wheelchair users and present an exciting way to "power walk" or wheel. Visit the Exerstrider website at www.walkingpoles.com for an example of how this inexpensive equipment is used.

### CHAIR EXERCISE

When feeling too tired or fatigued to perform your regular exercise routine in a standing position, try a few different variations of chair exercises. Numerous chair exercise videos on the market can be used by individuals with varying levels of movement. Several exercise videos allow you to work out in a wheelchair or regular chair. Many of these videos have been adapted for individuals at various levels of fitness. Visit the NCPAD website to access two videoclip series: *Quick Seated Stretching Exercises* and *Strengthening Exercises*.

### IMPORTANT REMINDERS

*Fatigue.* Obviously, you know all about fatigue and how much of an impact it can have on your day-to-day activity. Don't assume that exercise is going to cause you to become more fatigued. Some people have noticed that exercise helps them cope better with their fatigue and that they feel better overall after a good workout. However, many people have also expressed that they feel more fatigued after exercise, so make sure you include time to rest after your workout.

The key to avoiding and/or managing fatigue is to perform various types of exercise that are challenging yet do not totally exhaust you. Because everyone is different, experiment with various types of physical activities and select those that make you feel good and do not cause unusually high levels of fatigue. Keep in mind that everyone gets fatigued after a good workout, so expect some temporary fatigue immediately after you exercise. However, if the activity causes you to become excessively fatigued, find a better balance of activities that are more conducive to your ability level. The key is not to overdo it. One way to reduce fatigue is to break up your activity into small segments throughout the day. Most of the research indicates that you'll obtain the same benefits if you exercise three times a day for 10 minutes per session (i.e., 10 minutes before work, 10 minutes at lunchtime, and 10 minutes before dinner), or 30 minutes per day in one session. Find the program that is most suitable to you. On days when you are very tired, reduce the amount of exercise to a few minutes at a time and do light activities such as stretching or performing various balance exercises, rather than your more vigorous workout. Speak with your doctor if you are experiencing a high level of fatigue after exercising.

*Avoid the Heat.* Heat is clearly your nemesis when it comes to exercise. Make sure the environment you are exercising in is cool and that air circulation is good. Avoid stuffy, warm rooms. Find the right temperature that works for you. In general, temperatures in gyms and workout rooms should range between 67 and 72 degrees. If the facility is too warm, let the manager or owner know that it is too warm, and if he or she is unwilling to accommodate you, find another exercise facility. Also, avoid exercising outdoors when it is very warm and use air-conditioned facilities during hot and humid weather.

*Drink Plenty of Water.* Water intake is often avoided by many individuals who have difficulty controlling their bladder. Unfortunately, dehydration and lack of fluid intake can be a problem for individuals who are sensitive to the heat and cold. During the warmer months, the body needs an adequate balance of water to dissipate heat and cool the body, and during the colder months, adequate hydration is needed to keep the body warm and insulated. Before embarking on an outdoor recreational activity or joining a gym, make sure adequate bathroom facilities are available, which, of course, should be accessible.

*Vision.* If you are experiencing blurred vision in one or both eyes, make sure you exercise in a seated position to avoid a fall, or switch to an aquatics program where there is no risk of falling and injuring yourself. If you are participating in a fitness program in a health club, make sure the instructor is aware of your condition so that objects are not left in your path of travel.

*Bladder.* Exercise can often bring about a spontaneous need to void your bladder. Sometimes certain positions place pressure on the bladder, causing it to empty. Don't worry about accidents. These things are common and should in no way prevent you from exercising. If you are exercising in a facility or a class, let the instructor know that you may have an accident or may need to leave the class on a couple of occasions.

## A One-Stop Resource: The National Center on Physical Activity and Disability (NCPAD)

Out of the need for more information on physical activity for persons with various types of disabilities including MS, NCPAD was established through a cooperative agreement with the Centers for Disease Control and Prevention. NCPAD is an information and resource center that offers you the latest information on fitness, recreation, and sports programs. Questions related to specific topics are answered by qualified information specialists who are available during working hours (800-900-8086) or by e-mail (ncpad@uic.edu). The Center also publishes a monthly electronic newsletter and sends out monthly features via email on new topics and information related to physical activity and disability. You can subscribe to a listserv and receive this information for free by calling the hotline or by e-mailing the staff.

## General Exercise Tips

- Keep a close record of performance on static and dynamic balance tasks and make balance an important part of the exercise prescription.
- Avoid embarrassing situations related to urinary incontinence by having a plan before you start exercising.
- Make sure the pool temperature is adequately cool for you (i.e., under 84 degrees).
- Monitor fatigue closely.
- Maintain proper hydration.
- Avoid excessive overheating and workout in comfortable temperatures.
- Use appropriate gloves, straps, ace bandages, etc., to keep feet and hands on exercise machines.
- Use various types of adaptive equipment for your specific needs.

# Chapter 20
# Making Your Home Safer and More Accessible
Thomas D. Davies, AIA and Carol Peredo Lopez, AIA

HOW CAN YOU MAKE your home safer and more accessible through minor renovations or even new construction? The first step is to determine your home environment needs. Does your existing home satisfy the current needs of you and your family? Will it present more serious barriers in the future if you have less mobility and stamina? What changes should you plan for?

To answer these questions, identify the activities in which you engage when you are at home and identify changes that would facilitate them. Once you have established your family's needs, options can be developed. Depending on your home and circumstances, only minor physical modifications may be required to support your activities and provide a safer environment. On the other hand, it may be appropriate, for example, to add a new first-floor master bedroom suite with an accessible bath. This project could consolidate more of your activities on one level and also provide an accessible bath that is tailored to your specific needs.

Accessible home design is a complex subject that is impossible to address in this short chapter. A number of comprehensive publications are available, including PVA's *Accessible Home Design*. If you want more information, we recommend this resource. It is also useful to consult with therapists and other medical professionals who have experience in home modifications. They can make suggestions and recommend products based on other clients with similar needs. Complex construction projects require professional design services. If you are contemplating a major project, we recommend the use of an architect for a design that succeeds both functionally and aesthetically.

## ENTERING YOUR HOME
If your mobility is sometimes impaired, the first challenge is often gaining entrance to your home. Most homes have multiple entrances including front, garage, kitchen, and patio doors. Multistory homes may have entrances on two or even three levels depending on the house plan and lot slope. Your first objective is to access at least one house entrance. If your home has an elevator or stair lift, access can be to any floor. If not, access should be to the main living level.

If you can negotiate steps, the most helpful modification may be the addition of a handrail at your entry. Long exterior stair runs usually have handrails, but short runs of two, three, or four steps may not. Your new railing can be constructed of wood or metal, but be sure that the top rail's profile is easy to grip and set at the proper height. Rail height is usually governed by building codes, but it is prudent to test other stairs to decide what is right for you. If you find railings that function well, replicate the height when possible.

If you use a wheelchair or scooter, a gently sloped walk is the best access alternative when your lot is relatively flat and the adjacent driveway is approximately on the same level as the home's entry floor. Walks can connect a driveway drop-off point or public sidewalk with the home's front door to provide an accessible entrance. The walk's practicality depends on the vertical relationship between these locations. If the house entry and driveway are situated at approximately the same elevation, a gently inclined walk (less than 5%) can provide wheelchair access. If your entry door is elevated significantly above ground, you will need to find another means of access that is suitable for your mobility.

Ramps are practical alternatives if the height difference between the home's entry floor and yard grade is approximately 24 inches or less. The rule for determining accessible ramp slopes is 1 foot of run for each inch of rise. Thus, an 18-inch rise would require an 18-foot long run. As height difference increases, ramps must be lengthened to maintain an accessible slope (less than 1:12). Long ramps are problematic for manual wheelchair users and those who use walkers because of the strength and stamina necessary to ascend them. The descent can also be dangerous. Electric wheelchairs and scooters can climb and descend slightly steeper ramps.

For entrances where there is a substantial height difference between the yard and entry floor, an outdoor platform lift can be installed. Using architectural elements like screen walls, a mechanical lift can be visually integrated into the home's exterior facade. Lifts should be covered with a large enough roof to protect the occupant and mechanism from inclement weather.

Vehicular access is critical to every homeowner's independence, so an accessible garage entrance is important. The garage roof protects wheelchair users from inclement weather as they transfer to or from the driver's seat. Transfer can be time-consuming because it is necessary to load or unload the wheelchair or scooter. To facilitate transfer, garages must be wide enough to allow the wheelchair to be positioned beside the driver's door. Garages should ideally include a 5-foot access aisle. Lift- or ramp-equipped vans may require an 8-foot wide aisle. In many instances, those clearances will require that your two-car garage is used as a single-car facility. If you drive a raised-top van, garage door height is another design consideration. A standard door is

7 feet high, which may not be adequate for your vehicle.

## ELEVATORS AND STAIR LIFTS FOR ACCESS BETWEEN FLOORS

If you already own a multistory home or elect to purchase one, three alternatives are available to provide access to two or more interior floor levels. These are: 1) residential elevators, 2) stair lifts, and 3) inclined platform lifts. Of these choices, a residential elevator is the most accessible. Installing an elevator, however, can be expensive, so consider all options. Many factors affect the cost and practicality of any option for your specific installation.

Residential elevators are an increasingly affordable way to provide access between floor levels without stairs. Elevators can access multiple floor levels with a maximum vertical rise of 50' and as many as 6 stops. These elevators are either cable operated or hydraulic. They typically travel on a single, side-mounted rail. Hydraulic models are more expensive, but provide smoother and slightly faster operation. Two-speed elevators slow down as they arrive or depart floors in order to avoid abrupt movement as they stop and start, an important benefit for ambulatory passengers who must maintain their balance during operation. Elevator models vary in their weight capacity, cab size, and cab configuration. Most manufacturers offer stock cabs that have sufficient size and load capacity to accommodate wheelchairs and motorized scooters.

Stair lifts are a less expensive, but less accessible alternative to residential elevators. In many existing homes, a stair lift may be the most practical option due to space restrictions or budget limitations. Stair lifts can be retrofitted to most stair configurations, although installation costs increase exponentially for complex stair layouts. If you have a single, straight stair run, installation costs are relatively low. If you have multiple runs with turns and intermediate landings, costs increase significantly.

Stair lifts have several functional disadvantages when compared to elevators. Most important is that users must be capable of transferring to the lift seat. The transfer is difficult because lift seats must be swiveled in order to allow the user to sit or rise, and then swiveled back for the ascent and descent. Furthermore, the wheelchair must be precariously positioned at the upper landing's very edge to make the transfer. For independent lift use, an extra wheelchair must be kept at the top or bottom stair landing within reach from the lift seat. For many homeowners, however, these limitations are acceptable, and the chair lift may be the best alternative.

Inclined platform lifts are another alternative for access between floors. Platform lifts do not require that wheelchair users transfer from their chairs. They are very difficult, however, to retrofit into existing homes.

If you can use conventional stairs, it may be helpful to add or modify your railings to help you maintain your balance. For this purpose railings should be as continuous as possible without interruptions at intermediate landings. The rail profile should be sized to allow a firm, but comfortable grip, and the mounting brackets should not interfere with your grasp. If your stairs are narrow, it may be useful to install railings on both sides for simultaneous use during ascent and descent.

## MODIFYING YOUR BATHROOM OR DESIGNING A NEW ONE

Accessible bathrooms are complex spaces to design because they support a wide variety of activities. People with impaired mobility each have a different method of accomplishing their personal hygiene; this is particularly true of bathing. If you are designing a new bathroom or renovating an existing

one, it is critical that designers and homeowners engage in direct discussions regarding the details of the bathroom's use. Together, they should also carefully review all bathroom components including lighting, electrical switches, and towel bars to ensure that each functions as well as possible.

Bathroom lighting should be installed to suit specific needs and circumstances. The highest illumination is required at vanity mirrors for close activities such as applying makeup and shaving. Incandescent or full-spectrum fluorescent light is best suited for this purpose. Because this lighting is intense, light sources should be baffled to reduce glare. Vanity lighting for wheelchair or seated users requires minor adjustments to conventional arrangements. Most wheelchair users, for example, cannot get close enough to the wall mirror for focused activities such as shaving or applying makeup. A portable self-illuminated mirror that is set on the vanity top is helpful for this purpose.

Shower interiors are dark, particularly when curtains are closed, so a waterproof light installation is recommended inside stalls and tub/shower enclosures. If you have a large roll-in shower, two fixtures may be required for even lighting levels.

Light and fan wall switches should be installed in accessible locations that are a safe distance from water sources. Electrical outlets should be provided in locations that serve bathroom appliances such as hair dryers and razors. The vanity wing wall is an excellent outlet location for wheelchair users because it is easy to reach from the sink without repositioning their chairs. A bathroom telephone extension can be helpful if an occupant needs assistance.

Residential toilets are floor-mounted rather than wall-hung. Seat height is therefore determined by your fixture. If you are ambulatory, toilet seat height affects the ease of sitting and rising; both are easier if the seat is higher. If it is too high, however,

**Figure 20.1**
The Accessible Bathroom

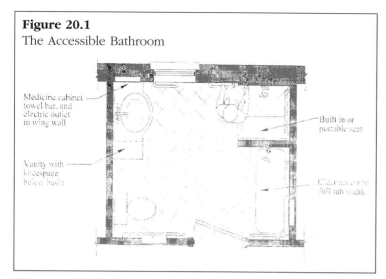

This accessible bathroom includes a shower stall, bathtub, toilet, and vanity. Accessories mounted on the vanity wing wall include a recessed medicine cabinet, electric outlet, and towel bar. They are all within reach of a user seated at the basin.

**Figure 20.2**
The Accessible Bathroom

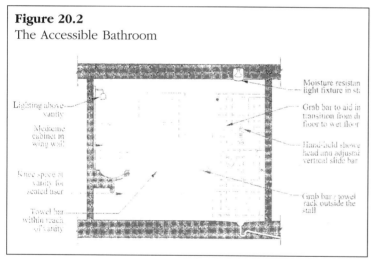

For seated showering, a hand spray attachment is particularly helpful. It can be clipped to the adjustable vertical side bar to provide a low water source that can be aimed and adjusted from a seated position. Wall-mounted grab bars inside and outside the stall aid ambulatory bathers to enter or exit.

chair seat level. With this vertical relationship, the transfer is neither up nor down, but straight across. Toilet seat height can be raised by installing special seat extenders. The seat cannot be lowered, but it may be necessary to remove it completely to accommodate a portable commode chair, or a foot stool can be used to raise the knees to a better position to facilitate bowel evacuation.

Vanity basins should be located adjacent to side walls so that electric outlets, medicine cabinets, and towel bars can be installed. The maximum counter height for most wheelchairs users is 34 inches, although a lower surface is usually preferred. Available knee space under the basin effectively controls the counter height, so both dimensions should be evaluated together. If you plan to be seated in a chair at a vanity, a lower counter top and knee space may be appropriate. Basins should be located horizontally at least 15 feet from side walls. If the bowl is too close, wheelchair users can't center themselves on the basin. If they are too far away, seated users cannot reach the wall. Front-to-back countertop depth should be sufficient to provide rear faucet clearance, but not deeper. Extra counter depth increases distance between users and the vanity mirror and light source. The mirror should be mounted as low as is practical, even if the back splash is eliminated.

## SELECTING OR MODIFYING A BATH FIXTURE

There is great variance between the techniques that individuals with mobility impairments employ to bathe themselves. If you are building a new bathroom, it is very important that your designer fully understands the method you utilize. Safety should be a primary concern because many bathing activities are difficult to perform and accidental falls often result in injuries. Bathing

users' feet do not touch the floor, which makes balance difficult to maintain. High seats also inhibit bowel muscles' natural contraction. For wheelchair users, seat height affects the ease of transfer and commode chair use. For wheelchair users who transfer to toilets, the most convenient seat height approximately matches their wheel-

fixtures are also used by other family members, so their needs should be considered.

The first step is to decide whether to install or modify fixtures for showering, bathing, or both. In general, showering is a less time-consuming way to bathe, and body cleaning and rinsing are more thorough. Showering is viewed as safer because of the difficulty of getting in and out of bathtubs. Medical authorities consider showering more hygienic. For many people, however, there are therapeutic and psychological benefits to soaking in a hot bathtub. Several techniques can be employed, but seated showering is the most common for bathers with impaired mobility.

Seated showering can be performed using a portable seat in a stall or a bench positioned over a bathtub. Seated showering is easier and safer than bathing because it is not necessary to recline in a tub or to maintain balance while standing in a shower. Portable shower seats allow wheelchair users to use conventional tubs or stalls for showering. The portable seat must be positioned within easy reach of the mixing valve or hot and cold faucets.

For seated showering, a hand spray attachment is very useful. This can be installed on your existing shower head by inserting a diverter valve. The hand spray can then be clipped to a vertical slide bar for adjustment to any convenient level. The spray allows the water to be turned off and on for soaping your body and then rinsing it.

For wheelchair users who cannot transfer to a seat, roll-in showers are the best alternative. Showering is performed while seated either in manual wheelchairs or special shower chairs. These chairs have four small-diameter caster wheels rather than two rear drive wheels so they must be pushed by a spouse or attendant. Because all four wheels caster independently, shower chairs require less maneuvering space than conventional wheelchairs.

In roll-in showers, bathers remain in their wheelchairs and bathe either independently or with assistance. A 36-inch × 54-inch roll-in stall accommodates bathers seated in most conventional wheelchairs or special shower chairs. A roll-in shower's most critical feature is a flush threshold curb instead of a raised dam. To provide this flush transition, roll-in stall bases are recessed down into the floor. To accommodate roll-in bases, homes with concrete floor slabs must have a depressed area under the stall. Homes with wood floors must include a lowered section constructed with shallower joists. These structural requirements increase roll-in shower costs and make retrofitting them difficult.

The design of a new accessible bathroom and the selection of appropriate fixtures require extensive research and discussion. If possible, try to visit manufacturers' showrooms to inspect fixtures before purchasing them. Review all the available options and accessories. The designer and client should review each step in the fixture's use and ensure that small details are not overlooked. The project drawings should include very detailed information on all aspects of the bathroom construction, including locations and height for accessories such as mirrors and towel bars.

## INSTALLING GRAB BARS IN YOUR BATHROOM

Grab bars aid users in three types of activities: 1) to maintain their balance; 2) to pull themselves laterally across a bench or seat; or 3) to assist them to sit down or rise up. They are commonly installed at toilets, bathtubs, and showers. In your project, you can elect either to install grab bars or to make provisions for future installations. The best location is determined by the bar's intended use and the individual user's body size and capabilities. A grab bar for a standing bather's use is mounted higher, for example, than one intended for a seated bather.

Many grab bars are installed to assist users who are seated on a toilet, shower bench, or tub seat. These grab bars are used primarily for balance. When the seated user is in a position without armrests on both sides, he or she holds a grab bar to maintain his or her balance. If they are seated over a bathtub, for example, they also use grab bars to steady themselves as they reach down to pick up a soap bar or across to adjust water temperature.

Grab bars can also assist users to move themselves laterally while seated. For this purpose, a long horizontal bar is the best configuration. To help ambulatory people to pull themselves up from a seated position, vertical wall installations are most useful. It is easier, however, to both sit and rise if you can assist yourself with two hands, rather than one. For this purpose, you can install pairs of low grab bars on toilet seats that function like chair armrests. If you are

**Figure 20.4**
Grab Bars

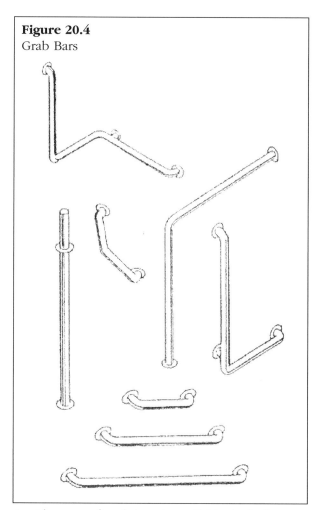

A wide array of grab bars is available, including fixed models that can be wall-mounted or installed between a room's floor and ceiling or between a wall and the floor. Bars that are integral to the toilet seat are also available to assist ambulatory users to sit and to rise.

**Figure 20.3**
Techniques to Install Grab Bars

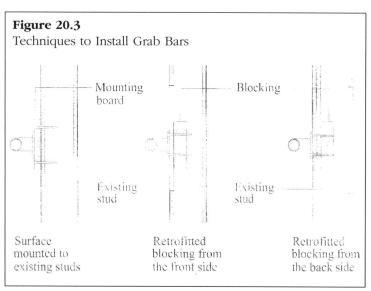

Mounting board     Blocking

Existing stud     Existing stud

Surface mounted to existing studs     Retrofitted blocking from the front side     Retrofitted blocking from the back side

The best method for wall-mounting a grab bar depends on its location and the existing finish material. The surface mounting detail provides anchorage without removing the existing wall finish. If the finish is removed, concealed blocking can be retrofitted between the studs. An alternative technique for a ceramic tile will is to remove the finish material from the wall's rear face and then install the concealed blocking from behind.

standing, either a vertical or horizontal grab bar can help you to steady yourself.

For ambulatory people, maintaining balance is very important when they are changing levels or moving between different floor surfaces. This is why handrails are provided at steps and grab bars are provided at shower stalls and tubs. For many wall installations, the proper mounting location is important to the bar's usefulness. It is therefore helpful if the location can be tested and adjusted to find the optimum position. The difficulty in adjusting the position is the availability of adequate structure for wall anchorage. In new construction, you can install blocking between wall studs to serve as anchorage points. Since the blocking is inexpensive and easy to install, allow sufficient latitude to adjust the grab bar's final location.

In existing construction, anchorage may need to be retrofitted in existing walls. Before going to this expense, it is ideal if you can test the installation. One way is to install the bar on a 1-foot × 6-foot wood board that is longer at both ends. The board can then be screw-mounted directly to the wall's stud framing. This arrangement typically provides sufficiently strong attachment points and also offers flexibility in selecting the eventual mounting location. This technique is useful in dry areas such as walls around toilets or outside shower entrances. Mounting boards work for ceramic tile walls, but test installations are impractical because drilled holes in ceramic tile are difficult to repair.

## MAKING YOUR KITCHEN MORE ACCESSIBLE

If you are building or renovating a kitchen, this can offer an opportunity to make it more functional and accessible. For wheelchair users, accessibility requirements that you establish before design begins will guide decisions related to counter arrangements and appliance selection. For example, if a wheelchair user resides alone and cooks for him- or herself, the kitchen layout can respond exclusively to the user's needs and preferences. On the other hand, if the wheelchair user lives with family members who do not have a disability, the arrangement should also respond to their needs. If future home resale is important, or if there are project budget limitations, homeowners may elect not to make kitchen modifications that are too customized or too expensive.

Whichever course you select, however, the kitchen plan should provide adequate wheelchair maneuvering clearances throughout.

Kitchen work sequences can be accommodated efficiently in several counter arrangements including U-shaped, L-shaped, and galley plans. Kitchens with island counters are variations of these basic arrangements. Each option offers both advantages and disadvantages for accessibility. The U-shaped kitchen, for example, is efficient for wheelchair users because the countertop surfaces are continuous. This allows items to be slid, rather than carried, between workstations. It is difficult for wheelchair users to move items between unconnected counters unless they have a lapboard on which to carry them. In this aspect, the galley kitchen's arrangement is perhaps the least appropriate. On the other hand, the two inside corners in U-shaped counters are difficult to reach when seated in a wheelchair. Galley kitchens do not have inside corners, so all counter space is easily accessible. Since none of the basic configurations is ideal, select the counter arrangement that is the best fit for your home.

Appliances should be carefully selected and located within your kitchen plan. Often, appliance models that the homeowner selects determine proper installation locations. A side-by-side model refrigerator/freezer, for example, should be located to accommodate both door swings. On the other hand, top or bottom freezer models have a single door swing, so clearance is only required on one side.

## CONCLUSIONS AND RECOMMENDATIONS

This chapter has only touched on a few aspects of residential accessible design. More information is available from resources such as instructive design publications and manufacturers' product literature. When using this information, however, bear in mind that your specific circumstances may not be addressed by generic design solutions. To sort through this material, keep in mind the reason for the specific design recommendation. If the design rationale does not apply to your circumstances, then the prototypical design may not meet your needs. Similarly, components of a generic solution may be unnecessary or even detrimental for your project. For example, a large roll-in shower stall is appropriate for someone who bathes while seated in a wheelchair. A smaller stall, however, may be more suitable for an ambulatory bather who uses walls or grab bars to maintain balance. Accessible design should be tailored specifically to each individual homeowner to best suit his or her needs as efficiently as possible.

# Chapter 21
# Managing Financial Resources
Thomas E. Stripling and Dorothy E. Northrop, MSW, ACSW

## SET THE STAGE

EVERY LIFESTYLE, whether it is jester, warrior, magician, or king, has real and implied costs. Purchasing the juggling cubes, stabling the warhorse, tuning the hourglass, or furnishing that summer castle are generally considered the direct costs of a chosen lifestyle; missing all those other bookings that one just can't get the time to perform could be called lost opportunities or indirect costs. Economists, who probably don't fit any of the four preceding lifestyles, like to calculate the direct and indirect costs to determine the effects of a lifestyle on a person's finances or to estimate how much funding one might need to conduct a particular lifestyle successfully.

Living with multiple sclerosis (MS), or any chronic health condition, is a lifestyle with direct and indirect costs. But before one enumerates either of the two cost categories, it is essential to make an important distinction. Life has usual and customary costs that every "style" has to address. Money for food, clothing, and shelter challenge the jester, warrior, magician, and king alike. Now, it is certain that "style" might dictate differences in the amount of costs, but one can assume that our four lifestyles have at least these costs in common. Living with MS is no different. Food, clothing, and shelter costs must be addressed adequately to provide a secure, if not comfortable, style in which one wishes to live. Living with MS presents some special or "incremental" costs that might be said to go beyond the basic life costs. For the following discussion, we'll label the MS costs as incremental in that these costs are often specific to the presence of MS in a person's life.

Expenses that are incremental costs of MS often include, but may not be limited to:

- Physician visits
- Hospitalizations
- Outpatient clinic visits other than to the doctor's office
- Prescriptions
- Over-the-counter medications
- Medical supplies
- Therapeutic visits or sessions, e.g., PT, OT, speech, etc.
- Equipment (e.g., mobility aids, assistive technology for health or work)
- Home nursing care visits
- Home modifications
- Vehicle modifications
- Aide or attendant services/home care
- Household assistance (e.g., housework or yard work)
- Copayments for medical visits or medications

It should be noted that not all direct costs are those paid by you or your spouse or family, but they might also be paid by insurance or other such programs. It is important to identify all costs when they happen and how often they happen regardless of who pays for them. This record will be handy for organizing a plan to meet such costs.

Indirect costs primarily are "missed opportunity" costs. The most obvious "missed opportunity" cost is lost wages due to changes in employment status. These losses might be total or partial, as some people with MS can work, but perhaps they are not working at a previous level or they do not receive advancements that might have occurred had their job performance not been compromised by aspects of their MS condition. Additionally, lost opportunities may represent financial changes for other family members, such as a spouse who has to alter his or her employment pattern in order to provide caregiver assistance at home, or children who have to change school placements or selections due to changes in household income that make tuition payments impossible. "Change of plans" costs may be subtle or even vague, but one should be watchful of such changes because they are real costs.

## WHAT ARE ECONOMIC CONSEQUENCES?

In the middle 1980s, Paralyzed Veterans of America (PVA) initiated a research agenda on the economic consequences of spinal cord injury and MS. The goal of this ambitious agenda was to document that "costs" for either spinal cord injury or MS could be identified and estimated for a year and a lifetime. The work was completed under contract to the Disability Income Systems, Inc. of Rutgers University, directed by Monroe Berkowitz, PhD and Carol Harvey, PhD. Three publications resulted from this agenda. See the references at the end of this chapter for these and other publications on this topic.

Economic consequences as used in this research were defined as the interaction between direct and indirect costs through the various stages of the condition (i.e., onset, sustaining, lifetime) and recognized the variety of payer participants in meeting the costs (e.g., Department of Veterans Affairs [VA], Medicare, Medicaid, private pay, private insurance, vocational rehabilitation, wages, etc.). The economic consequences recognized the interaction of costs and payers. It provided a conceptual framework by which one might understand the economic value of shifting costs and payers.

This framework provided an analytical mechanism by which healthcare delivery and reimbursement policies could be organized to maximize benefit to the individual and payers.

The analysis of PVA members with MS estimated that the average annual cost was $51,318 in healthcare items and services and lost earnings. Forty-seven percent of that total, or approximately $24,352, was direct costs for hospitalization, medical practitioner services, personal assistance and custodial care, durable medical equipment, and prescription medications. The aggregate cost for all 1,904 PVA members with MS in 1992 was $97.7 million. For anyone living with a chronic condition, it is important to understand that these studies show unequivocally that economic aspects can be quantified and that, over a lifetime, we are talking about serious amounts of money. You need to count your costs in order to understand your personal financial needs.

In 1998, Duke University researchers published a comprehensive assessment of the cost of MS in *Multiple Sclerosis*. Based on a study commissioned by the National Multiple Sclerosis Society (NMSS), these findings substantially support PVA findings. The only exception is that its model included "lost wages" as a direct cost. The combined costs for MS in this study were $34,103 annually. Adjusted for inflation today, this figure would be about $51,000.

The exactness of numbers is not the real issue for this discussion, but what is important is that costs can be estimated scientifically, and in the case of this immediate discussion, personally. You are encouraged to identify your personal costs either by daily journal or a monthly review of receipts. It is suggested that you track your financial experience for at least 3 months to be sure that a representative average can be obtained.

## PERSONAL FINANCIAL PLANNING

In 2003, PVA and the NMSS collaborated with the National Endowment for Financial Education (NEFE) to produce the book *Adapting: Financial Planning for a Life with Multiple Sclerosis.* This step-by-step personal financial planning guide is based on much of the preceding discussion. It asks one to identify the direct and indirect costs through a review of personal records or keeping a diary. It suggests ways to maximize a person's understanding of what it costs to live with MS, whether as an individual newly diagnosed or leaving work or retiring. The guide brings together a resource of thoughts and suggestions for organizing finances, building a spending plan, seeking expert assistance, and applying for governmental programs. The guide is not intended to replace expert advice or personal decision making, but it does go a long way toward stating that "it's only money," and everyone can gain a measure of mastery over their ability to pursue a lifestyle. You can obtain a copy of *Adapting* by contacting the PVA Distribution Center at 1-888-860-7244 or by calling the National MS Society at 1-800-FIGHT-MS.

*Adapting* presents outlines and worksheets for your MS journal, professional advisors, health-expense spreadsheet, job management, finding a new job, home assessment, home adaptations, income, expenses, and a financial plan. Each form is a suggestion and can be modified to address individual situations and experiences. At first glance, these worksheets might appear to be overkill, but experience has shown clearly that the more you know about these details, the stronger case you can make for yourself, your family, and benefit plans. You will find that the more you work with these details, the more refined your thinking will become, and thus, the more help these details will provide.

## PUBLIC BENEFIT PROGRAMS

Living with a chronic condition like MS often involves financial help beyond personal resources. Although there is no replacement for personal wages and income, public benefit programs can serve a critical role. *Adapting* lists a number of public benefits worthy of investigation. Whether you consider Medicare, Medicaid, or veterans benefits, there will be a need to use the organization of your income and expenses, as mentioned above. Most public benefits are based on "need," but you must be careful to understand that "need" is in the eye of the beholder. Programs have specific definitions either from legislation or regulations. It is wise to consider how best to present your need to any public program.

It is strongly recommended that you use professional help when applying for any public benefits. The U.S. Social Security Administration has benefit counselors and may provide you with a list of agencies and/or others who are certified to assist you in the application process. For VA benefits one should contact a "veterans service organization" such as PVA, Veterans of Foreign Wars, Disabled American Veterans, or Vietnam Veterans of America to request assistance from a "service officer." Each of these programs realizes the complex web of information required for application of benefits. Such information includes medical, employment, and financial records. In the case of VA, proof of honorable discharge from military service is required also. These programs have very detailed applications and appeals processes, and developing a competent record of information often is key. Professional help will be essential to securing appropriate benefits.

Last, it is noteworthy that if you are eligible to receive public benefits, they still are no replacement for personal wages and income. However, you must be sure that you are aware of any specific limits on personal income that might be a continuing condition for receiving public benefits. Maintaining a connection with your professional counselor might be necessary as you pursue your financial goals each year. It is appropriate to know income and/or financial limits so that you can balance your plans against your benefits.

## CONCLUSION

As this chapter opened with four possible lifestyles, we have attempted to provide some encouragement and tools to assist you to fully integrate financial aspects in living with MS. Like most personal skills, financial planning takes time and interest. Understanding "incremental costs" is the best way to realize the full extent and impact of living with MS. Whether you elect to be a jester, warrior, magician, or king, it is definitely possible to make finances work toward your independence now and into the future.

## REFERENCES

Whetten-Goldstein K, Sloan FA, Goldstein LB, Kulas ED. A Comprehensive assessment of the cost of multiple sclerosis in the United States. *Multiple Sclerosis* 1998;4:419–425.

*Adapting: Financial Planning for a Life with Multiple Sclerosis*. National Endowment for Financial Education, 2003.

*Economic Consequences of Spinal Cord Injury*. Washington, DC: Paralyzed Veterans of America; 1985.

*Economic Consequences of Severe Disabilities*. Washington, DC: Paralyzed Veterans of America; 1986.

*Economic Consequences of Traumatic Spinal Cord Injury*. New York: Demos Medical Publishing; 1990.

*Economic Consequences of Traumatic Spinal Cord Injury—Further Analysis*. Washington, DC: Paralyzed Veterans of America; 1991.

*The Economic Consequences of Multiple Sclerosis among PVA Members*. Washington, DC: Paralyzed Veterans of America; 1994.

*Economic Consequences of Traumatic Aging SCI*. New York: Demos Medical Publishing; 1995.

*Spinal Cord Injury: An Analysis of Medical and Social Costs*. New York: Demos Medical Publishing; 1998.

# Chapter 22
# Health Insurance Options
Dorothy E. Northrop, MSW, ACSW

IN THE SPRING OF 2003, a Kaiser Health Poll reported that more than twice as many people were concerned about healthcare costs than were worried about not being able to pay their rent or mortgage, losing money in the stock market, being a victim of a terrorist attack, or losing their job. Approximately 36 percent of Americans worried that the amount they paid for healthcare services or health insurance coverage would increase.

For people with a chronic disease or disability such as multiple sclerosis (MS), obtaining and maintaining health insurance coverage is crucial. The quality of one's health coverage determines the quality of one's healthcare, and having the necessary healthcare is a key factor in optimizing function and quality of life.

The most important "key" to getting needed healthcare services is to be a knowledgeable user of the healthcare system, which includes the following:

- Knowing all that you can about your disease
- Knowing about your own specific healthcare needs
- Knowing the details of your health plan

It also requires that you understand rights and protections that exist through legislation and regulation to help you obtain or maintain health insurance coverage. Twenty years ago, the landscape was vastly different. People with chronic conditions had few protections and faced blatant discrimination in their quest for coverage. This is not true today, but one must be informed and vigilant. Protections are only effective if they are understood and utilized. The purpose of this chapter is to make sure that you understand health insurance coverage and are knowledgeable of the options and protections that are available to you.

## SOURCES OF INSURANCE
The majority of Americans, and the majority of people with MS, receive their health insurance as a benefit from their employer. In the United States, unlike other industrialized nations, there is no universal health coverage for all citizens. Instead, the system is employment-based, and employers receive incentives and tax breaks to offer group health coverage to their employees. Employers are not required to offer health insurance benefits, but the majority of employers, approximately 66 percent, do offer it.

About half of employers offering health insurance coverage purchase the coverage from an insurance company. These employers are referred to as "fully insured." The other 50 percent of employers decide to become the insurer themselves. They collect the premiums, pay the claims, and assume the risk. They do not contract with insurance companies unless they choose to have them just administer the paperwork. These employers are referred to as "self-insured" or "self-funded." The kind of coverage your employer has is very important to know, as it determines the rights, protections, and appeal options available to you.

Some individuals must purchase policies on an individual basis if they are not part of an employer health plan. Individual policies are almost always more expensive than employer group coverage and insurers are usually selective as to whom they will insure. Since many people with chronic health conditions are rejected by individual insurance companies, 30 states have created an insurance option called "high risk pools." These pools can be a resource for those rejected in the individual insurance market, although coverage can be quite expensive.

Many Americans receive their health coverage from Medicare. Those over the age of 65 automatically become eligible for Medicare when they begin receiving Social Security. Traditional Medicare has two parts, Part A and Part B. Part A, which covers hospitalization and related expenses, is provided to all who are eligible without a premium. Part B, which provides coverage for physicians, lab costs, rehabilitation, etc., can be elected with the payment of a premium of $66.60/month, as of 2004.

Another group of individuals eligible for Medicare, other than those over 65, are those who are determined by the Social Security Administration to have a disability and are receiving Social Security Disability income. At present, there is a 2-year waiting period to receive Medicare once one starts receiving the disability income. This delay can present a hardship for people with disabilities, and advocacy efforts are addressing this issue.

Although Medicare is relatively comprehensive, its premiums, deductibles and co-insurances are quite expensive and, until the Medicare Prescription Drug, Improvement and Modernization Act of 2003, included no prescription coverage. Therefore, most recipients of traditional Medicare have purchased supplemental coverage to cover out-of-pocket expenses and additional benefits such as prescription drugs. These policies are called *Medigap* policies. The future of Medigap policies is currently uncertain in light of the changes to the Medicare program expected to be implemented in 2006.

There is currently also a *Medicare+ Choice* option, which is the managed care arm of Medicare. It is more restrictive in terms of providers, but generally includes additional benefits not covered by traditional Medicare and requires less out-of-pocket expenses. Beginning in 2006, a Medicare Part D is scheduled to be available, which will incorporate the prescription drug options that are to be part of the Medicare program.

Another source of insurance coverage, available to individuals with low-income who are blind, disabled, elderly, or are caring for dependent children, is *Medicaid*. This is a means-tested assistance program underwritten by a combination of federal and state funding. Most individuals who receive Supplemental Security Income (SSI) are covered by Medicaid. It can sometimes be difficult finding providers who will accept Medicaid, but benefits are relatively extensive and can often include coverage for such long-term care services as nursing home care, adult day programs, and/or home care.

The balance of healthcare coverage options derive from various governmental entities such as the Department of Veterans Affairs, TRICARE (active uniformed service members, and their families and retirees), the Federal Employee Health Benefits Program, state and local government employee programs, and State Child Health Insurance Programs.

## UNDERSTANDING YOUR HEALTH INSURANCE PLAN

Health insurance policies are complex and often very difficult to understand. However, it is important to be very clear about what your policy covers, what it does not, and how to appeal denials. Many plans make determinations of what they will cover based on "medical necessity." Appeals usually center around a difference of opinion between the physician or provider of care and the insurance company as to what intervention or treatment is medically necessary.

Most health plans today incorporate managed care to a varying degree. This means there will probably be some level of incentive and financial benefit for enrollees to use the particular network of providers associated with the plan. It is therefore important to review a plan's list of providers to see if specialists are included who are appropriate to your medical needs, and whether doctors with whom you have an established relationship are included in the plan.

The "Summary of Benefits" you receive when you enroll in a health plan is not a legal document. It is just what it says—a summary. Request the "Evidence of Coverage" document from your plan so that you have the exact details of your policy.

When reviewing your policy, pay particular attention to the following:

- Open versus restricted network of providers
- Required preauthorizations
- Access to specialists
- Coverage for hospitalization, major medical, and prescription drugs, particularly any MS treatments that are prescribed for you
- Amount of co-insurance, co-pays, and deductibles
- Pre-existing medical condition waiting periods
- Out-of-pocket maximums
- Levels of coverage for physical therapy, psychotherapy, rehabilitation, equipment, and home healthcare
- Specific coverage limitations and exclusions
- Yearly/lifetime maximums of coverage
- Options and procedures for appeal

If you find yourself in the position of having to select from a choice of plans, which is increasingly the case when selecting employer coverage these days, review each plan available to you using the above criteria in order to be sure you are selecting the plan most appropriate for you in terms of your particular medical concerns.

If you are applying for coverage, and you are asked questions about your health status, it is important that you not lie on the application and intentionally hide the fact that you have MS. You must respond honestly and fully to any question. However, you do not have to volunteer any information that is not requested directly or by implication.

## APPEALING A DENIAL

If a health plan does not cover a specific intervention or treatment, and it is explicit in the policy that this is the case, it is unlikely that an appeal to receive coverage will be successful. However, there are many instances when a denial is basically a difference of opinion as to the value of a treatment. When this is the case, proceeding with an appeal is not only recommended, it is often very successful.

The first thing you must do is review your policy and be absolutely clear about the appeal process. All health plans must specify the avenues to follow in order to have the plan reconsider its decision. This is true whether it be a private plan, Medicaid, or Medicare. It is important that these procedures be followed, particularly in terms of time limits, to be sure that your appeal is not summarily dismissed.

An important part of any appeal is documenting your position. The better you know MS and your particular disease course, the better you will be able to advocate on your own behalf. Use a health journal to document changes in your health status and your response to treatments and medications. Gather materials and peer-reviewed literature that can support your position. (Your National MS Society or

Paralyzed Veterans of America chapter can assist you with this.) Engage your physician as a partner in advocating for reconsideration of the denial.

If you complete your health plan's internal appeal process and continue to be dissatisfied, there are still other alternatives to pursue. Your next step will depend on the type of plan you have and what governmental entity oversees the plan. At this point, it is very important for you to know, if you have employment-based insurance, whether your plan is "fully insured" or "self-insured," as described on page 153.

If you have a "fully insured" employer group health plan, your plan is regulated by your state's Department of Insurance and is subject to state regulation and legislation with regard to patient rights. Questions about your protections and rights can be addressed to your state Insurance Department. If you have a fully insured plan, and you have exhausted the internal review process, most states have an external review option, which you can pursue.

Federal legislation, called the Employee Retirement Income Security Act (ERISA), prevents states from legislating "self-funded" employer plans. It says that states can regulate insurers but cannot regulate employers. Therefore, these plans are not subject to state overview or external review. They are regulated by the U.S. Department of Labor. Although these plans must provide an internal appeals process, the only recourse following an internal appeal is the filing of a lawsuit.

It is important to remember that it is ultimately the employer who determines the health insurance plan that is offered to employees. Therefore, it might also be appropriate to appeal directly to your employer to make sure that he understands the hardship of a particular decision or denial.

Medicare has its own external review option that is described in your Medicare handbook. It begins with an independent

contractor, proceeds to an administrative law judge, and then on to the Department of Health and Human Services Appeals Board. For those covered by Medicaid, state external review does not apply, but the right to a fair hearing is in place.

Although the process of appeal may seem daunting, and you may require assistance in going through the process, it can often be a worthwhile effort and result in the reversal of a denial.

## MAINTAINING HEALTH INSURANCE

Maintaining health insurance is extremely important to people with chronic conditions or diseases such as MS. Many express fear that leaving the workforce or changing from full-time to part-time employment will result in loss of health coverage, not only for themselves but for their families.

Concern is also expressed that people who change jobs may not be able to get health insurance coverage from their new employer because of their pre-existing condition.

Two pieces of federal legislation provide important protections to people with MS who have employment-related concerns about health insurance coverage.

### CONTINUATION COVERAGE (COBRA)

The Consolidated Omnibus Budget Reconciliation Act (COBRA) of 1985 applies to all companies with 20 or more employees. When an individual leaves a job for any reason other than gross misconduct, or converts from full-time to part-time employment, she must be given the opportunity to purchase continued health coverage under the employer plan for an additional 18 months at the group rate. The employer no longer must contribute to the plan, however, so the employee must pay for the full cost of coverage. Although this option can be expensive, it is important to remember that employer group plans are generally more comprehensive and less costly than insurance in the individual market.

If a person purchases COBRA coverage and it is determined that he/she has a disability according to the Social Security Administration, the length of time for continuation of coverage can be extended to 29 months. COBRA also requires employers to offer continuation coverage, up to 36 months, in the event of divorce, separation, a child leaving dependent status, or the death of an employee.

If a person is employed by a company with less than 20 employees and is not covered by this COBRA legislation, many states have passed mini-COBRA laws that can provide similar protections, though usually less extensive.

### PROTECTIONS REGARDING PRE-EXISTING CONDITIONS (HIPAA)

The Health Insurance Portability and Accountability Act (HIPAA) was passed by Congress in 1996 to protect health insurance coverage for Americans who move from one job to another or who have pre-existing medical conditions. Employer plans must cover all employees, regardless of health status. No employee can be dropped from coverage if he becomes ill. The longest an employer can delay coverage of a pre-existing condition is 1 year. Once that exclusion period is met, employees do not have to meet it again, even if they change jobs, provided they do so within 63 days. Therefore, people with pre-existing medical conditions can move from one group plan to another without jeopardizing their health insurance coverage.

HIPAA also protects those who lose group coverage, including COBRA, and must purchase an individual policy. As long as the individual has had continuous group coverage for 18 months and is not eligible for another group plan, Medicare, or Medicaid, he is guaranteed access to the individual market.

## VIGILANT ADVOCACY

The healthcare arena is constantly changing and people with chronic conditions and disabilities must aggressively promote their healthcare and be watchful of trends and changes in coverage that could compromise the quality of that care. Some plans may be less expensive in terms of premiums, but could be more expensive when it comes to getting the care that is needed. Prescription formularies change and can stop covering specific medications or introduce prohibitive co-pays. Some plans that employers are offering now, such as the Defined Contribution Plan, tend to shift the burden of care from employees that use little care to those who use more, and can result in significant gaps of coverage. Other potential barriers are cumbersome pre-authorizations, increasing reduction of benefits, larger co-pays, and the tiering of plans and formularies to induce members to go to a particular hospital or buy only generic drugs.

You are your own best advocate. Be an "educated consumer." Know your disease. Know your health plan. Know the protections that are out there for you. Engage your physician. Fight for what you need. Don't give up. You bring an important voice to your own healthcare and to the needs of people who share your concerns. Communicate the issues that you identify to those responsible for regulations and policy. Advise organizations such at the National MS Society and Paralyzed Veterans of America of inequities you are experiencing that need to be addressed on a broader level. It is only through education, and helping people to understand the personal impact of healthcare decisions, that change will happen. You can definitely contribute to making that difference.

# Chapter 23
# Community Living Options
Debra Frankel, MS, OTR

HIRING PERSONAL ASSISTANTS, as described in the following chapter, frequently meets the needs for people who require assistance with activities of daily living, and enables them to continue living in their own homes. However, other obstacles, such as an inaccessible home environment or the need for more hours of help and supervision than can be provided, may lead you to consider other community-based living options.

## ADULT DAY CARE

Adult day centers provide a daytime program that includes health, social, and support services in a supervised setting. This community-based service allows individuals to continue living at home and supplement the services they might need during the day in a setting outside of the home. You may still require home-based personal assistant services to help you get ready in the morning, get ready for bed at night, and for care on the weekends. However, an adult day program may be right for you if you need more hours of help each day than can be provided and if you would like opportunities for social interaction and other activities outside your home. Specific services offered in adult day programs might include: social and recreational activities, meals, rehabilitation, nursing care, personal care, and counseling. Most adult day health programs are geared to elders, although some serve a mixed-age population. Some even specialize in providing services to people with MS. There are several types of adult day care: social day care offers minimal personal care assistance and emphasizes social activities and mental stimulation; adult day health care offers moderate personal care assis-

tance, health monitoring, and rehabilitation therapies. There are also special programs that are specifically geared to those with cognitive impairments.

The staff of the adult day health program will work with you to develop an individualized plan that meets your social, recreational, and health needs. In general, when looking at a program, be sure that it:

- Provides the range of services you need.
- Offers a flexible schedule of full- or part-time care.
- Has well-trained staff and volunteers and a low staff to participant ratio.
- Adheres to state and national standards and guidelines.

You can often determine whether a program is right for you by asking about the types of activities offered and the age and disability range of the participants. It is also important to check a program's references and talk to two or three participants about their experiences. The National Adult Day Services Association (www.nadsa.org) can provide information about choosing a program.

Fees for adult day care vary, with daily fees ranging from $40 to $200 and more per day. Medicaid, in most states, provides funding for adult day care, including transportation to and from the program, for eligible individuals. Some private insurance or health maintenance organizations (HMOs) may partially cover adult day care or cover specific services provided as part of a program (e.g., occupational or speech therapy). Medicare may also cover some components of the program (e.g., rehabilitation therapies), but does not cover the cost of the program in full. Some private long-term care insurance policies cover adult day care. If you do not have coverage and are paying privately, the center might offer a sliding fee scale. Contact the National MS Society at 1-800-FIGHT MS for referrals to local adult day programs.

## ASSISTED LIVING

Assisted living is a community-based living option that combines housing, supportive services, and healthcare designed to meet the needs of people who require assistance with their daily activities. The types of services offered usually include: meals served in a common dining area (apartments may also have their own kitchens or kitchenettes), housekeeping services, transportation, personal care assistance, emergency call systems, medication management, health promotion programs, social activities, and laundry services. Assisted living programs may offer single rooms, double rooms, studio apartments, or one or two bedroom apartments. The facility may be free standing or housed with other residential options such as nursing homes or independent living units.

Today, most residents of assisted living facilities are elderly. However, more and more younger, disabled individuals and couples are seeking out these programs. It is very important to obtain enough information to determine whether assisted living is a good option for you. Many programs have specific admission criteria with regard to the amount of assistance you require with transfers and personal assistance. Also, ask about what your options are if your need for personal assistance increases significantly while you are living there. Determine exactly what services are offered and if they can be supplemented by your hiring additional help, if necessary.

Costs vary with the program and the types of services needed by the residents. Monthly fees (including rent and services) range from $1,500 to more than $6,000 per month. Some programs offer a basic fee with additional charges for special services. Most residences offer month-to-month arrangements, although some may require a long-term commitment. Make sure you fully understand the costs and services available.

Regulations and licensing requirements for assisted living programs vary from state to state. Residences must comply with local building codes and fire safety regulations, and some states require that staff be certified and receive special training. When considering a particular program, you will want to look into: state licensure and certification requirements, staff credentials and ratios of staff to residents, services and activities offered, costs, contracts, accessibility of the physical plant, availability of common areas, security, quality and size of living space, menus, and special dietary requirements. Be a cautious consumer! Marketing brochures may be misleading or unclear as to costs and availability of services. Contact the Assisted Living Facilities Association (ALFA) at www.alfa.org for a directory of facilities in your area.

## CARE MANAGEMENT

Care management is a process that involves hiring and working with a professional care manager who can help you figure out what you need and how to access the services that are available in your community. A care manager can help you navigate an often confusing healthcare and social service delivery system, arranging services, helping you apply for financial benefits, and planning for contingencies. The role of care management has been described as accessing the right care, at the right time, in the right place, by the right provider.

The manager may charge a flat fee or an hourly rate. Before you engage a manager, obtain his or her credentials, check references, and develop a written agreement regarding fees and work to be performed. Be sure to clarify whether expenses (e.g., phone charges, mileage) are included in the fee or will be charged separately. Most third-party payers do not cover the costs of care management (check with your insurance provider); however, you may find that the cost of hiring a professional is well worth the benefit you may realize in terms of coordinated, reliable support in helping you remain at home or in your community.

## OTHER COMMUNITY-BASED LIVING OPTIONS

Some communities offer other options, such as congregate or group homes that are specifically geared toward people with disabilities. Some individuals with MS in a given community have come together to share personal care services, forming personal assistance cooperatives or other creative ways to get the services they need and stay in their own homes. Contact your local chapter of the National MS Society to find out if such options are available in your area or for support and information in creating your own options.

Other community services, such as home-delivered meals, chore services, "paratransit" transportation services, and friendly visitor programs may also enable you to live more independently and safely in the community. Again, contact your local chapter of the National MS Society for more information about whether these services are available in your community and whether you meet eligibility requirements.

Healthcare policy regarding long-term care is beginning to reflect consumer preferences to stay at home and receive services in the home and community. Grants to states, called Home and Community Based Waivers, allow states to provide services that will enhance access to services that promote independent living in the community, as well as facilitate the transition from nursing homes to the community for some individuals. These programs encourage consumer direction and promote participation in community life. With these new programs, as well as with more and more providers responding to growing consumer demand, new options for community-based living options should become more available in the coming years.

## A NOTE ABOUT NURSING HOMES

Should you come to need nursing home care, that is, if the resources available in your home and community exceed your needs and/or if you require medical supervision and care that cannot be provided at home, work with the National MS Society to help you and your family select an appropriate facility. Nursing homes are licensed by each state to provide nursing care, personal assistance, rehabilitation, social/recreational activities, medical services, and more. While most nursing homes are geared toward caring for seniors, many have special programs for younger residents, some specifically for residents with MS.

Many people cannot conceive of a high quality of life in a nursing facility and may think of them as "the last stop." To the contrary, many individuals with severe MS who were socially isolated in their own homes, or whose needs were not being adequately met at home, find that their life improves significantly once admitted to a nursing home. Opportunities for socialization, stimulating activities, trips into the community, safety and peace of mind, and attention to personal care and medical needs may all contribute to a considerably improved quality of life. The National MS Society is working with many nursing facilities across the country to be sure their staff are well trained to care for younger residents with MS, and in turn, this is leading to better care and increased sensitivity to the unique needs of the resident with MS.

# Chapter 24
# Obtaining Personal Assistance
Debra Frankel, MS, OTR and Pamela Cavallo, MSW, CSW

## CONSIDERING INDEPENDENCE, DEPENDENCE, AND INTERDEPENDENCE

IN WESTERN SOCIETY, most people cherish independence. We often feel that adulthood doesn't begin until a measure of personal freedom has been established. Of course, no one is entirely free or totally independent, nor would we want to be. As social animals, we are really interdependent and generally happier for it.

Still, any threat to personal independence is serious. In the face of major changes in life, being able to remain in your own home, direct your own care, and make choices independently can be key to retaining a sense of control—your independence. Fortunately, health policy and the provision of health and personal care services for people with disabilities is becoming more consumer-directed and is beginning to favor community and home-based care over institutional care. For instance, The New Freedom Initiative, introduced by George W. Bush in 2001, consists of a series of efforts (and funding!) by the federal government to encourage consumer choice, maximize the participation of people with disabilities in their communities, and reduce barriers to community integration. Over the coming years, we should see more and more home and community-based initiatives that make living independently a greater reality for people with disabilities and elders, and provide for easier access to personal assistance and other home and community-based services. Also, as part of their efforts to comply with the 1999 Supreme Court ruling in *Olmstead vs. L.C. and E.W.*, policymakers in many states have passed or are considering legislative proposals designed to promote home and community-based service initiatives. (*Olmstead* held that unjustified isolation and segregation of persons with disabilities in institutional settings is a form of discrimination under the Americans with Disabilities Act.) An integral part of all these health policy initiatives is the availability of personal assistance services in the home.

Services such as personal assistance, nursing care, physical therapy, occupational therapy, counseling, and assistance with household cleaning, chores, and errand services can allow many people with multiple sclerosis (MS) to live at home safely and independently. Some of these services are covered by insurance; some you will have to pay for privately. We'll address these financial issues later.

## DETERMINING YOUR NEEDS

The first step in getting help at home is determining your needs. These may be:

- *Medical* (for example, medication management, bowel and bladder management, range-of-motion exercises, occupational therapy, etc.)
- *Personal care* (help with bathing, dressing, shaving, toileting, transferring, hair care, meal preparation, wheelchair and scooter maintenance, transportation, etc.)
- *Housework and chores* (help with shopping, errands, house cleaning, laundry, household paperwork and bill paying, etc.)
- *Companionship* (conversation, safety, social activities, etc.)

- *Emotional* (psychological support, counseling to address depression and assist in developing new life goals, etc.)
- *Environmental* (removal of barriers, e.g., stairs, narrow doorways, thresholds, inaccessible faucets, switches and controls, safe egress, etc.)

It's a good idea for you and your family members to discuss and identify the needs together and discuss how they might be met. Can a family member, friend, or volunteer be relied on for some needs? Could a personal emergency response system alleviate some worries about safety? Perhaps an adult day program could alleviate social isolation. It usually takes time to clarify what is needed and who is the best person to meet the needs. For now, we will primarily focus on personal assistance, rather than other home services.

TIPS FOR CONDUCTING A NEEDS ASSESSMENT

- You're the expert about what you need.
- Nonetheless, ask for feedback from others to help you "reality test."
- Prioritize how you want to spend your energy, particularly if it is limited and fatigue is a problem.
- Determine exactly what tasks you want your personal assistant to do.
- Consider the needs of those you live with.
- Think about your personality and how this influences whom you might select as an assistant.
- Determine hours and schedules that are realistic and convenient for you as well as that take into account what is reasonable to expect from an assistant.
- Consider needs beyond your usual daily schedule (e.g., help with special activities, holiday shopping, cultural outings, family events, etc.)
- Reassess your needs periodically, particularly following physical or other major changes.

## HIRING SOMEONE PRIVATELY ON YOUR OWN

If you decide to hire someone on your own, as opposed to going through an agency, you will be the employer, supervisor, evaluator, and consumer. The first step in hiring someone on your own is to describe the job in writing. This is essential. The job description should include the following elements:

- Specific duties
- Time required
- Expected daily routine
- Travel, if any
- Whether personal transportation is required
- Any special skills required, including medical and physical capabilities
- Salary (including method and frequency of payments) and benefits (including time off, sick days, etc.) All legal requirements must be met, including withholding income and Social Security taxes.

The next step is to get the word out that you are looking for an assistant. You may have to find more than one person, because your primary employee may get sick or need time off. You may also need holiday or vacation coverage. Some personal attendants may prefer part-time or intermittent assignments, so it may be possible to find back-up assistants who only want periodic or part-time work.

Ask your friends and acquaintances to help spread the word. In addition to your chapter of the National MS Society, contact senior centers, community centers, clergy and church organizations, and college employment offices. Try hospital-based schools for nurses, medical technicians, or therapists, as many of these students like health-related jobs. Post flyers at these locations. Contact the Independent Living Center in your area, as it may keep a roster of potential personal assistants. Contact service organizations such as the Knights of Columbus, Elks, Volunteers of America, and ethnic clubs. Consider advertising in the daily paper as well as in free neighborhood news and advertising weeklies, community bulletin boards, college newspapers, and local church bulletins. Some people have used the Internet with good results. For your own protection, omit your address and name in the ad. If you live alone and have the space, you might consider finding a roommate who, in exchange for rent, can offer some personal care assistance and/or companionship.

Hiring privately offers you greater control. You decide who comes to your home and you negotiate schedules, salaries, and responsibilities. In most cases, this option is less costly because the arrangements are made without the involvement of a third party. While it is unlikely that insurance will cover someone you hire on your own, Medicaid (in many states) will pay for personal care assistants hired independently through Independent Living or Personal Assistant Programs. Contact the Independent Living Center in your area for more information on Personal Assistant Programs.

When hiring someone who is a stranger, screening is very important. In some states, you can conduct a criminal background check on a potential employee. Check with your state government as to whether they have a Criminal History Systems Board that enables you to conduct a Criminal Offender Record Information check. Before interviewing applicants, prepare a checklist based on the most important requirements in the job description that you can use to screen and interview prospective candidates. Conducting interviews will help you assess whether the individual has the skills and personal characteristics for the job. If you're worried about your privacy or security, hold the interview in a public place (e.g., a coffee shop). Try to set a relaxed,

welcoming tone. Help applicants to feel comfortable sharing information about themselves. Take notes and be sure to write down all the essentials—basic identification data, telephone number, and address. You may find the presence of a friend or family member to be helpful. That person could help you to recall responses and provide his or her impressions.

Be sure to obtain:

- A written job application, complete with character and work references
- A completed W-4 form for payroll deductions, if the person is hired
- Any other forms needed (if you feel uncertain, call the local state employment office or other reliable source).

Check references! Be clear that you will adhere to a probation period (usually 90 days) during which time either you or your assistant may decide that the fit is not right.

When the personal assistant begins:

- Be sure you have established and agreed upon all the necessary terms and conditions. Both of you should sign a written agreement.
- Be sure you have discussed hours, a regular schedule, predictable variations in the schedule, time off, the pay schedule, the end of probation, periodic evaluations, and changes. The fee you will pay your help is determined by both your available resources and the community's "going rate." Rates vary from community to community. Use resources such as community social services, your National MS Society chapter, and people you respect who have employed help to establish the going rate. If you are offering other benefits, such as room and board or access to a vehicle for personal use, adjust the assistant's salary accordingly.

## HIRING SOMEONE THROUGH AN AGENCY

There are advantages to using professional home health agencies to hire a personal assistant. Agencies select and train home health aides, homemakers, physical therapists, occupational therapists, social workers, and nurses. The agency handles recordkeeping, scheduling, and coordinating care, and it bills insurance carriers directly, all of which can lift a burden off an overwhelmed family. Agency administrators are usually familiar with community services and know insurance requirements and limitations.

When looking for an agency, ask the following questions:

- Does the agency work with your insurance company, with Medicare, with Medicaid, etc.? Usually agency administrators process claims with Medicare and/or private insurance and the insured is responsible for some co-payment. However, keep in mind, while some insurance covers skilled care in the home or home health aides for a limited period, very few payers cover ongoing personal assistance. Plan to have to cover most of these costs privately.
- What services does the agency provide?
- Will the same person provide the home health services each day?
- Does the agency supply references for the professionals it sends?
- Are these professionals bonded?
- What are the fees? Is there a sliding scale for private payers?
- How do the fees compare with those of other agencies?
- Is there a backup system for emergencies, holidays, or sick days?
- How long has the agency been in business?
- Is the agency licensed and accredited by appropriate governmental agencies?

It is daunting to invite a stranger into your home and the intimate parts of your life. You and your family can make the situation less anxiety provoking by doing your homework well. Whether you use an agency or hire on your own, consider these cautions:

- Keep track of how much cash you have and where you have put it.
- Keep checkbooks, credit cards, and valuables out of site.
- If you need help writing checks, give them out one at a time.
- If an employee shops for you, always ask for and read the receipts.
- If possible, don't give an employee your credit cards. Rely on family members or trusted financial advisors.
- Don't discuss your finances with anyone except family and financial advisors.
- Keep track of your supply of medications by writing down how much you order and when.
- Don't borrow from or lend money to an employee.
- Arrange for periodic, unannounced visits by friends or relatives while your employee is on duty.
- Arrange a few code words with a close family member or spouse. In the event of a bad situation, you may want to telephone for help.

## FINANCING PERSONAL ASSISTANCE

Medicare, Medicaid, and private insurance cover some home care services. However, there are usually strict eligibility criteria and limitations on coverage.

*Medicare.* Medicare requires that certain services be provided by a licensed, certified home healthcare agency. Medicare provides 80 percent reimbursement for skilled nursing care and aides, physical therapy, speech therapy, occupational therapy, and medical social services. Medicare will only pay for personal care or homemaker services if there is also a need for skilled care (nursing or rehabilitation services). You cannot hire someone on your own for these services and receive any Medicare reimbursement. In addition, Medicare does not provide reimbursement for homemaker services, home-delivered meals, or for 24-hour nursing care in the home. All of this is subject to change.

*Medicaid.* Medicaid will cover personal care services on an ongoing basis for eligible persons in many states. Some states offer personal care assistance programs that allow you to hire someone on your own and receive Medicaid funds to pay your helpers.

*Private insurance.* Private insurance and HMOs may cover some home care services through an agency, usually for a limited period. They, like Medicare, may require that you need a skilled service, along with personal care or homemaker services.

*Veterans.* If you are a veteran, you might also want to check with the Department of Veterans Affairs to see if you are covered for home healthcare.

*Long-term care insurance.* Some long-term care insurance policies also provide coverage of home health services. Each policy is different, so if you have a policy, check your policy document or call your insurance agent for details.

*Other.* Some people over the age of 60 might find that their local Council on Aging offers assistance with home care.

If you are paying privately for agency assistance, some home health agencies offer a sliding fee scale, allowing individuals to pay according to their ability to do so. Generally, the cost of hiring a helper privately will come out of your own pocket. You are well advised to comply with Social Security regulations in hiring household help. The Social Security Administration can explain your responsibilities when paying assistants in your home.

## OTHER WAYS TO FEEL SAFER AT HOME

An emergency response system (ERS) can offer a sense of safety and security to many people who live by themselves. An ERS usually consists of a call button (worn as a necklace or bracelet) that can be pushed if you fall or need emergency help. Once activated, the system alerts an attendant at the system headquarters who will try to contact you to determine your needs. The attendant will then contact predetermined family members, neighbors, or local fire/emergency services to respond to your call. The call device can be worn in the shower and to bed, and the system is in operation 24 hours a day.

Home modifications might also help you feel safer and more independent. Widening doorways, creating an accessible bathroom, building a ramped entrance, and installing a porch lift can often enable someone to stay at home safely and more independently and get out in case of an emergency. A consultation with an occupational therapist, architect, or home modification specialist will help you identify your options. For referrals, contact the National Multiple Sclerosis Society (1-800-FIGHT-MS) or the Paralyzed Veterans of America (800-424-8200).

## NEEDS ASSESSMENT WORKSHEET

Use this worksheet as a tool to help you and your family identify your needs and how they will be met. You may have more than one name for some needs. Be very specific regarding *medical* needs, as some can only be met by a *trained* person. Keep in mind that needs may change as your condition changes. Reassess from time to time.

List of Needs   Who Will Help

| | Self | Family Member | Friend (Volunteer)/ Companion (Paid) | House-keeper/ Homemaker | Health Aide | Nurse/ Therapist |
|---|---|---|---|---|---|---|
| Laundry | | | | | | |
| Dust furniture | | | | | | |
| Vacuum | | | | | | |
| Make beds | | | | | | |
| Meal preparation | | | | | | |
| Dishwashing | | | | | | |
| Recordkeeping | | | | | | |
| Errands | | | | | | |
| Grocery shopping | | | | | | |
| Reading | | | | | | |
| Letter writing | | | | | | |
| Hobbies | | | | | | |
| Safety | | | | | | |
| Bathing | | | | | | |
| Dressing | | | | | | |
| Hair care | | | | | | |
| Nail care | | | | | | |
| Bowel program | | | | | | |
| Bladder program | | | | | | |
| Exercise | | | | | | |
| Transfers | | | | | | |
| Transportation for self—weekdays | | | | | | |
| Transportation for self—weekends | | | | | | |
| Transportation for children/others—weekdays | | | | | | |
| Transportation for children/others—weekends | | | | | | |

## Job Description Worksheet

**INSTRUCTIONS:** Use this worksheet to create your job description. Carefully consider all of your activities and needs and obtain input from others in your household.

**A. Job title:** This should reflect the major emphasis of the job. Personal assistance? Housekeeping? Other? Be flexible.

_____

**B. List of major duties:** Spell out what you need. You may think mopping and vacuuming is "light housekeeping" while someone else thinks "light housekeeping" means tidying up. Do you plan to go shopping yourself with someone to drive and carry for you? Or do you plan to send your helper with money and a list? Remember, "assist in shopping" could mean either one. Personal-care issues also need specifics. Do you need help using the toilet? Do you bathe alone, but need help transferring in and out of the tub? Use your Needs Assessment Worksheet as a reference.

_____

_____

_____

_____

**C. Hours:** Include expectations regarding holidays and weekends, sick time and vacation.

_____

_____

_____

_____

**D. Requirements:** Include all your personal "must haves" such as a driver's license, ability to lift 150 lb. person, willingness to be bonded. Also list language needs, smoking preference, and if you have pets or children.

_____

_____

_____

_____

**E. Experience desired:** Think through how much direction you feel willing or able to give. Don't discourage the right person by making requirements too high. On the other hand, don't discount the value of experience. Do you want someone with first aid certification or training in transferring? (When you check references, ask about experience your applicant claims.)

_____

_____

_____

_____

# Applicant Information Form

(Make copies for use when interviewing a job applicant.)

Name _____ SS # _____

Address                                    Telephone

_____       Day: _____

_____       Night: _____

_____       Cell: _____

Previous Employers/Experience

_____

_____

_____

_____

_____

References (must list 3)

| Name | Telephone | Relationship |
|------|-----------|--------------|
| _____ | _____ | _____ |
| _____ | _____ | _____ |

| Name | Telephone | Relationship |
|------|-----------|--------------|
| _____ | _____ | _____ |
| _____ | _____ | _____ |

| Name | Telephone | Relationship |
|------|-----------|--------------|
| _____ | _____ | _____ |
| _____ | _____ | _____ |

Comments

# Employment Agreement

Agreement between: _____ and _____

Date of Contract: _____ Job Title: _____

Specific Duties

_____

_____

_____

_____

_____

Hours

| Monday | Tuesday | Wednesday | Thursday | Friday | Saturday | Sunday |
|--------|---------|-----------|----------|--------|----------|--------|
|        |         |           |          |        |          |        |

Holiday Policy:

Vacation Policy:

Sick Policy:

Payment                                    Payment Schedule

$ _____          _____
(Indicate if Hourly, Daily, Weekly)

Personal Requirements

_____

_____

_____

_____

_____

Employer Signature                         Employee Signature

_____              _____

## Appendix A
# Helpful Resources for People with MS
Deborah Hertz, MPH and Nancy J. Holland, EdD, RN, MSCN

ONE OF THE FIRST STEPS in learning to cope with MS is gathering accurate, up-to-date information about the illness. Because knowledge is power, this information can help you make informed decisions, become aware of your needs, and take control of an unpredictable and complicated disease.

There are a great many resources available to help you and your family live with the diagnosis. The books and organizations described here are only part of what exists. To find out exactly what is available in your state as well as in your local community, you will need to be resourceful, to ask questions, and to be persistent. The results will be richly rewarding.

## FOR VETERANS: THE DEPARTMENT OF VETERANS AFFAIRS

Your ability to access benefits and services relating to multiple sclerosis from the Department of Veterans Affairs (VA) is based on whether the diagnosis is considered to be service-connected or not. The U.S. Congress passed legislation defining a diagnosis of multiple sclerosis as service-connected when there is documented evidence that initial signs and symptoms occurred within 7 years of discharge. Because the definition of service-connected multiple sclerosis is based on the evidence of symptoms, it is essential for veterans to have proper documentation in their medical records.

If your case of MS is determined to be service-connected, consult the booklet, *Federal Guide to Benefits for Veterans and Dependents*, which is updated annually. This is the most useful source of information about benefits and services available to veterans.

## MEDICAL SERVICES

The VA medical care system is organized into 21 regional networks, called Veterans Integrated Services Networks (VISNs). The system is based on the primary care provider model, in which primary care physicians are supported by specialists.

Many neurologists within the VA have experience treating people with multiple sclerosis. However, every veteran must question his or her primary care physician to ensure that the referral is to a neurologist with experience in MS.

Most MS clinics in the VA system are located in neurology departments. A few, however, are located in physical rehabilitation departments. You may wish to find out about the VA MS clinics in your network. If complicating health conditions arise during the course of your MS, you may wish to ask your primary care provider about MS specialty centers in other networks.

In December 2002, the VA medical system established two Centers of Excellence in research, education, and clinical treatment of multiple sclerosis. These MS Centers of Excellence (MSCoE) are resources to all the VA medical centers around the country. The two sites were selected because of their leadership in the areas of MS clinical care, research, education and training.

*MSCoE—West:*
**VA Puget Sound Health Care System**
1660 South Columbian Way
Seattle, WA 98108

**Portland VA Medical Center**
3710 SW US Veterans Hospital Road
Portland, OR 97201

*MSCoE—East:*
**VA Maryland Health Care System**
10 North Greene Street
Baltimore, MD 21201

OTHER VA RESOURCES

Social workers can play an important role in helping you to access resources. They can advise you about a variety of available services:

- Physical therapy, available with a prescription from your physician.
- Any necessary orthotic devices, including canes and walkers, from the prosthetics department.
- Exercise equipment, depending on whether the condition is considered service-connected or not and if requested by a health-care provider; examples include cycle equipment, a lifestyle standing wheelchair, a power trainer designed to fit in front of a wheelchair, and equipment for working the arms and legs for individuals who can transfer.
- Equipment such as a scooter or lift following a hospitalization, if it is part of your discharge plan.

In addition, if your MS is determined to be service-connected, you may be eligible to receive grants for several other types of services.

TRANSPORTATION

You may be eligible for cost-sharing on a handicap-equipped van.

HOME ADAPTATIONS

You may be eligible to receive a grant for as much as $48,000 toward the cost of adapting your home, buying an accessible home, or building a new one. However, that amount is not to exceed 50 percent of the cost. Other restrictions apply as well, so you need to speak with a case social worker. You may

also receive a grant for up to $9,250 toward home adaptations if the modifications are considered reasonable and necessary.

*Home improvements and structural alterations.*  A grant for as much as $4,100 may be available to build a ramp or redesign a bathroom if your situation is considered service-connected. If your condition is considered to be nonservice-connected, a grant for $1,200 may be available.

HOME CARE

You may be eligible for an aide or attendant to visit you following hospitalization, if you have a written prescription from your physician or if you need constant care in a nursing home. The *level* of home care services will depend upon your benefit level, income, health status, and number of hospitalizations.

## COMMUNITY RESOURCES: FOR VETERANS

Many nonprofit organizations provide free benefits counseling and can help you navigate through the VA system. Some also advocate for benefits and provide other services not available through VA. As a start in gathering information about the services available in your area, ask your local Veterans Affairs office for the names and addresses of local service agencies. Besides providing representation for veterans, some give nonmedical services. Finally, you may want to explore state veterans agencies, which are listed in your local telephone directory.

All of the following organizations have regional offices or chapters that can tell you about the resources available in your area.

**The American Legion**
1608 K Street, NW
Washington, DC 20006
202-861–2700

800-433–3318
www.legion.org

**AMVETS**
4647 Forbes Boulevard
Lanham, MD 20706
301-459–9600
877-7AMVETS (877-726-8387)
www.amvets.org

**Disabled American Veterans**
807 Maine Avenue, SW
Washington, DC 20024
202-554–3501
www.dav.org

**Paralyzed Veterans of America**
801 Eighteenth Street, NW
Washington, DC 20006
202-872–1300
800-424-8200
www.pva.org

**Veterans of Foreign Wars of the United States**
406 West 34th Street
Kansas City, MI 64111
816-756-3390
www.vfw.org

## COMMUNITY RESOURCES: FOR ALL PEOPLE WITH MS AND THEIR FAMILIES

### National Multiple Sclerosis Society
733 Third Avenue, Sixth Floor
New York, NY 10017
800-FIGHT-MS
800-344-4867
www.nationalmssociety.org

The National Multiple Sclerosis Society (NMSS) is the only nonprofit organization in the country that supports national and international research into the prevention, cure, and treatment of MS, as well as offer-ing programs and educational materials to people with MS and their families. Its goal is to end the devastating effects of the disease. The Society is committed to empowering people with MS to live to the maximum of their capabilities within the least restrictive environment.

NMSS provides nonmedical services to people with MS and their families through a network of approximately 138 chapters and branches across the United States. The Society also provides information about MS to people who have the disease and their families, to healthcare and other professionals, and to members of the public. Chapters and branches provide a variety of programs and services designed to help individuals with MS learn about health issues and maintain their independence. You can reach your local chapter by calling (800) FIGHT–MS.

Some of the resources available include:

- Educational publications on medical, psycho-social, and wellness issues (some available in Spanish)
- Educational programs including programs for people newly diagnosed
- Referrals to help you find physicians, rehabilitation specialists, home care agencies, long-term care facilities, psychologists, and other professionals
- Newsletter and lending library
- Self-help groups
- Crisis intervention
- Recreational opportunities
- Advocacy

### Paralyzed Veterans of America (PVA)
801 18th Street, NW
Washington, DC 20006
202-872-1300
800-424-8200 (toll-free)
888-860-7244 (publication orders)
www.pva.org

PVA, a congressionally chartered veterans service organization since 1946, has developed unique expertise on the special needs of its members—veterans with spinal cord injury or disease—that is also applicable to anyone with spinal cord dysfunction. PVA is a leading advocate for research and education, quality healthcare, veterans' benefits, sports and recreation opportunities, accessible architecture, and civil rights to maximize the independence of those with spinal cord dysfunction.

PVA represents over 21,000 members and has 120 employees at its national headquarters, 34 local chapters and 56 field service office around the country. Approximately 20 percent of PVA members have MS. PVA has published an extensive array of consumer guides and professional clinical practice guidelines on issues such as fatigue management, spasticity, disease-modifying therapies, urinary dysfunction, wheel chair use, managing personal assistants, accessible home design, and accessible travel (see "Books" section. Many are also available for download from the Web (www.pva.org) and some are available in Spanish. PVA has also promoted the development of MS Centers of Excellence within the Department of Veterans Affairs and engages with other organizations in vigorous efforts to promote MS program building.

**United Spinal Association (formerly called Eastern Paralyzed Veterans Association)**
75–20 Astoria Boulevard
Jackson Heights, NY 11370–1177
718-803–3782
800-444–0120
www.unitedspinal.org

This organization's mission is to enhance the lives of all individuals with spinal cord injuries or diseases by ensuring quality health care, promoting research, and advocating for civil rights and independence. The organization continues to remain committed to veterans but has expanded services to all people with spinal cord injuries or diseases, MS being one of them. The United Spinal Association has programs to assist members to improve accessibility of their homes. It also publishes the *MS Quarterly Report*.

SUPPORT PROGRAMS FOR PEOPLE ON DISEASE MODIFYING DRUGS
In the United States, the makers of the disease modifying drugs sponsor support programs for patients and their families. These programs offer information about the treatments, side effects, how to access medications, issues about remaining on therapy and financial assistance.

**Shared Solutions™, sponsored by Teva Neuroscience**
800-887-8100
www.copaxone.com or
www.sharedsolutions.com

**MS ActiveSource℠, sponsored by Biogen Idec**
800-456-2255
www.avonex.com or
www.msactivesource.com

**MS Pathways℠, sponsored by Berlex Laboratories**
800-788-1467
www.betaseron.com or
www.mspathways.com

**MS Lifelines™, sponsored by Serono, Inc.**
877-447-3243
www.rebif.com or www.mslifelines.com

CENTERS FOR INDEPENDENT LIVING
Every state has Centers for Independent Living. These community-based, nonresidential organizations provide programs and services to promote independent living for

people with disabilities. You can call (713) 520-0232 to obtain a copy of the *Directory of Independent Living Centers and Related Organizations.*

VOCATIONAL REHABILITATION SERVICES

The U.S. Department of Education requires that all states have a vocational and rehabilitation agency. These agencies offer a variety of counseling, evaluation and job placement services specifically for people with disabilities. In order to qualify for services you must demonstrate that your disability has affected your employment ability. Check with your state agency about eligibility and services available since there is considerable variation from state to state. While variation between states exists, all state agencies offer assessment of eligibility and need, some counseling and job placement services, training, rehabilitation technology services (including modification of vehicles) and occupational licenses and equipment. You can find your state vocational rehabilitation agency on the web at www.bcol02.ed.gov/Programs/EROD/.

## Complementary and Alternative Medicine (CAM)

www.ms-cam.org

This website is a service of the Rocky Mountain MS Center in Denver, a nonprofit corporation. They collect and share information from people with MS about their experiences with CAM. They also review and summarize published literature on CAM.

## RESOURCES FOR CAREGIVERS

It is critical that your spouse or loved one who may be attending to your needs is also taking care of his or herself. The two national organizations below offer a variety of support services and information for care-providers of people with chronic conditions.

## Well Spouse Foundation

P.O. Box 801
New York, NY 10023
212-685-8815 or 800-838-0879
www.wellspouse.org

Services include advocacy for home health and long-term care, peer support, and a newsletter.

## The National Family Caregivers Association (NFCA)

10400 Connecticut Avenue, #500
Kensington, MD 20895-3944
800-896-3650
www.nfcacares.org

NFCA promotes self-advocacy and self-care, offers education and information, and provides support services.

## GENERAL RESOURCES

## American Association of Sex Educators, Counselors, and Therapists (AASECT)

P.O. Box 238
Mount Vernon, IA 52314
319-895-8407
www.aasect.org

AASECT can provide you with a list of AASECT certified sex therapists in your area.

## American Automobile Association (AAA)

www.aaapublicaffairs.com

The AAA has an online (only) publication called "Disabled Driver's Mobility Guide." It includes information about adaptive equipment, vehicle modifications, driver training and related services, as well as contact information.

## American Cancer Society

1599 Clifton Rd.
Atlanta, GA 30329
800-ACS-2345 (800-227-2345)
www.cancer.org

The American Cancer Society (ACS) is a nationwide, community-based voluntary health organization with over 3,400 local offices. You can receive information about all types of cancer, risk factors, prevention, treatment options, decision making tools and other services such as support groups, information and referral and educational programs. ACS also offers professional education and administers research and medical grants, and clinical fellowships.

## The American Heart Association (AHA)

7272 Greenville Avenue
Dallas, TX 75231-4596
800-AHA-USA-1 (800-242-8721)
www.americanheart.org

The American Heart Association is a national voluntary health agency whose mission is to reduce disability and death from cardiovascular diseases and stroke. The association provides a wide array of educational materials and programs on heart disease and stroke for the public and for healthcare professionals.

## The American Lung Association®

61 Broadway, 6th Floor
NY, NY 10006
212-315-8700
800-LUNGUSA
www.lungusa.org

The American Lung Association® is a great resource for individuals wanting information about lung disease in all its forms, with special emphasis on asthma, tobacco control and environmental health.

## National Mobility Equipment Dealers Association (NMEDA)

800-833-0427
www.nmeda.org

NMEDA is an association of dealers who modify vehicles for people with disabilities. The website provides information about where to find these car/van dealers, funding resources, and news from the industry. Locations within the United States and Canada are included.

## Rehabilitation Engineering and Assistive Technology Society of North America (RESNA)

1700 N. Moore Street, Suite 1540
Arlington, VA 22209
703-524-6686
www.resna.org/taproject/

RESNA is an association that assists people with disabilities through advancement of rehabilitation and assistive technologies. The website offers a link to your state's assistive technology projects. Many states also have financial loan programs, and RESNA can link you to local resources at www.resna.org/AFTAP/.

## Sexuality Information and Education Council of the United States (SIECUS)

130 W. 42nd Street, Suite 350
New York, NY 10036
212-819-9770
www.siecus.org

SIECUS has a resource center and library at its New York office and publishes an annotated bibliography on sexuality and disability.

## FEDERAL RESOURCES

Many programs and services are available through the United States government. Some of the most relevant for people with MS are listed below.

## Equal Employment Opportunity Commission (EEOC)

Office of Communication and
Legislative Affairs
1801 L Street, NW
9th Floor
Washington, DC 20507

800-669–4000
800-669–3362 (publications)
202-663–4900
www.eeoc.gov

EEOC handles questions and concerns about employment discrimination.

## Federal Trade Commission (FTC)

Correspondence Branch
6th Street and Pennsylvania Avenue, NW
Room 692
Washington, DC 20580
202-326-2222
www.ftc.gov

The FTC's Bureau of Consumer Protection protects consumers against false advertising or other fraudulent practices. They investigate and offer information about false advertising.

## Library of Congress

Division for the Blind and Physically Handicapped
1291 Taylor Street, NW
Washington, DC 20542
800-424–8567
800-424–9100
202-707–5100
www.loc.gov

The Library of Congress provides a variety of services for people with visual impairments, including free books on tape, along with the loan of listening equipment; library services through 140 cooperating libraries; and a free booklet, Information for Handicapped Travelers.

## National Cancer Institute (NCI)

NCI Public Inquiries Office
6116 Executive Boulevard
Room 3036A
Bethesda, MD 20892-8322
800-4-CANCER (800-422-6237)
TTY: 800-332-8615
www.nci.nih.gov or www.cancer.gov

NCI offers information about all types of cancers, cancer prevention, diagnosis, treatment statistics, research clinical trials and news. You can receive information through NCI's website by phone or e-mail. Information specialists are available to receive calls, and there is also the opportunity to have a confidential "chat" online with NCI information specialists, Monday through Friday 9:00 AM–10:00 PM Eastern time. The 800-4-CANCER number can also provide a list of accredited mammography centers.

## National Center for Complementary and Alternative Medicine (NCCAM)

National Institutes of Health
NCCAM Clearinghouse
P.O. Box 7923
Gaithersburg, MD 20898-7923
888-644-6226 – English and Spanish
TTY: 866-464-3616 (for hearing impaired)
www.nccam.nih.gov

Information specialists are available to answer questions about the Center and complementary and alternative medicines.

## National Council on Disability

1331 F Street, NW
Suite 1050
Washington, DC 20004
202-272–2004
www.ncd.gov

The National Council on Disability studies and makes recommendations about public policy for people with disabilities. The council also publishes Focus, a free newsletter.

## National Highway Traffic Safety Administration (NHTSA)

400 7th Street SW, Room 6240
Washington, DC 20590
www.nhtsa.dot.gov

NHTSA is the federal government agency with the authority to regulate the manufacture of automotive adaptive equipment and modified vehicles used by persons with disabilities.

**National Park Service**
1849 C Street, NW
Washington, DC 20240
202-208-6843
www.nps.gov

The National Park Service provides information about accessible trails and lodging at national parks and monuments throughout the United States.

**Office of Disability Employment Policy—U.S. Department of Labor**
Frances Perkins Building
200 Constitution Avenue, NW
Washington, DC 20210
866-633-7365
www.dol.gov/odep

The Office of Disability Employment Policy sponsors a job accommodation network (JAN) and publishes information on employment issues for people with disabilities and their employers. You can reach the JAN directly by calling:

800-526–7234
800-ADA WORK/(800) 232-9675
304-293–7186

**Social Security Administration (SSA)**
6401 Security Boulevard
Baltimore, MD 21235
800-772–1213
www.ssa.gov

Contact the Social Security Administration to determine if you are entitled to receive benefits, based on your level of disability.

**U.S. Department of Justice**
Civil Rights Division
Office on the Americans with
Disabilities Rights Section

Civil Rights Division
P.O. Box 66738
Washington, DC 20035-6738
202-514–0301
www.usdoj.gov/crt

The Department of Justice, Civil Rights Division is responsible for enforcement of the Americans with Disabilities Act (ADA). Copies of the ADA can be obtained from that office.

**U.S. Food and Drug Administration (FDA)**
Office of Consumer Affairs
Consumer Inquiry Section
5600 Fishers Lane (HFED88)
Rockville, MD 20857
301-827-4420
888-INFO-FDA (888-463-6332)
www.fda.gov

The FDA assures the safety, efficacy, and security of human and veterinary drugs, biological products, medical devices, our nation's food supply, cosmetics, and products that emit radiation. The FDA is also responsible for advancing the public health by helping to speed innovations that make medicines and foods more effective, safer, and more affordable; and helping the public get the accurate, science-based information they need to use medicines and foods to improve their health.

**U.S. Postal Inspection Service**
Office of Criminal Investigation
Washington, DC 20260-2168
202-268-4293
www.usps.com/postalinspectors/

The US Postal Inspection Service protects the public against misuse of mail. It monitors products purchased by mail.

# BOOKS

A large number of publications are available to assist people with multiple sclerosis and their families. Some of these publications contain extensive resource sections.

*Adapting: Financial Planning for a Life with Multiple Sclerosis.* A joint publication of the National Endowment for Financial Education, National Multiple Sclerosis Society, and Paralyzed Veterans of America. 2003.

This guide will assist persons with MS to manage their money wisely and meet the financial challenges that they may encounter. It includes a comprehensive list of resources available to MS patients, as well as information on employment rights, accessibility issues, financial worksheets, and helpful tips for handling the financial burdens associated with the disease.

Axelson, P. et al. *The Manual Wheelchair Training Guide.* Minden, NV. Pax Press. 1998.

This manual can teach wheelchair users and their helpers to access the world with a full range of manual wheelchair skills. Clear instructions accompanied by detailed illustrations of each skill show the readers how to negotiate terrain as mundane as indoor floors and as challenging as escalators.

Axelson, P. et al. *The Powered Wheelchair Training Guide.* Minden, NV. Pax Press. 2002.

This book will help powered wheelchair users and their training assistants develop the skills to negotiate commonly encountered environments such as ramps, tight spaces, and curb ramps. Also includes tips on how to use public transportation, traveling in inclement weather, and how to handle emergencies.

Bowling, AC. *Alternative Medicine and Multiple Sclerosis.* New York: Demos Medical Publishing, 2001.

This book offers an unbiased review of the complementary and alternative therapy approaches considered by people with MS. It discusses the use and evidence available to support (or not) treatments like acupuncture, herbal medicine, vitamins, and others.

Cassileth, B. *Alternative Medicine Handbook.* New York. WW Norton, 2000.

This book discusses 53 different complementary and alternative therapies. It does not make recommendations, however, it describes what is known about each, including risks and benefits, notes any research done to support evidence and provides information to help make consumers informed decision makers. This book is not specific to multiple sclerosis.

Coyle, P.K., Halper J. *Meeting the Challenges of Progressive Multiple Sclerosis.* New York: Demos Medical Publishing. 2001.

Designed for people with progressive MS, this book addresses important topics related to worsening disease and disability.

Ernst, E., et al. *Complementary and Alternative Medicine: A Desktop Reference.* London, UK: Mosby, 2001.

This book is used as a reference for health care professionals and includes evidence-based information about complementary and alternative therapies. It provides objective information.

Holland, N., Murray T.J., and Reingold S. *Multiple Sclerosis: A Guide for the Newly Diagnosed,* 2nd edition. New York: Demos Medical Publishing, 2000.

(En español: *Esclerosis Múltiple: Guía Practica Para El Recién Diagnosticado,* 2002.)

This book for people with MS, as well as their families and friends, is an excellent guide to learning about the illness. The authors cover disease management, treatment options, and current research. A list of recommended reading is included.

Kalb, R. *Multiple Sclerosis: A Guide for Families*. New York: Demos Medical Publishing.

In this comprehensive guide, professionals in the fields of neurology, psychology, obstetrics/gynecology, social work, health economics, and law provide information designed to help families understand and cope effectively with the challenges posed by this chronic, unpredictable illness.

Kalb, R. *Multiple Sclerosis: Questions You Have, Answers You Need*, 3rd edition. New York: Demos Medical Publishing, 2004.

Written in a question-and-answer format, this descriptive and very thorough guide covers a wide range of topics, including commonly used medications. Sections covering MS literature and resources are excellent.

Kraft, GH, Catanzaro M. *Living with Multiple Sclerosis*, 2nd edition. New York: Demos Medical Publishing, 2000.

This book presents an adapted version of the questions-and-answer portion of a National Multiple Sclerosis Society national teleconference titled Taking Care: Options to Maximize Your Health. The book includes information on exercise and nutrition.

Northrop, D.E., Cooper S. *Health Insurance Resource Manual: Options for People with a Chronic Disease or Disability*. New York: Demos Medical Publishing, 2003

This is a comprehensive resource for individuals who are uninsured or underinsured and who need a place to begin seeking assistance. You'll find information about a wide variety of options to assist people who want to better understand the healthcare system.

Schapiro, R.T. *Managing the Symptoms of Multiple Sclerosis*, 4th edition. New York: Demos Medical Publishing, 2003.

This informative book explores the symptoms of MS and provides effective management strategies. including personal management strategies.

Spero, D. *The Art of Getting Well: A Five-Step Plan for Maximizing Health When You Have a Chronic Illness*. Alameda, CA: Hunter House Publishers. 2002.

David Spero, R.N., is a nurse, journalist and health educator who was diagnosed with MS 12 years before he wrote this book. The book explains how people can recover their health and improve their lives despite chronic problems for which medicine has no cure. In his five-step plan, he describes how to slow down, make changes, get help, value your body and take responsibility, and thus to master "the art of embracing wellness."

PVA PUBLICATIONS ON MS AND RELATED TOPICS

The following books are available from the Paralyzed Veterans of America (PVA) Distribution Center. Call (toll-free) 1-888-860-7244 to place your order or to request a complete catalog of PVA publications, or check out the PVA website at www.pva.org (click on "PVA Store") to download copies.

*Accessible Transit and the Law*. Washington, DC: Paralyzed Veterans of America. Free; available by download *only* from the PVA website www.pva.org (click on "PVA Store").

This booklet outlines the types of transportation facilities covered by the Americans with Disabilities Act (in essence, any system that serves the public except air travel, which is covered by the Air Carrier Access Act), what they must do to become accessible under the law, and the dates by which they must have achieved accessibility.

*The ADA: Tax Incentives: Assisting Accessibility.* Washington, DC: Paralyzed Veterans of America. Free (plus cost of shipping and handling).

The Americans with Disabilities Act provides tax credits and deductions for businesses that incur expenses in making accommodations to be become accessible. This brochure describes what business expenses are covered and how to claim these special tax incentives. Free; available by download *only* from the PVA website www.pva.org (click on "PVA Store").

*The Air Carrier Access Act: Common Questions and Answers about Air Travel for Wheelchair Users.* Washington, DC: Paralyzed Veterans of America. Free; available by download *only* from the PVA website www.pva.org (click on "PVA Store").

This pamphlet responds to the most frequently asked questions concerning the implications of the Air Carrier Access Act.

*The Air Carrier Access Act: Make It Work for You.* Washington, DC: Paralyzed Veterans of America. 2002.

In 1990, the U.S. Department of Transportation issued regulations to enforce the Air Carrier Access Act, which guarantees that people with disabilities receive consistent and nondiscriminatory treatment when traveling by air. This brochure explains some of those regulations and provides information about what to do in case you are discriminated against by an air carrier. Free (plus cost of shipping and handling).

*The Americans with Disabilities Act: Your Personal Guide to the Law.* Washington, DC:

Paralyzed Veterans of America. Available in English or Spanish. 2002.

An overview of the provisions of the Americans with Disabilities Act. This guide provides information on the provisions covering employment regulations, state and local governments, public accommodations, transportation, telecommunications, and tax incentives. Free (plus cost of shipping and handling).

Axelson, P. et al. *A Guide to Wheelchair Selection: How to Use the ANSI/RESNA Wheelchair Standards to Buy a Wheelchair.* Washington, DC: Paralyzed Veterans of America.

This book provides useful information on wheelchair standards and test procedures in a consumer-friendly format. By explaining how to use the information disclosed by test procedures, the book can help wheelchair users be more informed when selecting a wheelchair.

Davies, Jr., TD, and K. Beasley. *Accessible Home Design: Architectural Solutions for the Wheelchair User.* Washington, DC: Paralyzed Veterans of America. 1999.

This book explains and illustrates practical and economical architectural designs that will help make new and renovated single-family homes accessible. Chapters focus on such critical areas as kitchens, bathrooms, and multiple levels.

*Disease Modifying Therapies in Multiple Sclerosis: Evidence-Based Management Strategies for Disease Modifying Therapies in Multiple Sclerosis.* Washington, DC: Multiple Sclerosis Council for Clinical Practice Guidelines, with administrative and financial support from PVA. Free (plus cost of shipping and handling). 2001.

Over the last decade there has been a considerable increase in the number of agents available for treatment of MS, particularly those designed to prevent or postpone future neurological injury. This guideline considers the available evidence for the clinical use of these disease-modifying agents, including anti-inflammatory, immunomodulatory, and immunosuppressive treatments.

*Fair Housing: How to Make the Law Work for You (3rd edition)*. Washington, DC: Paralyzed Veterans of America. 1998.

The Fair Housing Amendments Act of 1988, which became effective in 1989, protects people with disabilities from discrimination in the purchase or rental of housing. PVA has created this publication to explain the rights of individuals with disabilities when they seek housing and the remedies they can pursue of they encounter discrimination because of their disability.

*Fatigue and Multiple Sclerosis: Evidence-Based Management Strategies for Fatigue in Multiple Sclerosis*. Washington, DC: Multiple Sclerosis Council for Clinical Practice Guidelines, with administrative and financial support from PVA. Free (plus cost of shipping and handling). 1998.

Fatigue is now recognized as the most common symptom of MS. This clinical practice guideline provides an algorithm intended to guide clinicians in the evaluation and treatment of MS-related fatigue.

*Fatigue: What You Should Know*. Washington, DC: Multiple Sclerosis Council for Clinical Practice Guidelines, with administrative and financial support from PVA. Free; available by download *only* from the PVA website www.pva.org (click on "PVA Store"). 2000.

This guide for people with MS, their caregivers, and their families is the companion consumer guide to the Council's professional clinical practice guideline on fatigue and MS.

*A Guide to Managed Care, for People with Spinal Cord Injury or Disease (2nd edition)*. Washington, DC: Paralyzed Veterans of America. 1997.

What is managed care? How does managed care affect people with spinal cord dysfunction? What are unique needs of people with spinal cord dysfunction in managed care? This brochure will answer these questions and help you better understand how you can choose a plan that will meet your particular health-care needs.

*The Keys to Managed Care: A Guide for People with Physical Disabilities*. Washington, DC: Washington, DC: National Rehabilitation Hospital Center for Health and Disability Research, Paralyzed Veterans of America, and Eastern Paralyzed Veterans Association (now the United Spinal Association). 2000.

This guide has been developed to help people with physical disabilities who are already in managed care plans learn how they can get the best health care possible. The information in this guide was collected by talking to people with disabilities. In speaking with these individuals, it became clear that they were all using a small set of specific strategies to get the services they needed from their managed care plans. These strategies are described in this guide as the keys to getting better health care.

*Kitchen Design for the Wheelchair User*. Paralyzed Veterans of America. Free; available by download *only* from the PVA website www.pva.org (click on "PVA Store").

For most wheelchair users, no room presents more complex design challenges than the kitchen. This pamphlet tells how this important room can be tailored to meet the needs of its users. Free; available by download *only* from the PVA website www.pva.org (click on "PVA Store").

*Managing Personal Assistants: A Consumer Guide.* Washington, DC: Paralyzed Veterans of America. 2000.

This consumer guide features information on recruiting, hiring, training, keeping, and firing personal assistants, as well as on funding sources and taxes. It contains forms that guide the consumer through the process of managing personal assistants.

*Preventing Discrimination in the Workplace.* Washington, DC: Paralyzed Veterans of America. Free; available by download *only* from the PVA website www.pva.org (click on "PVA Store").

The Americans with Disabilities Act contains requirements and guidelines for employers to follow in removing barriers to employment for people with disabilities. The goal is to ensure that people with disabilities do not encounter discrimination in the employment process or environment. This brochure provides information useful for both employers and employees concerning measures to ensure accessible, discrimination-free workplaces. Free; available by download *only* from the PVA website www.pva.org (click on "PVA Store").

*Questions and Answers About the Americans With Disabilities Act.* Paralyzed Veterans of America. Free; available by download *only* from the PVA website www.pva.org (click on "PVA Store").

This pamphlet responds to the most frequently asked questions concerning the implications of the Americans with Disabilities Act. Free (plus cost of shipping and handling).

*Spasticity Management in Multiple Sclerosis: Evidence-Based Management Strategies for Spasticity Treatment in Multiple Sclerosis.* Washington, DC: Multiple Sclerosis Council for Clinical Practice Guidelines, with administrative and financial support from PVA and the Consortium of Multiple Sclerosis Centers. Free (plus cost of shipping and handling). 2003.

When properly treated, the immediate symptoms of spasticity as well as secondary complications can be avoided. This guideline synthesizes the currently available literature and identifies many key questions that remain to be investigated.

*Urinary Dysfunction and Multiple Sclerosis.* Washington, DC: Multiple Sclerosis Council for Clinical Practice Guidelines, with administrative and financial support from PVA. Free (plus cost of shipping and handling). 1999.

This guideline offers a sequential pathway for management of bladder dysfunction in an office or clinic setting.

*Wheelchairs: Your Options and Rights, A Guide to Department of Veterans Affairs Eligibility.* Washington, DC: Paralyzed Veterans of America. Available in English or Spanish. 1997.

This booklet describes the eligibility criteria for veterans who need to obtain wheelchairs from the U.S. Department of Veterans Affairs. It also discusses the prescription and issuance process, as well as the types of wheelchairs that can be provided. Free (plus cost of shipping and handling).

# Appendix B
# Medications Commonly Used in Multiple Sclerosis

THE INFORMATION CONTAINED in these pages will help you to be more informed about the medications you are taking and therefore more able to discuss your questions and concerns with your physician. This information should never be used as a substitute for your own physician's instructions and recommendations.

The following guidelines apply to the use of any and all the medications that you take:

- Make sure that your physician knows your medical history, including all medical conditions for which you are currently being treated and any allergies you have.
- Tell your physician if you are breastfeeding, currently pregnant, or planning to become pregnant in the near future.
- Make a list of all the drugs you are currently taking—including both prescription and over-the-counter medications—and provide your physician with a copy for your medical chart.
- Take your medications only as your physician prescribes them for you. If you have questions about the recommended dosage, ask your physician.

- Unless otherwise instructed, store medications in a cool, dry place; exposure to heat or moisture may cause the medication to break down. Liquid medications that are stored in the refrigerator should not be allowed to freeze.
- Unless otherwise directed by your physician or pharmacist, the general instructions concerning a missed dose of medication are as follows: If you miss a dose, take it as soon as possible. However, if it is almost time for your next dose, skip the one you missed and go back to the regular dosing schedule. Do not double dose.
- Keep all medications out of the reach of children.

The following table lists all of the products described in this appendix. For each product, the table gives the generic or chemical name, the brand name, and the common usage in MS, as well as its availability in the United States and Canada. Products available without a prescription are so indicated.

| GENERIC NAME | BRAND NAME | USAGE IN MS |
|---|---|---|
| Alprostadil | Prostin VR | Erectile dysfunction |
| Alprostadil | MUSE | Erectile dysfunction |
| Amantadine | Symmetral | Fatigue |
| Amitriptyline | Elavil | Pain (dysesthesias) |
| Baclofen | | Spasticity |
| Baclofen (intrathecal) | Baclofen Intrathecal | Spasticity |
| Bisacodyl | Dulcolax (U.S.) Bisacolax (Canada) | Constipation |
| Carbamazepine | Tegretol | Pain (trigeminal neuralgia) |
| Ciprofloxacin | Cipro | Urinary tract infections |
| Clonazepam | Klonopin (U.S.) Rivotril (Canada) Syn-Clonazepam (Canada) | Tremor; pain; spasticity |
| Desmopressin | DDAVP | Bladder dysfunction |
| Desmopressin | DDAVP Nasal Spray | Bladder dysfunction |
| Dexamethasone | Decadron | Acute exacerbations |
| Diazepam | Valium | Spasticity (muscle spasms) |
| Docusate[1] | Colace | Constipation |
| Docusate[1] | Enemeez Mini Enema | Constipation |
| Duloxetine hydrochloride | Cymbalta (U.S./Canada) | Depression; pain |
| Fluoxetine | Prozac | Depression; fatigue |
| Gabapentin | Neurontin | Pain (dysesthesias; spasticity) |
| Glatiramer acetate | Copaxone | Disease modifying agent |
| Glycerin[1] | Sani-Supp suppository (U.S.) | Constipation |
| Imipramine | Tofranil | Bladder dysfunction; pain |
| Interferon beta-1a | Avonex | Disease modifying agent |
| Interferon beta-1a | Rebif | Disease modifying agent |
| Interferon beta-1b | Betaseron | Disease modifying agent |
| Magnesium hydroxide | Phillips' Milk of Magnesia | Constipation |
| Meclizine | Antivert (U.S.) Bonamine (Canada) | Nausea; vomiting; dizziness |
| Methenamine | Hiprex, Mandelamine (U.S.) Hip-rex, Mandelamine (Canada) | Urinary tract infections (preventative) |
| Methylprednisolone | Solu-Medrol | Acute exacerbations |

| GENERIC NAME | BRAND NAME | USAGE IN MS |
|---|---|---|
| Mineral oil | | Constipation |
| Mitoxantrone | Novantrone | Disease modifying agent |
| Modafinil | Provigil | Fatigue |
| Nitrofurantoin | Macrodantin | Urinary tract infection |
| Nortriptyline | Pamelor (U.S.) Aventyl (Canada) | Depression |
| Oxybutynin | Ditropan | Bladder dysfunction |
| Oxybutynin (extended release formula) | Ditropan XL | Bladder dysfunction |
| Oxybutynin (transdermal patch) | Oxytrol | Bladder dysfunction |
| Papaverine | | Erectile dysfunction |
| Paroxetine | Paxil | Depression; anxiety |
| Pemoline | Cylert | Fatigue |
| Phenazopyridine | Pyridium | Urinary tract infections (symptom relief) |
| Phenytoin | Dilantin | Pain (parasthesias) |
| Prednisone | Deltasone | Acute exacerbations |
| Propantheline bromide | Pro-Banthine | Bladder dysfunction |
| Psyllium hydrophilic mucilloid | Metamucil | Constipation |
| Sertraline | Zoloft | Depression; anxiety |
| Sildenafil | Viagra | Erectile dysfunction |
| Sodium phosphate | Fleet Enema | Constipation |
| Solifenacin succinate | Vesicare (U.S.) | Bladder dysfunction |
| Sulfamethoxazole | Bactrim; Septra | Urinary tract infections |
| Tadalafil | Cialis (U.S.) | Erectile dysfunction |
| Tizanidine hydrochloride | Zanaflex | Spasticity |
| Tolterodine | Detrol (U.S.) | Bladder dysfunction |
| Topiramate | Topamax | Pain; tremor |
| Trospium chloride | Sanctura (U.S.) | Bladder dysfunction |
| Vardenafil | Levitra (U.S.) | Erectile dysfunction |
| Venlafaxine | Effexor | Depression |

**Chemical Name:** Alprostadil (al-*pross*-ta-dill); also called Prostaglandin E1

*Brand Name:* Prostin VR (U.S. and Canada)

*Generic Available:* No

*Description:* Alprostadil belongs to a group of medicines called vasodilators, which cause blood vessels to expand, thereby increasing blood flow. When alprostadil is injected into the penis, it produces an erection by increasing blood flow to the penis.

PROPER USAGE

- Alprostadil should never be used as a sexual aid by men who are not impotent. If improperly used, this medication can cause permanent damage to the penis.
- Alprostadil is available by prescription and should be used only as directed by your physician, who will instruct you in the proper way to give yourself an injection so that it is simple and essentially pain-free.
- Alprostadil is sometimes used in combination with a medicine called phentolamine (Regitine®—U.S.; Rogitine®—Canada).

PRECAUTIONS

- Do not use more of this medicine or use it more often than it has been prescribed for you. Using too much of this medicine will result in a condition called priapism, in which the erection lasts too long and does not resolve when it should. Permanent damage to the penis can occur if blood flow to the penis is cut off for too long a period of time.

POSSIBLE SIDE EFFECTS

- Side effects that you should report to your physician so he or she can adjust the dosage or change the medication: pain at the injection site; burning or aching during erection.
- Rare side effects that require immediate attention: erection continuing for more than 4 hours. If you cannot be seen immediately by your physician, you should go to the emergency room for prompt treatment.

**Chemical Name:** Alprostadil (al-*pross*-ta-dill); also called Prostaglandin E1

*Brand Name:* MUSE (U.S. and Canada) [suppository form]

*Generic Available:* No

*Description:* Alprostadil belongs to a group of medicines called vasodilators, which cause blood vessels to expand, thereby increasing blood flow. MUSE is a semisolid pellet of medication in the form of a suppository. When the suppository is inserted into the urethra, it produces an erection by increasing blood flow to the penis.

PROPER USAGE

- Alprostadil should never be used as a sexual aid by men who are not impotent. If improperly used, this medication can cause permanent damage to the penis.
- Alprostadil is available by prescription and should be used only as directed by your physician, who will instruct you in the proper way to insert the suppository.

PRECAUTIONS

- Do not use more of this medicine or use it more often than it has been prescribed for you. Using too much of this medicine will result in a condition called priapism, in which the erection lasts too long and does not resolve when it should. Permanent damage to the penis can occur if blood flow to the penis is cut off for too long a period of time.

POSSIBLE SIDE EFFECTS

- Side effects that you should report to your physician so he or she can adjust the dosage or change the medication: burning or aching during erection.

- Rare side effects that require immediate attention: erection continuing for more than 4 hours. If you cannot be seen immediately by your physician, you should go to the emergency room for prompt treatment.

**Chemical Name:** Amantadine (a-*man*-ta-deen)

*Brand Name:* Symmetrel (U.S. and Canada)

*Generic Available:* Yes (U.S.)

*Description:* Amantadine is an antiviral medication used to prevent or treat certain influenza infections; it is also given as an adjunct for the treatment of Parkinson's disease. It has been demonstrated that this medication, through some unknown mechanism, is sometimes effective in relieving fatigue in multiple sclerosis.

PROPER USAGE

- The usual dosage for the management of fatigue in MS is 100 to 200 mg daily, taken in the earlier part of the day in order to avoid sleep disturbance. Doses in excess of 300 mg daily usually cause livedo reticularis, a blotchy discoloration of the skin of the legs.

PRECAUTIONS

- The precautions listed here pertain to the use of this medication as an antiviral or Parkinson's disease treatment. There are no reports at this time concerning the precautions in the use of the drug to treat fatigue in MS.
- Drinking alcoholic beverages while taking this medication may cause increased side effects such as circulation problems, dizziness, lightheadedness, fainting, or confusion. Do not drink alcohol while taking this medication.
- This medication may cause some people to become dizzy, confused, or lightheaded, or to have blurred vision or trouble concentrating.

- Amantadine may cause dryness of the mouth and throat. If your mouth continues to feel dry for more than 2 weeks, check with your physician or dentist since continuing dryness may increase the risk of dental disease.
- This medication may cause purplish red, net-like, blotchy spots on the skin. This problem occurs more often in females and usually occurs on the legs and/or feet after amantadine has been taken regularly for a month or more. The blotchy spots usually go away within 2 to 12 weeks after you stop taking the medication.
- Studies of the effects of amantadine in pregnancy have not been done in humans. Studies in some animals have shown that amantadine is harmful to the fetus and causes birth defects.
- Amantadine passes into breast milk. However, the effect of amantadine in newborn babies and infants is not known.

POSSIBLE SIDE EFFECTS

- The side effects listed here pertain to the use of amantadine as an antiviral or Parkinson's disease treatment. There are no reports at the present time of the side effects associated with the use of this drug in the treatment of MS-related fatigue.
- Side effects that may go away as your body adjusts to the medication and do not require medical attention unless they continue or are bothersome: difficulty concentrating; dizziness; headache; irritability; loss of appetite; nausea; nervousness; purplish red, net-like, blotchy spots on skin; trouble sleeping or nightmares; constipation*; dryness of the mouth; vomiting.
- Rare side effects are side effects that should be reported as soon as possible to your physician: blurred vision*; confu-

sion; difficult urination*; fainting; hallucinations; convulsions; unusual difficulty in coordination*; irritation and swelling of the eye; mental depression; skin rash; swelling of feet or lower legs; unexplained shortness of breath.

*Since it may be difficult to distinguish between certain common symptoms of MS and some side effects of amantadine, be sure to consult your healthcare professional if an abrupt change of this type occurs.

**Chemical Name:** Amitriptyline (a-mee-*trip*-ti-leen)

*Brand Name:* Elavil (U.S. and Canada)

*Generic Available:* Yes (U.S. and Canada)

*Description:* Amitriptyline is a tricyclic antidepressant used to treat mental depression. In multiple sclerosis, it is frequently used to treat painful paresthesias in the arms and legs (e.g., burning sensations, pins and needles, stabbing pains) caused by damage to the pain regulating pathways of the brain and spinal cord.

*Note:* Other tricyclic antidepressants are also used for the management of neurologic pain symptoms. Clomipramine (Anafranil®—U.S. and Canada), desipramine (Norpramin®—U.S. and Canada), doxepin (Sinequan®—U.S. and Canada), imipramine (Tofranil®—U.S. and Canada), nortriptyline (Pamelor®—U.S.; Aventyl®—Canada), trimipramine (U.S. and Canada). While each of these medications is given in different dosage levels, the precautions and side effects listed for amitriptyline apply to these other tricyclic medications as well.

PRECAUTIONS

- Amitriptyline adds to the effects of alcohol and other central nervous system depressants (e.g., antihistamines, sedatives, tranquilizers, prescription pain medications, seizure medications, muscle relaxants, sleeping medications), possibly causing drowsiness. Be sure that your physician knows if you are taking these or other medications.
- This medication causes dryness of the mouth. Because continuing dryness of the mouth may increase the risk of dental disease, alert your dentist that you are taking amitriptyline.
- This medication may cause your skin to be more sensitive to sunlight than it is normally. Even brief exposure to sunlight may cause a skin rash, itching, redness or other discoloration of the skin, or severe sunburn.
- This medication may affect blood sugar levels of diabetic individuals. If you notice a change in the results of your blood or urine sugar tests, check with your physician.
- Do not stop taking this medication without consulting your physician. The physician may want you to reduce the amount you are taking gradually in order to reduce the possibility of withdrawal symptoms such as headache, nausea, and/or an overall feeling of discomfort.
- Studies of amitriptyline have not been done in pregnant women. There have been reports of newborns suffering from muscle spasms and heart, breathing, and urinary problems when their mothers had taken tricyclic antidepressants immediately before delivery. Studies in animals have indicated the possibility of unwanted effects in the fetus.
- Tricyclics pass into breast milk. Only doxepin (Sinequan®) has been reported to cause drowsiness in the nursing baby.

POSSIBLE SIDE EFFECTS

- Side effects that may go away as your body adjusts to the medication and do not require medical attention unless they continue for more than 2 weeks or are bothersome: dryness of mouth; constipation*; increased appetite and weight gain; dizziness; drowsiness*; decreased sexual ability*; headache; nausea; unusual tiredness or weakness*; unpleasant taste; diarrhea; heartburn; increased sweating; vomiting.

- Uncommon side effects that should be reported to your physician as soon as possible: blurred vision*; confusion or delirium; difficulty speaking or swallowing*; eye pain*; fainting; hallucinations; loss of balance control*; nervousness or restlessness; problems urinating*; shakiness or trembling; stiffness of arms and legs*.

- Rare side effects that should be reported to your physician as soon as possible: anxiety; breast enlargement in males and females; hair loss; inappropriate secretion of milk in females; increased sensitivity to sunlight; irritability; muscle twitching; red or brownish spots on the skin; buzzing or other unexplained sounds in the ears; skin rash, itching; sore throat and fever; swelling of face and tongue; weakness*; yellow skin.

- Symptoms of acute overdose: confusion; convulsions; severe drowsiness*; enlarged pupils; unusual heartbeat; fever; hallucinations; restlessness and agitation; shortness of breath; unusual tiredness or weakness; vomiting.

*Since it may be difficult to distinguish between certain common symptoms of MS and some side effects of amitriptyline, be sure to consult your healthcare professional if an abrupt change of this type occurs.

Chemical Name: Baclofen (*bak*-loe-fen)

*Brand Name:* None

*Generic Available:* Yes

*Description:* Baclofen acts on the central nervous system (CNS) to relieve spasms, cramping, and tightness of muscles caused by spasticity in multiple sclerosis.

PROPER USAGE

- People with MS are usually started on an initial dose of 5 mg every 6 to 8 hours. If necessary, the amount is increased by 5 mg per dose every 5 days until symptoms improve. The goal of treatment is to find a dosage level that relieves spasticity without causing excessive weakness or fatigue. The effective dose may vary from 15 mg to 160 mg per day or more.

PRECAUTIONS

- If you are taking more than 30 mg daily, do not stop taking this medication suddenly. Stopping high doses of this medication abruptly can cause convulsions, hallucinations, increases in muscle spasms or cramping, mental changes, or unusual nervousness or restlessness. Consult your physician about how to reduce the dosage gradually before stopping the medication completely.

- This drug adds to the effects of alcohol and other CNS depressants (such as antihistamines, sedatives, tranquilizers, prescription pain medications, seizure medications, other muscle relaxants), possibly causing drowsiness. Be sure that your physician knows if you are taking these or other medications.

- Studies of birth defects with baclofen have not been done with humans. Studies in animals have shown that baclofen, when given in doses several times higher than the amount given to humans, increases the chance of hernias, incomplete or slow development of bones in the fetus, and lower birth weight.

- Baclofen passes into the breast milk of nursing mothers but has not been reported to cause problems in nursing infants.

## POSSIBLE SIDE EFFECTS

- Side effects that typically go away as your body adjusts to the medication and do not require medical attention unless they continue for several weeks or are bothersome: drowsiness or unusual tiredness*; increased weakness*; dizziness or lightheadedness; confusion; unusual constipation*; new or unusual bladder symptoms*; trouble sleeping; unusual unsteadiness or clumsiness*.

- Unusual side effects that require immediate medical attention: fainting; hallucinations; severe mood changes; skin rash or itching.

- Symptoms of overdose: sudden onset of blurred or double vision*; convulsions; shortness of breath or troubled breathing; vomiting.

*Since it may be difficult to distinguish between certain common symptoms of MS and some side effects of baclofen, be sure to consult your healthcare professional if an abrupt change of this type occurs.

**Chemical Name:** Baclofen (intrathecal)

*Brand Name:* Intrathecal Baclofen (ITB Therapy)

*Generic Available:* No

*Description:* Baclofen acts on the central nervous system to relieve spasms, cramping, and tightness of muscles caused by spasticity in multiple sclerosis. Intrathecal baclofen therapy (ITB) consists of long-term delivery of baclofen to the intrathecal space in the spinal column. It is used in MS for those individuals with severe spasticity whose symptoms are not sufficiently relieved with oral baclofen and other oral medications. Because ITB is administered directly into the intrathecal space, it provides better spasticity reduction at lower doses than can be achieved with oral medications that, at higher doses, can produce sedation, sleepiness, and imbalance.

## PROPER USAGE

- Individuals who are considered candidates for intrathecal baclofen are given a test dose via lumbar puncture. Those who respond positively to the test dose can be considered for ongoing ITB therapy.

- The SynchroMed® Infusion System consists of: a small titanium disk, about 3 inches in diameter and 1 inch thick, which contains a refillable reservoir for the liquid, and a computer chip that regulates the battery-operated pump; a flexible silicone catheter that serves as the pathway from the pump to the intrathecal space.

- Implantation of the pump requires two incisions—one in the lower abdomen to create a pocket for the pump, and another one in the lower back for inserting the catheter that is looped around the torso, inside the body, connecting the pump to the intrathecal space.

- The dose of medication delivered by the pump is programmed, and subsequently adjusted if necessary, by noninvasive radiotelemetry. The pump is refilled every 4 to 12 weeks by injection, in a procedure lasting about 20 minutes.

- To prevent the baclofen supply from running out, the pump contains a programmable alarm that sounds whenever the reservoir need to be refilled, the battery is low, or the pump is malfunctioning in some way. In the event that the alarm sounds, you should contact your physician immediately.

## PRECAUTIONS

- As with any surgical procedure, the implantation of the pump carries with it the risk of infection, and the risks associated with general anesthesia. There is an additional risk of spinal fluid leakage.

- Your doctor should check your progress at regular visits, especially during the first few weeks of treatment with this medicine. During this time, the amount of medicine you are using may have to be changed often to meet your individual needs.

- Make sure to keep all appointments to refill the pump. If the pump is not refilled on time, you may experience return of your muscle tightness and early withdrawal symptoms that might include: itching of the skin; decreased blood pressure (blurred vision*, confusion, dizziness, faintness or lightheadedness when rising from a lying or sitting position, sweating, unusual tiredness or weakness*); burning; crawling; itching; numbness; prickling; "pins and needles;" or tingling feelings*; seizures.
- Abruptly stopping intrathecal baclofen can result in serious medical problems and in rare cases has been fatal.

POSSIBLE SIDE EFFECTS

- Side effects that typically go away as your body adjusts to the medication and do not require medical attention unless they continue for several weeks or are bothersome: drowsiness or unusual tiredness*; increased weakness*; dizziness or lightheadedness; confusion; unusual constipation*; new or unusual bladder symptoms*; trouble sleeping; unusual unsteadiness or clumsiness*.
- Unusual side effects that require immediate medical attention: high fever; altered mental status; spasticity that is worse than was experienced prior to starting ITB therapy; muscle rigidity.
- Symptoms of overdose: drowsiness; lightheadedness; sudden onset of blurred or double vision*; shortness of breath or troubled breathing; vomiting; seizures; loss of consciousness; coma.

*Since it may be difficult to distinguish between certain common symptoms of MS

and some side effects of intrathecal baclofen, be sure to consult your healthcare professional if an abrupt change of this type occurs.

**Chemical Name:** Bisacodyl (bis-a-*koe*-dill)

*Brand Name:* Dulcolax—tablet or suppository (U.S.); Bisacolax—tablet or suppository (Canada)

*Generic Available:* Yes (U.S. and Canada)

*Description:* Bisacodyl is an over-the-counter stimulant laxative that can be used in either oral or suppository form. Stimulant laxatives encourage bowel movements by increasing the muscle contractions in the intestinal wall that propel the stool mass. Although stimulant laxatives are popular for self-treatment, they are more likely to cause side effects than other types of laxatives.

PROPER USAGE

- Laxatives are to be used to provide short-term relief only, unless otherwise directed by the nurse or physician who is helping you to manage your bowel symptoms. A regimen that includes a healthy diet containing roughage (whole grain breads and cereals, bran, fruit, and green, leafy vegetables), six to eight full glasses of liquids each day, and some form of daily exercise is most important in stimulating healthy bowel function.
- If your physician has recommended this laxative for management of constipation, follow his or her recommendations for its use. If you are treating yourself for constipation, follow the directions on the package insert.
- The tablet form of this laxative is usually taken on an empty stomach to speed results. The tablets are coated to allow them to work properly without causing stomach irritation or upset. Do not chew or crush the tablets or take them within an hour of drinking milk or taking an antacid.

- A bedtime dose usually produces results the following morning. Be sure to consult your physician if you experience problems or do not get relief within a week.

PRECAUTIONS

- Do not take any laxative if you have signs of appendicitis or inflamed bowel (e.g., stomach or lower abdominal pain, cramping, bloating, soreness, nausea, or vomiting). Check with your physician as soon as possible.
- Do not take any laxative for more than 1 week unless you have been told to do so by your physician. Many people tend to overuse laxatives, which often leads to dependence on the laxative action to produce a bowel movement. Discuss the use of laxatives with your healthcare professional to ensure that the laxative is used effectively as part of a comprehensive, healthy bowel management regimen.
- Do not take any laxative within 2 hours of taking other medication because the desired effectiveness of the other medication may be reduced.
- If you are pregnant, discuss with your physician the most appropriate type of laxative for you to use.
- Some laxatives pass into breast milk. Although it is unlikely to cause problems for a nursing infant, be sure to let your physician know if you are using a laxative and breast-feeding at the same time.

POSSIBLE SIDE EFFECTS

- Side effects that may go away as your body adjusts to the medication and do not require medical attention unless they persist or are bothersome: belching; cramping; diarrhea; nausea.
- Unusual side effects that should be reported to your physician as soon as possible: confusion; irregular heartbeat; muscle cramps; skin rash; unusual tiredness or weakness.

**Chemical Name:** Carbamazepine (kar-ba-*maz*-e-peen)

*Brand Name:* Tegretol (U.S. and Canada)

*Generic Available:* Yes (U.S.)

*Description:* Carbamazepine is used to relieve shock-like pain, such as the facial pain caused by trigeminal neuralgia (tic douloureux).

PROPER USAGE

- It is very important that you take this medicine exactly as directed by your physician in order to obtain the best results and lessen the chance of serious side effects.
- Carbamazepine is not an ordinary pain reliever. It should be used only when your physician prescribes it for certain types of pain. Do not take this medication for other aches or pains.
- If you miss a dose of this medication, take it as soon as possible. If it is almost time for your next dose, skip the missed dose and go back to your regular dosing schedule. Do not double dose. If you miss more than one dose in a day, check with your physician.
- It is very important that your physician check your progress at regular intervals. Your physician may want to have certain tests done to see if you are receiving the correct amount of medication or to check for certain side effects of which you might be unaware.

PRECAUTIONS

- Carbamazepine adds to the effects of alcohol and other central nervous system depressants that may cause drowsiness (e.g., antihistamines, sedatives, tranquilizers, prescription pain medications, seizure medications, muscle relaxants). Be sure that your physician knows if you are taking these or other medications.
- Some people who take carbamazepine may become more sensitive to sunlight

than they are normally. Exposure to sunlight, even for brief periods of time, may cause a skin rash, itching, redness or other discoloration of the skin, or severe sunburn.

- Oral contraceptives (birth control pills) that contain estrogen may not work properly while you are taking carbamazepine. You should use an additional or alternative form of birth control while taking this drug.
- Carbamazepine affects the urine sugar levels of diabetic patients. If you notice a change in the results of your urine sugar tests, check with your physician.
- Before having any medical tests or any kind of surgical, dental, or emergency treatment, be sure to let the healthcare professional know that you are taking this medication.
- Carbamazepine has not been studied in pregnant women. There have been reports of babies having low birth weight, small head size, skull and facial defects, underdeveloped fingernails, and delays in growth when their mothers had taken carbamazepine in high doses during pregnancy. Studies in animals have shown that carbamazepine causes birth defects when given in large doses.
- Carbamazepine passes into breast milk, and the baby may receive enough of it to cause unwanted effects. In animal studies, carbamazepine has affected the growth and appearance of nursing babies.

POSSIBLE SIDE EFFECTS

- Side effects that typically go away as your body adjusts to the medication and do not require medical attention unless they continue for several weeks or are bothersome: clumsiness or unsteadiness*; mild dizziness*; mild drowsiness*; lightheadedness; mild nausea or vomiting; aching joints or muscles; constipa-

tion*; diarrhea; dryness of mouth; skin sensitivity to sunlight; irritation of mouth or tongue; loss or appetite; loss of hair; muscle or abdominal cramps; sexual problems in males*.

- Check with your physician as soon as possible if any of the following side effects occur: blurred or double vision*; confusion; agitation; severe diarrhea, nausea, or vomiting; skin rash or hives; unusual drowsiness; chest pain; difficulty speaking or slurred speech*; fainting; frequent urination*; unusual heartbeat; mental depression or other mood or emotional changes; unusual numbness, tingling, pain, or weakness in hands or feet*; ringing or buzzing in ears; sudden decrease in urination; swelling of face, hands, feet, or lower legs; trembling; uncontrolled body movements; visual hallucinations.
- Check with your physician immediately if any of the following occur: black tarry stools or blood in urine or stools; bone or joint pain; cough or hoarseness; darkening of urine; nosebleeds or other unusual bleeding or bruising; painful or difficult urination; tenderness, swelling, or bluish color in leg or foot; pale stools; pinpoint red spots on skin; shortness of breath or cough; sores, ulcers, or white spots on lips or in the mouth; sore throat, chills, and fever; swollen glands; unusual tiredness or weakness*; wheezing, tightness in chest; yellow eyes or skin.
- Symptoms of overdose that require immediate attention: unusual clumsiness or unsteadiness*; severe dizziness or fainting; fast or irregular heartbeat; unusually high or low blood pressure; irregular or shallow breathing; severe nausea or vomiting; trembling, twitching, and abnormal body movements.

*Since it may be difficult to distinguish between certain common symptoms of MS and some side effects of carbamazepine, be sure to consult your healthcare professional if an abrupt change of this type occurs.

**Chemical Name:** Ciprofloxacin (sip-roe-*flox*-a-sin) combination

*Brand Name:* Cipro (U.S. and Canada)

*Generic Available:* No

*Description:* Ciprofloxacin is one of a group of antibiotics (fluoroquinolones) used to kill bacterial infection in many parts of the body. It is used in multiple sclerosis primarily to treat urinary tract infections.

PROPER USAGE

- This medication is best taken with a full glass (8 ounces) of water. Additional water should be taken each day to help prevent some unwanted effects.
- Ciprofloxacin may be taken with meals or on an empty stomach.
- Finish the full course of treatment prescribed by your physician. Even if your symptoms disappear after a few days, stopping this medication prematurely may result in a return of the symptoms.
- This medication works most effectively when it is maintained at a constant level in your blood or urine. To help keep the amount constant, do not miss a dose. It is best to take the doses at evenly spaced times during the day and night.

PRECAUTIONS

- This medication may cause some people to become dizzy, lightheaded, drowsy, or less alert.
- If you are taking antacids that contain aluminum or magnesium, be sure to take them at least 2 hours before or after you take ciprofloxacin. These antacids may prevent the ciprofloxacin from working properly.
- This medication may cause your skin to become more sensitive to sunlight. Stay out of direct sunlight during the midday hours, wear protective clothing, and apply a sun block product that has a skin protection factor (SPF) of at least 15.
- Studies of birth defects have not been done in humans. This medication is not recommended during pregnancy since antibiotics of this type have been reported to cause bone development problems in young animals.
- Some of the antibiotics in this group are known to pass into human breast milk. Since they have been reported to cause bone development problems in young animals, breast-feeding is not recommended during treatment with this medication.

POSSIBLE SIDE EFFECTS

- Side effects that may go away as your body adjusts to the medication and do not require medical attention unless they continue or are bothersome: abdominal or stomach pain; diarrhea; dizziness; drowsiness*; headache; lightheadedness; nausea or vomiting; nervousness; trouble sleeping.
- Rare side effects that should be reported to your physician immediately: agitation; confusion; fever; hallucinations; peeling of the skin; shakiness or tremors*; shortness of breath; skin rash; itching; swelling of face or neck.

*Since it may be difficult to distinguish between certain common symptoms of MS and some side effects of ciprofloxacin, be sure to consult your healthcare professional if an abrupt change of this type occurs.

**Chemical Name:** Clonazepam (kloe-*na*-ze-pam)

*Brand Name:* Klonopin (U.S.); Rivotril; Syn-Clonazepam (Canada)

*Generic Available:* No

*Description:* Clonazepam is a benzodiazepine that belongs to the group of medications called central nervous system depressants, which slow down the nervous system. Although clonazepam is used for a variety of medical conditions, it is used in multiple sclerosis primarily for the treatment of tremor, pain, and spasticity.

PROPER USAGE
- Keep this medication out of the reach of children. An overdose of this medication may be especially dangerous for children.

PRECAUTIONS
- During the first few months taking clonazepam, your physician should check your progress at regular visits to make sure that this medicine does not cause unwanted effects.
- Take this medication only as directed by your physician; do not increase the dose without a prescription to do so.
- Clonazepam adds to the effects of alcohol and other central nervous system depressants (e.g., antihistamines, sedatives, tranquilizers, prescription pain medications, seizure medications, muscle relaxants, sleeping medications). Consult your physician before taking any of these CNS depressants while you are taking clonazepam. Taking an overdose of this medication or taking it with alcohol or other CNS depressants may lead to unconsciousness and possibly death.
- Stopping this medication suddenly may cause withdrawal side effects. Reduce the amount gradually before stopping completely.
- Clonazepam frequently causes people to become drowsy, dizzy, lightheaded, clumsy, or unsteady. Even if taken at bedtime, it may cause some people to feel drowsy or less alert on awakening.
- Studies in animals have shown that clonazepam can cause birth defects or other problems, including death of the animal fetus.
- Overuse of clonazepam during pregnancy may cause the baby to become dependent on it, leading to withdrawal side effects after birth. The use of clonazepam, especially during the last weeks of pregnancy, may cause breathing problems, muscle weakness, difficulty in feeding, and body temperature problems in the newborn infant.
- Clonazepam may pass into breast milk and cause drowsiness, slow heartbeat, shortness of breath, or troubled breathing in nursing babies.

POSSIBLE SIDE EFFECTS
- Side effects that may go away during treatment as your body adjusts to the medication and do not require medical attention unless they continue for several weeks or are bothersome: drowsiness or tiredness; clumsiness or unsteadiness*; dizziness or lightheadedness; slurred speech*; abdominal cramps or pain; blurred vision or other changes in vision*; changes in sexual drive or performance*; gastrointestinal changes, including constipation* or diarrhea; dryness of mouth; fast or pounding heartbeat; muscle spasm*; trouble with urination*; trembling.
- Unusual side effects that should be discussed as soon as possible with your physician: behavior problems, including difficulty concentrating and outbursts of anger; confusion or mental depression; convulsions; hallucinations; low blood pressure; muscle weakness; skin rash or itching; sore throat, fever, chills; unusual bleeding or bruising; unusual excitement or irritability.
- Symptoms of overdose that require immediate emergency help: continuing confusion; severe drowsiness; shakiness; slowed heartbeat; shortness of breath;

slow reflexes; continuing slurred speech*; staggering*; unusual severe weakness*.

*Since it may be difficult to distinguish between certain common symptoms of MS and some side effects of clonazepam, be sure to consult your healthcare professional if an abrupt change of this type occurs.

**Chemical Name:** Desmopressin acetate (des-moe-*press*-in)

*Brand Name:* DDAVP Tablets (U.S. and Canada)

*Generic Available:* No

*Description:* Desmopressin is a synthetic analogue of the natural pituitary hormone 8-arginine vasopression (ADH), that works on the kidneys to control urination. It is used in MS to block the kidney's production of urine for brief periods of time, e.g., to treat nocturia by reducing nighttime awakening to urinate.

PROPER USAGE

- Keep this medication in the refrigerator but do not allow it to freeze.

PRECAUTIONS

- Let your physician know if you have heart disease, blood vessel disease, or high blood pressure. Desmopressin can cause an increase in blood pressure.
- Studies have not been done in pregnant women. It has been used before and during pregnancy to treat diabetes mellitus and has not been shown to cause birth defects.
- It is not known whether desmopressin passes into breast milk and should therefore be used with caution by women who are breastfeeding.

POSSIBLE SIDE EFFECTS

- Side effects that typically go away as your body adjusts to the medication and do not require medical attention unless they

continue for several weeks or are bothersome: runny or stuffy nose; abdominal or stomach cramps; flushing of the skin; headache; nausea; pain in the vulva.
- Unusual side effects that require immediate medical attention: confusion; convulsions; unusual drowsiness*; continuing headache; rapid weight gain; markedly decreased urination.

*Since it may be difficult to distinguish between certain common symptoms of MS and some side effects of desmopressin, be sure to consult your healthcare professional if an abrupt change of this type occurs.

**Chemical Name:** Desmopressin acetate (des-moe-*press*-in)

*Brand Name:* DDAVP Nasal Spray (U.S. and Canada)

*Generic Available:* No

*Description:* Desmopressin is a synthetic analogue of the natural pituitary hormone 8-arginine vasopression (ADH), that works on the kidneys to control urination. It is used in MS to block the kidney's production of urine for brief periods of time, e.g., to treat nocturia by reducing nighttime awakening to urinate.

PROPER USAGE

- Keep this medication in the refrigerator but do not allow it to freeze.

PRECAUTIONS

- Let your physician know if you have heart disease, blood vessel disease, or high blood pressure. Desmopressin can cause an increase in blood pressure.
- Studies have not been done in pregnant women. It has been used before and during pregnancy to treat diabetes mellitus and has not been shown to cause birth defects.
- Desmopressin passes into breast milk but has not been reported to cause problems in nursing infants.

- Side effects that typically go away as your body adjusts to the medication and do not require medical attention unless they continue for several weeks or are bothersome: runny or stuffy nose; abdominal or stomach cramps; flushing of the skin; headache; nausea; pain in the vulva.
- Unusual side effects that require immediate medical attention: confusion; convulsions; unusual drowsiness*; continuing headache; rapid weight gain; markedly decreased urination.

*Since it may be difficult to distinguish between certain common symptoms of MS and some side effects of desmopressin, be sure to consult your healthcare professional if an abrupt change of this type occurs.

**Chemical Name:** Dexamethasone (dex-a-*meth*-oh-zone)

*Brand Name:* Decadron (U.S. and Canada)

*Generic Available:* Yes (U.S. and Canada)

*Description:* Dexamethasone is one of a group of corticosteroids (cortisone-like medicines) that are used to relieve inflammation in different parts of the body. Corticosteroids are used in MS for the management of acute exacerbations because they have the capacity to close the damaged blood–brain barrier and reduce inflammation in the central nervous system. Although dexamethasone is among the most commonly used corticosteroids in MS, it is only one of several possibilities. Other commonly used corticosteroids include prednisone, betamethasone, and methylprednisolone. The following information pertains to all the various corticosteroids.

PROPER USAGE

- Most neurologists treating MS believe that high-dose corticosteroids given intravenously are the most effective treatment for an MS exacerbation, although the exact protocol for the drug's use may differ somewhat from one treating physician to another. Patients generally receive a 4-day course of treatment (either in the hospital or as an outpatient), with doses of the medication spread throughout the day (see Methylprednisolone). The high-dose, intravenous dose is typically followed by a gradually tapering dose of an oral corticosteroid (usually ranging in length from 10 days to 5 or 6 weeks). Dexamethasone is commonly used for this oral taper. Oral dexamethasone may also be used instead of the high-dose, intravenous treatment if the intravenous treatment is not desired or is medically contraindicated.

PRECAUTIONS

- This medication can cause indigestion and stomach discomfort. Always take it with a meal and/or a glass or milk. Your physician may prescribe an antacid for you to take with this medication.
- Take this medication exactly as prescribed by your physician. Do not stop taking it abruptly; your physician will give you a schedule that gradually tapers the dose before you stop it completely.
- Since corticosteroids can stimulate the appetite and increase water retention, it is advisable to follow a low-salt and/or a potassium-rich diet and watch your caloric intake.
- Corticosteroids can lower your resistance to infection and make any infection that you get more difficult to treat. Contact your physician if you notice any sign of infection, such as sore throat, fever, coughing, or sneezing.
- Avoid close contact with anyone who has chicken pox or measles. Tell your physician immediately if you think you have been exposed to either of these illnesses. Do not have any immunizations

after you stop taking this medication until you have consulted your physician. People living in your home should not have the oral polio vaccine while you are being treated with corticosteroids since they might pass the polio virus on to you.

- Corticosteroids may affect the blood sugar levels of diabetic patients. If you notice a change in your blood or urine sugar tests, be sure to discuss it with your physician.

- The risk of birth defects in women taking corticosteroids during pregnancy has not been studied. Overuse of corticosteroids during pregnancy may slow the growth of the infant after birth. Animal studies have demonstrated that corticosteroids cause birth defects.

- Corticosteroids pass into breast milk and may slow the infant's growth. If you are nursing or plan to nurse, be sure to discuss this with your physician. It may be necessary for you to stop nursing while taking this medication.

- Corticosteroids can produce mood changes and/or mood swings of varying intensity. These mood alterations can vary from relatively mild to extremely intense, and can vary in a single individual from one course of treatment to another. Neither the patient nor the physician can predict with any certainty whether the corticosteroids are likely to precipitate these mood alterations. If you have a history of mood disorders (depression or bipolar disorder, for example), be sure to share this information with your physician. If you begin to experience unmanageable mood changes or swings while taking corticosteroids, contact your physician so that a decision can be made whether or not you need an additional medication to help you until the mood alterations subside.

POSSIBLE SIDE EFFECTS

- Side effects that may go away as your body adjusts to the medication and do not require medical attention unless they continue or are bothersome: increased appetite; indigestion; nervousness or restlessness; trouble sleeping; headache; increased sweating; unusual increase in hair growth on body or face.

- Less common side effects that should be reported as soon as possible to your physician: severe mood changes or mood swings; decreased or blurred vision*; frequent urination*.

- Additional side effects that can result from the prolonged use of corticosteroids and should be reported to your physician: acne or other skin problems; swelling of the face; swelling of the feet or lower legs; rapid weight gain; pain in the hips or other joints (caused by bone cell degeneration); bloody or black, tarry stools; elevated blood pressure; markedly increased thirst (with increased urination indicative of diabetes mellitus); menstrual irregularities; unusual bruising of the skin; thin, shiny skin; hair loss; muscle cramps or pain. Once you stop this medication after taking it for a long period of time, it may take several months for your body to readjust.

*Since it may be difficult to distinguish between certain common symptoms of MS and some side effects of dexamethasone, be sure to consult your healthcare professional if an abrupt change of this type occurs.

**Chemical Name:** Diazepam (dye-*az*-e-pam)
*Brand Name:* Valium (U.S. and Canada)
*Generic Available:* Yes (U.S.)
*Description:* Diazepam is a benzodiazepine that belongs to the group of medicines called central nervous system depressants, which slow down the nervous system.

Although diazepam is used for a variety of medical conditions, it is used in multiple sclerosis primarily for the relief of muscle spasms and spasticity.

PROPER USAGE

- Keep this medication out of the reach of children. An overdose of this medication may be especially dangerous for children.

PRECAUTIONS

- Your physician should check your progress at regular visits to make sure that this medication does not cause unwanted effects.
- Take diazepam only as directed by your physician; do not increase the dose without a prescription to do so.
- Diazepam adds to the effects of alcohol and other central nervous system depressants (e.g., antihistamines, sedatives, tranquilizers, prescription pain medications, seizure medications, muscle relaxants, or sleeping medications). Consult your physician before taking any of these CNS depressants while you are taking diazepam. Taking an overdose of this medication or taking it with alcohol or other CNS depressants may lead to unconsciousness and possibly death.
- Stopping this medication suddenly may cause withdrawal side effects. Reduce the amount gradually before stopping completely.
- Diazepam may cause some people to become drowsy, dizzy, lightheaded, clumsy, or unsteady. Even if taken at bedtime, it may cause some people to feel drowsy or less alert on awakening.
- The use of diazepam during the first 3 months of pregnancy has been reported to increase the chance of birth defects.
- Overuse of diazepam during pregnancy may cause the baby to become depend-

ent on the medicine, leading to withdrawal side effects after birth. The use of diazepam, especially during the last weeks of pregnancy, may cause breathing problems, muscle weakness, difficulty in feeding, and body temperature problems in the newborn infant. When diazepam is given in high doses (especially by injection) within 15 hours before delivery, it may cause breathing problems, muscle weakness, difficulty in feeding, and body temperature problems in the newborn infant.

- Diazepam may pass into breast milk and cause drowsiness, slow heartbeat, shortness of breath, or troubled breathing in nursing babies.

POSSIBLE SIDE EFFECTS

- Side effects that may go away during treatment as your body adjusts to the medication and do not require medical attention unless they continue for several weeks or are bothersome: clumsiness or unsteadiness*; dizziness or lightheadedness; slurred speech*; abdominal cramps or pain; blurred vision or other changes in vision*; changes in sexual drive or performance*; constipation*; diarrhea; dryness of mouth; fast or pounding heartbeat; muscle spasm*; trouble with urination*; trembling*; unusual tiredness or weakness*.
- Unusual side effects that should be discussed with your physician as soon as possible: behavior problems, including difficulty concentrating and outbursts of anger; confusion or mental depression; convulsions; hallucinations; low blood pressure; muscle weakness*; skin rash or itching; sore throat, fever, chills; unusual bleeding or bruising; unusual excitement or irritability.
- Symptoms of overdose that require immediate emergency help: continuing confusion; unusually severe drowsiness;

shakiness; slowed heartbeat; shortness of breath; slow reflexes; continuing slurred speech; staggering; unusually severe weakness*.

*Since it may be difficult to distinguish between certain common symptoms of MS and some side effects of diazepam, be sure to consult your healthcare professional if an abrupt change of this type occurs.

**Chemical Name:** Docusate (*doe*-koo-sate)

*Brand Name:* Colace (U.S. and Canada)

*Generic Available:* Yes (U.S. and Canada)

*Description:* Docusate is an over-the-counter stool softener (emollient) that helps liquids to mix into dry, hardened stool, making the stool easier to pass.

PROPER USAGE

- Laxatives are to be used to provide short-term relief only, unless otherwise directed by the nurse or physician who is helping you to manage your bowel symptoms. A regimen that includes a healthy diet containing roughage (whole grain breads and cereals, bran, fruit, and green, leafy vegetables), six to eight full glasses of liquids each day, and some form of daily exercise is most important in stimulating healthy bowel function.
- If your physician has recommended this laxative for management of constipation, follow his or her recommendations for its use. If you are treating yourself for constipation, follow the directions on the package insert.
- Results usually occur 1 to 2 days after the first dose; some individuals may not get results for 3 to 5 days. Be sure to consult your physician if you experience problems or do not get relief within a week.

PRECAUTIONS

- Do not take any type of laxative if you have signs of appendicitis or inflamed bowel (e.g., stomach or lower abdominal pain, cramping, bloating, soreness, nausea, or vomiting). Check with your physician as soon as possible.
- Do not take any laxative for more than 1 week unless you have been told to do so by your physician. Many people tend to overuse laxatives, which often leads to dependence on the laxative action to produce a bowel movement. Discuss the use of laxatives with your healthcare professional to ensure that the laxative is used effectively as part of a comprehensive, healthy bowel management regimen.
- Do not take mineral oil within 2 hours of taking docusate. The docusate may increase the amount of mineral oil that is absorbed by the body.
- Do not take any laxative within 2 hours of taking another medication because the desired effectiveness of the other medication may be reduced.
- If you are pregnant, discuss with your physician the most appropriate type of laxative for you to use.
- Some laxatives pass into breast milk. Although it is unlikely to cause problems for a nursing infant, be sure to let your physician know if you are using a laxative and breast-feeding at the same time.

POSSIBLE SIDE EFFECTS

- Side effects that may go away as your body adjusts to the medication and do not require medical attention unless they persist or are bothersome: stomach and/or intestinal cramping.
- Unusual side effect that should be reported to your physician as soon as possible: skin rash.

**Chemical Name:** Docusate (*doe*-koo-sate) stool softener laxative

*Brand Name:* Enemeez® Mini Enema (U.S.)

*Generic Available:* Yes (Canada)

*Description:* Enemeez is an over-the-counter stool softener (emollient) that comes in a small, plastic, single-dose tube for insertion into the rectum. It works to produce bowel movements in a short time by introducing liquid into the stool to soften dry, hardened stool, making the stool easier to pass. The small size of this enema makes it easy to use without compromising its effectiveness.

PROPER USAGE

- Laxatives are to be used to provide short-term relief only, unless otherwise directed by the nurse or physician who is helping you to manage your bowel symptoms. A regimen that includes a healthy diet containing roughage (whole grain breads and cereals, bran, fruit, and green, leafy vegetables), six to eight full glasses of liquids each day, and some form of daily exercise, is most important in stimulating healthy bowel function.
- If your physician has recommended this laxative for management of constipation, follow his or her recommendations for its use. If you are treating yourself for constipation, follow the directions on the package insert.
- Results usually occur 15 minutes to 1 hour after insertion. Be sure to consult your physician if you experience problems or do not get relief within a day or two.

PRECAUTIONS

- Do not use any type of laxative if you have signs of appendicitis or inflamed bowel (e.g., stomach or lower abdominal pain, cramping, bloating, soreness, nausea, or vomiting). Check with your physician as soon as possible.
- Do not take any laxative for more than one week unless you have been told to do so by your physician. Many people tend to overuse laxatives, which often leads to dependence on the laxative action to produce a bowel movement. Discuss the use of laxatives with your healthcare professional to ensure that the laxative is used effectively as part of a comprehensive, healthy bowel management regimen.
- If you are pregnant, discuss with your physician the most appropriate type of laxative for you to use.

POSSIBLE SIDE EFFECTS

- Side effect that may go away as your body adjusts to the medication and does not require medical attention unless it persists or is bothersome: skin irritation surrounding the rectal area.
- Less common side effects that should be reported to your physician: rectal bleeding, blistering, burning, itching, or pain.

**Chemical Name:** Duloxetine hydrochloride Delayed-release (doo-*lox*-uh-teen)

*Brand Name:* Cymbalta (U.S. and Canada)

*Generic Available:* No

*Description:* Duloxetine hydrochloride is used in MS to treat mental depression and neuropathic pain. It belongs to a group of medications known as selective serotonin and norepinephrine reuptake inhibitors (SSNRI).

PROPER USAGE

- Duloxetine should be swallowed whole and not chewed or crushed. The medication can be taken with or without food.

PRECAUTIONS

- While a person with a major depressive disorder may experience some relief in 1 to 4 weeks, the medication should be continued as directed by your physician.
- Your physician should monitor your progress at regularly scheduled visits in

order to adjust the dose and help reduce any side effects.

- You and your family members should be alert to any abrupt emotional and/or behavioral changes (e.g., heightened anxiety, agitation, panic attacks, insomnia, irritability, hostility, impulsivity, undue excitement or hypomania, worsening of depression, or suicidal ideation) and report them to your physician.
- You should not take this medication if you are taking or have recently taken a monamine oxidase inhibitor (MAOI), are taking thioridazine, or have uncontrolled narrow-angle glaucoma.
- Any drug of this type can impair judgment, thinking, or motor skills. Although duloxetine has not been shown in clinical studies to impair these functions, it can cause sedation. Do not drive or operate any hazardous machinery until you know that the medication does not interefere with ability to engage in these activities.
- In animal studies, duloxetine has been shown to have adverse effects on pre- and postnatal development. Studies have not been done in pregnant women. Be sure to notify your physician as soon as possible if you become pregnant or intend to become pregnant.
- It is not known whether duloxetine is excreted into breast milk, but nursing while on duloxetine is not recommended.

POSSIBLE SIDE EFFECTS

- Side effects that may go away as your body adjusts to the medication and do not require medical attention unless they continue for several weeks or are bothersome: nausea, dry mouth, constipation, decreased appetite, fatigue, sleepiness, increased sweating, decreased sexual drive or ability, urinary hesitation.

**Chemical Name:** Fluoxetine (floo-*ox*-uh-teen)

*Brand Name:* Prozac (U.S. and Canada)

*Generic Available:* Yes

*Description:* Fluoxetine is used to treat mental depression and panic disorder. It is also used occasionally to treat MS fatigue.

PROPER USAGE

- This medication should be taken in the morning when used to treat depression because it can interfere with sleep. If it upsets your stomach, you may take it with food.

PRECAUTIONS

- It may take 4 to 6 weeks for you to feel the beneficial effects of this medication.
- Your physician should monitor your progress at regularly scheduled visits in order to adjust the dose and help reduce any side effects.
- There have been suggestions that the use of fluoxetine may be related to increased thoughts about suicide in a very small number of individuals. More study is needed to determine if the medicine causes this effect. If you have concerns about this, be sure to discuss them with your physician.
- Fluoxetine adds to the effects of alcohol and other central nervous system depressants (e.g., antihistamines, sedatives, tranquilizers, sleeping medicine, prescription pain medicine, barbiturates, seizure medication, and muscle relaxants). Be sure that your physician knows if you are taking these or any other medications.
- This medication affects the blood sugar levels of diabetic individuals. Check with your physician if you notice any changes in your blood or urine sugar tests.
- Dizziness or lightheadedness may occur, especially when you get up from a lying or sitting position. Change positions

slowly to help alleviate this problem. If the problem continues or gets worse, consult your physician.

- Fluoxetine may cause dryness of the mouth. If your mouth continues to feel dry for more than 2 weeks, check with your physician or dentist. Continuing dryness of the mouth may increase the chance of dental disease.
- Studies have not been done in pregnant women. Fluoxetine has not been shown to cause birth defects or other problems in animal studies.
- Fluoxetine passes into breast milk and may cause unwanted effects, such as vomiting, watery stools, crying, and sleep problems in nursing babies. You may want to discuss alternative medications with your physician.

POSSIBLE SIDE EFFECTS

- Side effects that may go away as your body adjusts to the medication and do not require medical attention unless they continue for several weeks or are bothersome: decreased sexual drive or ability*; anxiety and nervousness; diarrhea; drowsiness*; headache; trouble sleeping; abnormal dreams; change in vision*; chest pain; decreased appetite; decrease in concentration; dizziness; dry mouth; fast or irregular heartbeat; frequent urination*; menstrual pain; tiredness or weakness*; tremor*; vomiting.
- Unusual side effects that should be discussed with your physician as soon as possible: chills or fever; joint or muscle pain; skin rash; hives or itching; trouble breathing.
- Symptoms of overdose that require immediate medical attention: agitation and restlessness; convulsions; severe nausea and vomiting; unusual excitement.

*Since it may be difficult to distinguish between certain common symptoms of MS

and some side effects of fluoxetine, be sure to consult your healthcare professional if an abrupt change of this type occurs.

**Chemical Name:** Gabapentin (ga-ba-*pen*-tin)

*Brand Name:* Neurontin (U.S.)

*Generic Available:* Yes (Canada)

*Description:* Gabapentin is an antiepileptic used to control some types of seizures in epilepsy. It is used in multiple sclerosis to control dysesthesias (pain caused by MS lesions) and the pain caused by spasticity.

PROPER USAGE

- Gabapentin may be taken with or without food. You must wait 2 hours after taking an antacid to take gabapentin.
- If gabapentin is taken 3 times a day, do not allow more than 12 hours to elapse between any 2 doses.
- If you miss a dose of this medication, take it as soon as possible. However, if it is almost time for your next dose, skip the missed dose, then go back to your regular dosing schedule. Do not double dose.

PRECAUTIONS

- This medicine will add to the effects of alcohol and other central nervous system depressants that may cause drowsiness (e.g., antihistamines, sedatives, tranquilizers, prescription pain medications, seizure medications, and muscle relaxants). Be sure that your physician knows if you are taking these or any other medications.
- Before having any medical tests or surgical, dental, or emergency treatment of any kind, be sure to let the healthcare professional know that you are taking this medication.
- Consult your physician before stopping this medication because stopping abrupt-

ly may result in seizures. Depending on the dose you are taking, your physician may want you to decrease your dose gradually to avoid seizures.

- Gabapentin has not been studied in pregnant women. However, animal studies have shown possible bone and kidney problems in offspring. If you are pregnant or planning to become pregnant, discuss this with your physician before starting this medication.
- It is not known whether gabapentin passes into breast milk. Women who wish to breast-feed should consult with their physician.

POSSIBLE SIDE EFFECTS

- Side effects that typically go away as your body adjusts to the medication and do not require medical attention unless they continue for several weeks or are bothersome: blurred or double vision*; dizziness; drowsiness, muscle ache; swelling of hands or legs; tremor*; unusual tiredness*; weakness*; diarrhea, frequent urination*; indigestion; low blood pressure; slurred speech*; sleep difficulty; weakness*.
- Check with your doctor as soon as possible if any of the following side effects occur: clumsiness or unsteadiness*; continuous, uncontrolled eye movements; depression; mood changes; memory problems*; hoarseness; lower back pain; painful or difficult urination.
- Symptoms of overdose requiring immediate attention: double vision*; severe diarrhea, dizziness; drowsiness; slurred speech*.

*Since it may be difficult to distinguish between certain common symptoms of MS and some side effects of gabapentin, be sure to consult your healthcare professional if an abrupt change of this type occurs.

**Chemical Name:** Glatiramer acetate (gla-*teer*-a-mer *ass*-i-tate) (formerly called Copolymer-1)

*Brand Name:* Copaxone (U.S. and Canada)

*Generic Available:* No

*Description:* Glatiramer acetate is a synthetic protein that simulates myelin basic protein, a component of the myelin that insulates nerve fibers in the brain and spinal cord. Through a mechanism that is not completely understood, this drug seems to block myelin-damaging T-cells by acting as a myelin decoy. In controlled clinical trials with relapsing-remitting MS, those taking the drug had a significant reduction in annual relapse rate compared to control subjects who were given a placebo.

APPROVAL BY THE U.S. FOOD AND DRUG ADMINISTRATION (FDA)

- Glatiramer acetate is approved by the FDA to reduce the frequency of relapses in patients with relapsing-remitting MS.

PROPER USAGE

- Glatiramer acetate is injected subcutaneously (between the fat layer just under the skin and the muscles beneath) once a day. The physician or nurse will instruct you in correct injection procedures, using a specially designed set of training materials. Do not attempt to inject yourself until you are sure that you understand the procedures.
- Glatiramer acetate should be kept refrigerated at all times. If refrigeration is not available, the drug may be safely stored at room temperature for up to seven days.
- Glatiramer acetate is light-sensitive; protect it from light when not injecting.
- Use each pre-filled syringe for only one injection. Dispose of the syringes as directed by your physician and keep them out of the reach of children.

- Because injection-site reactions (swelling, redness, discoloration, or pain) are relatively common, it is recommended that the sites be rotated according to a schedule provided for you by your physician. Do not use any one site more than once per week.

PRECAUTIONS

- Do not use a pre-filled syringe that appears cloudy or contains particles.
- Do not change the dose or dosing schedule of this medication without consulting your physician.
- Glatiramer acetate is not recommended for use during pregnancy. Women who wish to become pregnant should discuss this medication, and all others they are taking, with their physician. If you become pregnant while on the medication, inform your physician. Glatiramer acetate is a Pregnancy Category B medication, meaning that although no adverse effects have been found in animal studies, no adequate, well-controlled studies have been done in pregnant women to demonstrate its safety in humans.
- It is not known whether glatiramer acetate passes into the breast milk. Nursing women should discuss the use of this medication with their physician.

POSSIBLE SIDE EFFECTS

- Side effects that generally resolve on their own and do not require medical attention unless they continue for several weeks or are bothersome: injection-site reactions (e.g., swelling, the development of a hardened lump, redness, tenderness, increased warmth of the skin, or itching at the site of the injection); runny nose; tremor*; unusual tiredness or weakness*; weight gain.
- Unusual side effects that should be discussed as soon as possible with your

doctor: hives (an itchy, blotchy swelling of the skin) or severe pain at the injection site.
- Possible immediate post-injection reaction: Approximately 13 percent of individuals using Copaxone will experience, at one time or another, a transient (very temporary) reaction immediately after injecting glatiramer acetate. This reaction, which usually occurs only once, includes flushing or chest tightness with heart palpitations, anxiety, and difficulty breathing. During the clinical trials, these reactions occurred very rarely, usually within minutes of an injection. They lasted approximately 15 minutes and resolved without further problem.

COPAXONE SUPPORT PROGRAM:
Shared Solutions®
1-800-887-8100
www.copaxone.com
www.sharedsolutions.com

*Since it may be difficult to distinguish between certain common symptoms of MS and some side effects of glatiramer acetate, be sure to consult your healthcare professional if an abrupt change of this type occurs.

**Chemical Name:** Glycerin (*gli*-ser-in)

*Brand Name:* Sani-Supp suppository (U.S.)

*Generic Available:* Yes (U.S. and Canada)

*Description:* A glycerin suppository is a hyperosmotic laxative that draws water into the bowel from surrounding body tissues. This water helps to soften the stool mass and promote bowel action.

PROPER USAGE

- Laxatives are to be used to provide short-term relief only, unless otherwise directed by the nurse or physician who is helping you to manage your bowel symptoms. A regimen that includes a healthy diet containing roughage (whole grain breads and cereals, bran, fruit, and green, leafy vegetables), six to eight full glasses of liquids each day, and some form of daily exercise is most important in stimulating healthy bowel function.

- If your physician has recommended this laxative for management of constipation, follow his or her recommendations for its use. If you are treating yourself for constipation, follow the directions on the package insert.
- If the suppository is too soft to insert, refrigerate it for 30 minutes or hold it under cold water before removing the foil wrapper.
- Glycerin suppositories often produce results within 15 minutes to 1 hour. Be sure to consult your physician if you experience problems or do not get relief within a week.

PRECAUTIONS

- Do not take any type of laxative if you have signs of appendicitis or inflamed bowel (e.g., stomach or lower abdominal pain, cramping, bloating, soreness, nausea, or vomiting). Check with your physician as soon as possible.
- Do not take any laxative for more than 1 week unless you have been told to do so by your physician. Many people tend to overuse laxatives, which often leads to dependence on the laxative action to produce a bowel movement. Discuss the use of laxatives with your healthcare professional to ensure that the laxative is used effectively as part of a comprehensive, healthy bowel management regimen.
- If you are pregnant, discuss with your physician the most appropriate type of laxative for you to use.
- Use only water to moisten the suppository prior to insertion in the rectum. Do not lubricate the suppository with miner-

al oil or petroleum jelly, which might affect the way the suppository works.

POSSIBLE SIDE EFFECTS

- Side effect that may go away as your body adjusts to the medication and does not require medical attention unless it persists or is bothersome: skin irritation around the rectal area.
- Less common side effects that should be reported to your physician as soon as possible: rectal bleeding; blistering, or itching.

**Chemical Name:** Imipramine (im-*ip*-ra-meen)

*Brand Name:* Tofranil (U.S. and Canada)

*Generic Available:* Yes (U.S. and Canada)

*Description:* Imipramine is a tricyclic anti-depressant used to treat mental depression. Its primary use in multiple sclerosis is to treat bladder symptoms, including urinary frequency and incontinence. Imipramine is also prescribed occasionally for the management of neurologic pain in MS.

PROPER USAGE

- To lessen stomach upset, take this medication with food, even for a daily bedtime dose, unless your physician has told you to take it on an empty stomach.

PRECAUTIONS

- Imipramine adds to the effects of alcohol and other central nervous system depressants (e.g., antihistamines, sedatives, tranquilizers, prescription pain medications, seizure medications, muscle relaxants, and sleeping medications), possibly causing drowsiness. Be sure that your physician knows if you are taking these or any other medications.
- This medication causes dryness of the mouth. Because continuing dryness of the mouth can increase the risk of den-

tal disease, alert your dentist if you are taking imipramine.

- Imipramine may cause your skin to be more sensitive to sunlight than it is normally. Even brief exposure to sunlight may cause a skin rash, itching, redness or other discoloration of the skin, or severe sunburn. Stay out of the sun during the midday hours. Wear protective clothing and a sun block that has a skin protection factor (SPF) of at least 15.

- This medication may affect blood sugar levels of diabetic individuals. If you notice a change in the results of your blood or urine sugar tests, check with your physician.

- Do not stop taking imipramine without consulting your physician. The physician may want you to reduce gradually the amount you are taking to reduce the possibility of withdrawal symptoms such as headache, nausea, and/or an overall feeling of discomfort.

- Studies of imipramine have not been done in pregnant women. There have been reports of newborns suffering from muscle spasms or heart; breathing or urinary problems when their mothers had taken tricyclic antidepressants immediately before delivery. Studies in animals have indicated the possibility of unwanted effects in the fetus.

- Imipramine passes into breast milk, but has not been reported to have any effect on the nursing infant.

POSSIBLE SIDE EFFECTS

- Side effects that may go away as your body adjusts to the medication and do not require medical attention unless they continue for more than two weeks or are bothersome: dizziness; drowsiness*; headache; decreased sexual ability*; increased appetite; nausea; unusual tiredness or weakness*; unpleasant taste; diarrhea; heartburn; increased sweating; vomiting.

- Uncommon side effects that should be reported to your physician as soon as possible: blurred vision*; confusion or delirium; constipation*; difficulty speaking or swallowing; eye pain*; fainting; fast or irregular heartbeat; hallucinations; loss of balance control*; nervousness or restlessness; problems urinating*; shakiness or trembling; stiffness of arms and legs*.

- Rare side effects that should be reported to your physician as soon as possible: anxiety; breast enlargement in males and females; hair loss; inappropriate secretion of milk in females; increased sensitivity to sunlight; irritability; muscle twitching; red or brownish spots on the skin; buzzing or other unexplained sounds in the ears; skin rash; itching; sore throat and fever; swelling of face and tongue; weakness*; yellow skin.

- Symptoms of acute overdose: confusion; convulsions; severe drowsiness*; enlarged pupils; unusual heartbeat; fever; hallucinations; restlessness and agitation; shortness of breath; unusual tiredness or weakness*; vomiting.

*Since it may be difficult to distinguish between certain common symptoms of MS and some side effects of imipramine, be sure to consult your healthcare professional if an abrupt change of this type occurs.

**Chemical Name:** Interferon (in-ter-*feer*-on) beta-1a

*Brand Name:* Avonex (U.S. and Canada)

*Generic Available:* No

*Description:* Avonex is a medication manufactured by a biotechnological process from one of the naturally occurring interferons (a type of protein). It is made up of exactly the same amino acids (major components of proteins) as the interferon beta found in the human body. In controlled clinical trials in relapsing MS, those taking the medication had a reduced risk of disability progression, experienced fewer exacerbations, and showed a reduction in number and size of active lesions in the brain (as shown on MRI) when compared with the group taking a placebo. In a subsequent study of patients who had experienced a single demyelinating event in the optic nerve, spinal cord, or brainstem, and had lesions typical of MS on brain MRI, Avonex significantly delayed the time to a second exacerbation, and thus to a clinically definite diagnosis of MS.

### APPROVAL BY THE U.S. FOOD AND DRUG ADMINISTRATION (FDA)

- Avonex is approved by the FDA for the treatment of patients with relapsing forms of MS to slow the accumulation of physical disability and decrease the frequency of clinical exacerbations. Patients with MS in whom efficacy has been demonstrated include those who have experienced a first clinical episode and have MRI features consistent with MS.

### PROPER USAGE

- Avonex is given as a once-a-week intramuscular (IM) injection, usually in the large muscles of the thigh, upper arm, or hip.
- You and your care partner will be instructed in safe and proper IM injection procedures. If you are unable to self-inject and have no family member or friend available to do the injections, your physician or nurse will administer the injections. Do not attempt to inject yourself until you are sure that you understand the procedures.
- Avonex is available in a pre-mixed syringe. Store all unused syringes in the refrigerator. Let each syringe come to room temperature (about 20 minutes) prior to injecting. Do not expose the medication to high temperatures (in a glove compartment or on a window sill, for example) and do not allow it to freeze.
- Do not reuse the pre-filled syringes. Dispose of the syringes as directed by your physician and keep them out of the reach of children.
- Since flu-like symptoms are a fairly common side effect during the initial weeks of treatment, it is recommended that the injection be given at bedtime. Taking acetaminophen (Tylenol®) or ibuprofen (Advil® or Motrin®) immediately prior to each injection and during the 24 hours following the injection will also help to relieve the flu-like symptoms.

### PRECAUTIONS

- Prior to taking Avonex, be sure to tell your physician if you have ever had any of the following medical problems:
  - Depression, anxiety, or trouble sleeping
  - Problems with your thyroid gland
  - Blood problems such as bleeding or bruising easily, anemia, low white cell count
  - Seizures
  - Heart problems
  - Liver disease
- Avonex should not be used during pregnancy or by any woman who is trying to become pregnant. Women taking Avonex should use birth control measures at all times. If you want to become pregnant while being treated with Avonex, discuss the matter with your physician. If you become pregnant while using Avonex, stop the treatment and contact your physician.
- There was no increase in depression reported by people receiving Avonex in the clinical trial. However, since depression and suicidal thoughts are known to occur with some frequency in MS, and depression and suicidal thoughts have

been reported with high doses of various interferon products, it is recommended that individuals with a history of severe depressive disorder be closely monitored while taking Avonex. Additionally, there have been post-marketing reports of depression, suicidal ideation, and/or development of new or worsening of pre-existing other psychiatric disorders, including psychosis. Some of these patients improve upon cessation of Avonex dosing.

- (Note: Post-marketing data include reports from patients and/or their doctors of clinical events that have occurred while the patient was taking the medication. Since these reports occur outside the context of a controlled clinical trial, there is no way to determine the relationship between the event and the medication. This is particularly true for the reported onset of depressive symptoms or other emotional changes, since these types of emotional symptoms are common in people with MS whether or not they are taking an interferon. Independent studies of the incidence of depression in people with MS taking interferon beta medications have not confirmed any relationship between depressive symptoms and the medications.)

- Avonex is to be used with caution in individuals with a seizure disorder. A few individuals with no prior history of seizures have experienced seizures while on Avonex. Since seizures are known to occur somewhat more frequently in people with MS than in the general population, it is not known whether these seizures were related to the MS, to the medication, or to some combination of the two.

- Patients with cardiac disease should be closely monitored for a worsening of their condition. While Avonex is not known to cause cardiac problems, there have been infrequent post-marketing reports of congestive heart failure and other cardiac problems in people with no prior history and no other factors predisposing them to heart problems.

- Because of the potential of Avonex to affect the functioning of the liver and thyroid gland, and to cause a drop in the levels of white blood cells, red blood cells, and platelets in a person's system, periodic blood tests are recommended.

POSSIBLE SIDE EFFECTS

- Common side effects include flu-like symptoms (fatigue, chills, fever, muscle aches, and sweating). Most of these symptoms will tend to disappear after the initial few weeks of treatment. If they continue, become more severe, or cause you significant discomfort, be sure to talk them over with your physician.

- Symptoms of depression, including ongoing sadness, anxiety, loss of interest in daily activities, irritability, low self-esteem, guilt, poor concentration, indecisiveness, confusion, and eating and sleep disturbances should be reported promptly to your doctor.

AVONEX SUPPORT PROGRAM
Avonex ActiveSource℠
1-800-456-2255
www.avonex.com
www.msactivesource.com

**Chemical Name:** Interferon (in-ter-*feer*-on) beta-1a

*Brand Name:* Rebif (U.S. and Canada)

*Generic Available:* No

*Description:* Rebif is a medication manufactured by a biotechnological process from one of the naturally occurring interferons (a type of protein). It is made up of exactly the same amino acids (major components of proteins) as the interferon beta found in the human body. A controlled clinical trial in relapsing-remitting MS compared three groups—those receiving 22 mcg (micrograms) three times per week, those receiving 44 mcg three times a week, and those receiving placebo. Over the 2-year study, the two experimental groups demonstrated a lower relapse rate, prolonged time to first relapse, a higher proportion of relapse-free patients, a lower number of active lesions on MRI, and delay in progression of disability when compared to the placebo group. Rebif is currently available at the 44 mcg dose in pre-filled syringes ready for subcutaneous injection.

### APPROVAL BY THE U.S. FOOD AND DRUG ADMINISTRATION (FDA)

- Rebif is approved for the treatment of patients with relapsing forms of MS to decrease the frequency of clinical exacerbations and delay the accumulation of physical disability.
- Reporting on the outcome of the evidence trial, which compared Rebif and Avonex (both interferon beta-1a), the FDA added the following information to the labeling of Rebif:
  - "Patients treated with Rebif 44 mcg sc (delivered subcutaneously) tiw (3 times per week) were more likely to remain relapse-free at 24 and 48 weeks than were patients treated with Avonex 30 mcg im (delivered intramuscularly) qw (once per week)."

### PROPER USAGE

- Rebif is given three times a week subcutaneously (between the fat layer just under the skin and the muscles beneath). The physician or nurse will instruct you in the injection procedure, using a specially designed set of training materials. Do not attempt to inject yourself until you are sure that you understand the procedures.

- When beginning treatment, it is recommended that you start at 8.8 mcg three times a week and gradually increase over a 4-week period to the 44 mcg dose in order to reduce the side effects. A starter kit with 22 mcg syringes is available to facilitate the gradual increase in dose.
- Rebif should be administered at the same time of day, on the same days of the week, preferably in the late afternoon. Doses must be at least 48 hours apart.
- Rebif should be stored in the refrigerator. Storage at room temperature without exposure to heat or light is permissible for up to 30 days. Do not allow the medication to freeze.
- Do not reuse needles or syringes. Dispose of the syringes as directed by your physician and keep them out of the reach of children.
- Since flu-like symptoms are a fairly common side effect during the initial weeks of treatment, it is recommended that the injection be given at bedtime. Taking acetaminophen (Tylenol®) or ibuprofen (Advil® or Motrin®) immediately prior to each injection and during the 24 hours following the injection will also help to relieve the flu-like symptoms.

### PRECAUTIONS

- Rebif should not be used during pregnancy or breast-feeding, or by any woman who is trying to become pregnant. Women taking Rebif should use birth control measures at all times. If you want to become pregnant while being treated with Rebif, discuss the matter with your physician. If you become pregnant while using Rebif, stop the treatment and contact your physician.
- There was no increase in depression reported by people receiving Rebif in the clinical trial. However, some patients

treated with interferons, including Rebif, have become seriously depressed, and depression and suicidal thoughts are known to occur with some frequency in MS. It is recommended that individuals with a history of severe depressive disorder be closely monitored while taking Rebif. Anyone who experiences significant feelings of sadness or helplessness, or feels like hurting him- or herself or others, should speak with a friend or family member right away and contact the physician as soon as possible.

- Rebif can affect liver function. Your physician may ask you to have regular blood tests to make sure that your liver is working properly. If you notice that your skin or the whites of your eyes become yellow, or if you are bruising more easily than usual, contact your physician. A post-marketing case of liver failure has been reported in a person taking Rebif along with another medication that was potentially toxic to the liver. While this type of problem is extremely rare, people must make sure that their physician is aware of any history of liver disease, alcoholism, or other liver problems, as well as of all the medications they are taking.

- Because of the potential of Rebif to affect the levels of white blood cells, red blood cells, and platelets in a person's system, blood tests are recommended at regular intervals. Thyroid function tests are recommended every 6 months in patients with a history of thyroid dysfunction.

## Possible Side Effects

- Common side effects include flu-like symptoms (fatigue, chills, fever, muscle aches, and sweating) and injection site reactions (swelling, redness, discoloration, and pain). Most of these symptoms tend to disappear over time. If they continue, become more severe, or cause significant discomfort, be sure to talk them over with your physician. Contact your physician if the injection sites become inflamed, hardened, or lumpy, and do not inject into any area that has become hardened or lumpy.

- Most of these symptoms will tend to disappear after the initial few weeks of treatment. If they continue, become more severe, or cause you significant discomfort, be sure to talk them over with your physician.

- Symptoms of depression, including ongoing sadness, anxiety, loss of interest in daily activities, irritability, low self-esteem, guilt, poor concentration, indecisiveness, confusion, and eating and sleep disturbances, should be reported promptly to your doctor.

REBIF SUPPORT PROGRAM:
MS LifeLines™
1-877-44-REBIF (1-877-447-3243)
www.rebif.com
www.mslifelines.com

**Chemical Name:** Interferon (in-ter-*feer*-on) beta-1b

*Brand Name:* Betaseron (U.S. and Canada)

*Generic Available:* No

*Description:* Betaseron is a medication manufactured by a biotechnological process from one of the naturally occurring interferons (a type of protein). In a clinical trial of 372 ambulatory patients with relapsing-remitting MS, those taking the currently recommended dose of the medication experienced fewer exacerbations, a longer time between exacerbations, and exacerbations that were generally less severe than those of patients taking a lower dose of the medication or a placebo. Additionally, patients on interferon beta-1b had no increase in total lesion area, as shown on MRI, in contrast to the placebo group, that had a significant increase.

APPROVAL BY THE U.S. FOOD AND DRUG ADMINISTRATION

- Betaseron is approved for the treatment of relapsing forms of MS to reduce the frequency of clinical exacerbations. Relapsing forms of MS include individuals with secondary-progressive MS who continue to experience relapses or acute attacks.

PROPER USAGE

- Betaseron is injected subcutaneously (between the fat layer just under the skin and the muscles beneath) every other day. The physician or nurse will instruct you in the injection procedure, using a specially designed set of training materials. Do not attempt to inject yourself until you are sure that you understand the procedures.
- Betaseron is supplied with a pre-filled diluant syringe to which the medication needs to be added prior to injection; no refrigeration is necessary.
- Do not reuse needles or syringes. Dispose of the syringes as directed by your physician and keep them out of the reach of children.
- Since flu-like symptoms are a common side effect associated with at least the initial weeks of taking Betaseron, it is recommended that the medication be taken at bedtime. Taking acetaminophen (Tylenol®) or ibuprofen (Advil®) thirty minutes before each injection will also help to relieve the flu-like symptoms.
- Because injection site reactions (swelling, redness, discoloration, or pain) are relatively common, it is recommended that the sites be rotated according to a schedule provided for you by your physician. Injection site necrosis (skin damage), which occurs in about 5 percent of patients during the first four months of therapy, has been reported in post-marketing studies even after a year

of treatment. To avoid infection and other complications, you should report promptly any break in the skin, which may be associated with blue-black discoloration, swelling, or drainage of fluid from the injection site. Your physician will determine whether to continue treatment while the skin lesions are being treated.

PRECAUTIONS

- Betaseron should not be used during pregnancy or by any woman who is trying to become pregnant. Women taking Betaseron should use birth control measures at all times.
- Because of the potential of Betaseron to affect the functioning of the liver and thyroid gland, and to alter the levels of white blood cells, red blood cells, and platelets in a person's system, blood tests are recommended at regular intervals.
- During the clinical trial of interferon beta-1b, there were four suicide attempts and one completed suicide among those taking interferon beta-1b. Although there is no evidence that the suicide attempts were related to the medication itself, it is recommended that individuals with a history of severe depressive disorder be closely monitored while taking Betaseron.

POSSIBLE SIDE EFFECTS

- Common side effects include flu-like symptoms (fatigue, chills, fever, muscle aches, and sweating) and injection site reactions (swelling, redness, discoloration, and pain). Most of these symptoms tend to disappear over time. If they continue, become more severe, or cause significant discomfort, be sure to talk them over with your physician. Contact your physician if the injection sites become inflamed, hardened, or lumpy, and do not inject into any area that has become hardened or lumpy.

- Depression, including suicide attempts, has been reported by patients taking Betaseron. Common symptoms of depression are sadness, anxiety, loss of interest in daily activities, irritability, low self-esteem, guilt, poor concentration, indecisiveness, confusion, and eating and sleep disturbances. If you experience any of these symptoms for longer than a day or two, contact your physician promptly.

BETASERON SUPPORT PROGRAM
MS Pathways<sup>SM</sup>
1-800-788-1467
1-800-948-5777 (financial issues)
www.betaseron.com
www.mspathways.com

**Chemical Name:** Magnesium hydroxide (mag-*nee*-zhum hye-*drox*-ide)

*Brand Name:* Phillips' Milk of Magnesia (available in granule form in Canada, in wafer form in the U.S., and in powder or effervescent powder in the U.S. and Canada) is one of several brands of bulk-forming laxatives that are available over-the-counter.

*Generic Available:* No

*Description:* Magnesium hydroxide is an over-the-counter hyperosmotic laxative of the saline type that encourages bowel movements by drawing water into the bowel from surrounding body tissue. Saline hyperosmotic laxatives (often called "salts") are used for rapid emptying of the lower intestine and bowel. They are not to be used for the long-term management of constipation.

PROPER USAGE

- Laxatives are to be used to provide short-term relief only, unless otherwise directed by the nurse or physician who is helping you to manage your bowel symptoms. A regimen that includes a healthy diet containing roughage (whole grain breads and cereals, bran, fruit, and green, leafy vegetables), six to eight full glasses of liquids each day, and some form of daily exercise is most important in stimulating healthy bowel function.
- If your physician has recommended this laxative for management of constipation, follow his or her recommendations for its use. If you are treating yourself for constipation, follow the directions on the package insert. Results are often obtained 90 minutes to 3 hours after taking a hyperosmotic laxative. Be sure to consult your physician if you experience problems or do not get relief within a week.
- Each dose should be taken with 8 ounces or more of cold water or fruit juice. A second glass of water or juice with each dose is often recommended to prevent dehydration. If concerns about loss of bladder control keep you from drinking this amount of water, talk it over with the nurse or physician who is helping you manage your bowel and bladder symptoms.

PRECAUTIONS

- Do not take any type of laxative if you have signs of appendicitis or inflamed bowel (e.g., stomach or lower abdominal pain, cramping, bloating, soreness, nausea, or vomiting). Check with your physician as soon as possible.
- Do not take any laxative for more than 1 week unless you have been told to do so by your physician. Many people tend to overuse laxatives, which often leads to dependence on the laxative action to produce a bowel movement. Discuss the use of laxatives with your healthcare professional to ensure that the laxative is used effectively as part of a comprehensive, healthy bowel management regimen.

- Do not take any laxative within 2 hours of taking another medication because the desired effectiveness of the other medication may be reduced.
- Although laxatives are commonly used during pregnancy, some types are better than others. If you are pregnant, consult your physician about the best laxative for you to use.
- Some laxatives pass into breast milk. Although it is unlikely to cause problems for a nursing infant, be sure to let your physician know if you are using a laxative and breast-feeding at the same time.

POSSIBLE SIDE EFFECTS

- Side effects that may go away as your body adjusts to the medication and do not require medical attention unless they continue or are bothersome: cramping; diarrhea; gas; increased thirst.
- Unusual side effects that should be reported to your physician as soon as possible: confusion; dizziness; irregular heartbeat; muscle cramps, unusual tiredness or weakness.

**Chemical Name:** Meclizine (*mek*-li-zeen)

*Brand Name:* Antivert (U.S.); Bonamine (Canada)

*Generic Available:* Yes (U.S.)

*Description:* Meclizine is used to prevent and treat nausea, vomiting, and dizziness.

PRECAUTIONS

- This drug adds to the effects of alcohol and other central nervous system depressants (e.g., antihistamines, sedatives, tranquilizers, prescriptions pain medications, seizure medications, muscle relaxants, and sleeping medications), possibly causing drowsiness. Be sure that your physician knows if you are taking these or any other medications.
- Meclizine may cause dryness of the mouth. If dryness continues for more than 2 weeks, speak to your physician or dentist, since continuing dryness of the mouth may increase the risk of dental disease.
- This medication has not been shown to cause birth defects or other problems in humans. Studies in animals have shown that meclizine given in doses many times the usual human dose causes birth defects such as cleft palate.
- Although meclizine passes into breast milk, it has not been reported to cause problems in nursing babies. However, since this medication tends to decrease bodily secretions, it is possible that the flow of breast milk may be reduced in some women.

POSSIBLE SIDE EFFECTS

- Side effects that typically go away as your body adjusts to the medication and do not require medical attention unless they continue for more than 2 weeks or are bothersome: drowsiness*; blurred vision*; constipation*; difficult or painful urination; dizziness; dryness of mouth, nose, and throat; fast heartbeat; headache; loss of appetite; nervousness or restlessness; trouble sleeping; skin rash; upset stomach.

*Since it may be difficult to distinguish between certain common symptoms of MS and some side effects of meclizine, be sure to consult your healthcare professional if an abrupt change of this type occurs.

**Chemical Name:** Methenamine (meth-**en**-a-meen)

*Brand Name:* Hiprex; Mandelamine (U.S.); Hip-Rex; Mandelamine (Canada)

*Generic Available:* No

*Description:* Methenamine is an anti-infective medication that is used to help prevent infections of the urinary tract. It is usually prescribed on a long-term basis for individuals with a history of repeated or chronic urinary tract infections.

PROPER USAGE

- Before you start taking this medication, check your urine with phenaphthazine paper or another test to see if it is acidic. Your urine must be acidic (pH 5.5 or below) for this medicine to work properly. Consult your healthcare professional about possible changes in your diet if necessary to increase the acidity of your urine (e.g., avoiding citrus fruits and juices, milk and other dairy products, antacids; eating more protein and foods such as cranberries and cranberry juice with added vitamin C, prunes, or plums).

PRECAUTIONS

- The effects of methenamine in pregnancy have not been studied in either humans or animals. Individual case reports have not shown that this medication causes birth defects or other problems in humans.
- Methenamine passes into breast milk but has not been reported to cause problems in nursing infants.

POSSIBLE SIDE EFFECTS

- Side effects that typically go away as your body adjusts to the medication and do not require medical attention unless they continue or are bothersome: nausea; vomiting.
- Unusual side effect that should be reported immediately to your physician: skin rash.

**Chemical Name:** Methylprednisolone (meth-ill-pred-*niss*-oh-lone)

*Brand Name:* Solu-Medrol (U.S. and Canada)

*Generic Available:* Yes (U.S. and Canada)

*Description:* Methylprednisolone is one of a group of corticosteroids (cortisone-like medications) that are used to relieve inflammation in different parts of the body. Corticosteroids are used in MS for the management of acute exacerbations because they have the capacity to close the damaged blood-brain barrier and reduce inflammation in the central nervous system. Although methylprednisolone is among the most commonly used corticosteroids in MS, it is only one of several possibilities. Other commonly used corticosteroids include dexamethazone, prednisone, betamethasone, and prednisolone. The following information pertains to all of the various corticosteroids.

PROPER USAGE

- Most neurologists treating MS believe that high-dose corticosteroids given intravenously are the most effective treatment for an exacerbation, although the exact protocol for the drug's use may differ somewhat from one treating physician to another. Patients generally receive a 4-day course of treatment (either in the hospital or as an outpatient), with doses of the medication spread throughout the day. This high-dose, intravenous steroid treatment is then typically followed by a gradually tapering dose of an oral corticosteroid (see Prednisone®).

PRECAUTIONS

- Since corticosteroids can stimulate the appetite and increase water retention, it is advisable to follow a low-salt and/or potassium-rich diet and watch your caloric intake. Your physician will make specific dietary recommendations for you.
- Corticosteroids can lower your resistance to infection and make any infection that you get more difficult to treat. Contact your physician if you notice any sign of infection, such as sore throat, fever, coughing, or sneezing.

- Avoid close contact with anyone who has chicken pox or measles. Tell your physician right away if you think you have been exposed to either of these illnesses. Do not have any immunizations after you stop taking this medication until you have consulted your physician. People living in your home should not have the oral polio vaccine while you are being treated with corticosteroids since they might pass the polio virus on to you.
- Corticosteroids may affect the blood sugar levels of diabetic patients. If you notice a change in your blood or urine sugar tests, be sure to speak to your physician.
- The risk of birth defects for women taking corticosteroids is not known. Overuse of corticosteroids during pregnancy may slow the growth of the infant after birth. Animal studies have demonstrated that corticosteroids cause birth defects.
- Corticosteroids pass into breast milk and may slow the infant's growth. If you are nursing or plan to nurse, be sure to discuss this with your physician. It may be necessary for you to stop nursing while taking this medication.
- Corticosteroids may produce mood changes and/or mood swings of varying intensity. These mood alterations can vary from relatively mild to extremely intense, and can vary in a single individual from one course of treatment to another. Neither the patient nor the physician can predict with any certainty whether the corticosteroids are likely to precipitate these mood alterations. If you have a history of mood disorders (depression or bipolar disorder, for example), be sure to share this information with your physician. If you begin to experience mood changes or swings that feel unmanageable, contact your physician so that a decision can be made about whether or not you need an additional medication to help you until the mood alterations subside.

POSSIBLE SIDE EFFECTS
- Side effects that may go away as your body adjusts to the medication and do not require medical attention unless they continue or are bothersome: increased appetite; indigestion; nervousness or restlessness; trouble sleeping; headache; increased sweating; unusual increase in hair growth on body or face.
- Less common side effects that should be reported as soon as possible to your physician: severe mood changes or mood swings; decreased or blurred vision*; frequent urination*.
- Additional side effects that can result from the prolonged use of corticosteroids and should be reported to your physician: acne or other skin problems; swelling of the face; swelling of the feet or lower legs; rapid weight gain; pain in the hips or other joints (caused by bone cell degeneration); bloody or black, tarry stools; elevated blood pressure; markedly increased thirst (with increased urination indicative of diabetes mellitus); menstrual irregularities; unusual bruising of the skin; thin, shiny skin; hair loss; muscle cramps or pain. Once you stop this medication after taking it for a long period of time, it may take several months for your body to readjust.

*Since it may be difficult to distinguish between certain common symptoms of MS and some side effects of methylprednisolone, be sure to consult your healthcare professional if an abrupt change of this type occurs.

**Chemical Name:** Mineral oil

Mineral oil is available in a variety of brands in the U.S. and Canada.

*Generic Available:* Yes

*Description:* Mineral oil is a lubricant laxative that is taken by mouth. It encourages bowel movements by coating the bowel and the stool with a waterproof film that helps to retain moisture in the stool.

PROPER USAGE

- Laxatives are to be used to provide short-term relief only, unless otherwise directed by the nurse or physician who is helping you to manage your bowel symptoms. A regimen that includes a healthy diet containing roughage (whole grain breads and cereals, bran, fruit, and green, leafy vegetables), six to eight full glasses of liquids each day, and some form of daily exercise is most important in stimulating healthy bowel function.
- If your physician has recommended this type of laxative for management of constipation, follow his or her recommendations for its use. If you are treating yourself for constipation, follow the directions on the package insert. Mineral oil is usually taken at bedtime because it takes 6 to 8 hours to produce results. Be sure to consult your physician if you experience problems or do not get relief within a week.
- Mineral oil should not be taken within 2 hours of mealtime because the mineral oil may interfere with food digestion and the absorption of important nutrients.
- Mineral oil should not be taken within two hours of taking a stool softener (see Docusate®) because the stool softener may increase the amount of mineral oil that is absorbed by the body.

PRECAUTIONS

- Do not take any type of laxative if you have signs of appendicitis or inflamed bowel (e.g., stomach or lower abdominal pain, cramping, bloating, soreness,

nausea, or vomiting). Check with your physician as soon as possible.
- Do not take any laxative for more than one week unless you have been told to do so by your physician. Many people tend to overuse laxative products, which often leads to dependence on the laxative action to produce a bowel movement. Discuss the use of laxatives with your healthcare professional to ensure that the laxative is used effectively as part of a comprehensive, healthy bowel management regimen.
- Mineral oil should not be used very often or for long periods of time. Its gradual build-up in body tissues can cause problems, and may interfere with the body's absorption of important nutrients and vitamins A, D, E, and K.
- Do not take any laxative within 2 hours of taking another medication because the desired effectiveness of the other medication may be reduced.
- Mineral oil should not be used during pregnancy because it may interfere with absorption of nutrients in the mother and, if used for prolonged periods, cause severe bleeding in the newborn infant.
- Be sure to let your physician know if you are using a laxative and breast-feeding at the same time.

POSSIBLE SIDE EFFECTS

- Uncommon side effect that usually does not need medical attention: skin irritation around the rectal area.

**Chemical Name:** Mitoxantrone for injection concentrate (mye-toe-*zan*-trone)

*Brand Name:* Novantrone (U.S. and Canada)

*Generic Available:* No

*Description:* Novantrone belongs to the general group of medicines called antineoplastics. Prior to its approval for use in MS, it was used only to treat certain forms of cancer. It acts in MS by suppressing the activity of T cells, B cells, and macrophages that are thought to lead the attack on the myelin sheath.

The use of Novantrone for the treatment of MS has been evaluated in a series of European studies over a period of ten years. In a randomized, placebo-controlled, multicenter clinical trial involving patients with secondary-progressive or progressive-relapsing disease, participants received 12mg/m² of Novantrone by short IV infusion once every three months for 24 months. Novantrone was found to delay the time to first treated relapse and time to disability progression. It also reduced the number of treated relapses and number of new lesions detected by magnetic resonance imaging.

### Approval by the U.S. Food and Drug Administration (FDA)

- Based on findings from these studies, the FDA approved Novantrone in for reducing neurologic disability and/or the frequency of clinical relapses (attacks) in:
  - Patients with secondary progressive MS (disease that has changed from relapsing-remitting to progressive at a variable rate)
  - Progressive-relapsing MS (disease characterized by gradual increase in disability from onset with clear, acute relapses along the way)
  - Worsening relapsing-remitting MS (disease characterized by clinical attacks without complete remission, resulting in a step-wise worsening of disability
  - *Novantrone has not been approved for the treatment of primary-progressive MS* (characterized by progression from disease onset with no acute attacks or remissions)

### Proper Usage

- *Evaluation of cardiac output is necessary before treatment is started.* The drug should be used only in those with normal cardiac function, once every three months at a dose of 12mg/m². Periodic cardiac monitoring is required throughout the treatment period.
- The lifetime cumulative dose is limited to 140 mg/m² (approximately 8 to 12 doses over two to three years) because of possible cardiac toxicity.
- Because Novantrone can increase the risk for infection by decreasing the number of protective white blood cells, blood counts and liver function should be evaluated prior to each dose.

### Precautions

- It is important that your doctor check your progress at regular intervals to make sure that this medicine is working properly and to check for unwanted effects.
- While being treated with this medication, and during the period following treatment, do not have any immunizations (vaccinations) with live virus vaccines without your doctor's approval. Mitoxantrone may lower your body's resistance to infection, making you susceptible to the infection that the immunization is designed to help you avoid. Neither you nor anyone in your household should take the oral polio vaccine.
- If possible, avoid people with infections. Contact your physician if you think you are getting an infection, or if you get a fever or chills, cough or hoarseness, lower back or side pain, or painful or difficult urination.
- When receiving Novantrone, it is important for your physician to know if you are taking any of the following:
  - Amphotericin B by injection
  - Antithyroid agents

- Azathioprine
- Chloramphenicol
- Colchicine
- Flucytosine
- Ganciclovir
- Plicamycin
- Probenecid
- Sulfinpyrazone
- Zidovudine

or if you have previously been treated with:
- radiation
- other cancer medications

- The presence of other medical problems may affect the use of Novantrone. Let your doctor know if you have any of the following:
  - chicken pox or recent exposure to it
  - herpes zoster (shingles)
  - gout or history of gout
  - kidney stones
  - heart disease
  - liver disease
- The fluid for infusion is dark blue and may cause your urine to become blue-green in color for a period of 24 hours after each administration. The whites of the eyes may also appear bluish in color.
- Tell your doctor if you are pregnant or intending to have children. This medicine may cause birth defects if either the man or woman is receiving it at the time of conception. A pregnancy test is recommended prior to each treatment for women of child-bearing age. Many medications of this type can cause permanent sterility. Be sure you have discussed this with your physician before taking this medication.
- Novantrone is excreted in human milk. Breastfeeding should be discontinued before a woman starts treatment.
- A higher incidence of leukemia has been reported in cancer patients, previously treated with chemotherapy, who were then treated with higher doses of Novantrone than is prescribed for treating MS.

POSSIBLE SIDE EFFECTS
- Side effects that may go away as your body adjusts to the medication and do not require medical attention unless they continue or are bothersome: nausea, temporary hair loss, and menstrual disorders in females.
- Side effects that should be reported to your physician as soon as possible: fever or chills, lower back or side pain; painful or difficult urination; swelling of feet and lower legs; black, tarry stools, cough or shortness of breath; sores in mouth and on lips, stomach pain.

NOVANTRONE SUPPORT PROGRAM:
1-800-566-8268
www.immunex.com

**Chemical Name:** Modafinil (moe-*daf*-i-nil)

*Brand Name:* Provigil (U.S.)

*Generic Available:* Alertec (Canada)

*Description:* Modafinil is a wakefulness-promoting agent approved for the treatment of narcolepsy. While it does not cure narcolepsy, it helps people stay awake during the day. In 2000, the manufacturer, Cephalon, conducted a study of modafinil in people with MS to evaluate it as a potential treatment for MS-related fatigue. Seventy-two people with different forms of MS took two different doses of modafinil and inactive placebo over 9 weeks, and self-evaluated their fatigue levels using standard fatigue and sleepiness scales. Participants reported feeling least fatigued while taking a lower dose of modafinil, and there was a statistically significant difference in fatigue scores for the lower dose versus placebo. The higher dose of modafinil was not reported to be effective.

## PROPER USAGE

- The usual dosage for the management of fatigue in MS is 100 to 200 mg daily, taken in the earlier part of the day to avoid sleep disturbance. If you miss a dose of modafinil and remember it before noon the next day, take the missed dose as soon as possible. If you remember it after noon, skip the missed dose so that the medication will not make it difficult for you to sleep at night.

## PRECAUTIONS

- The precautions listed here pertain to the use of this medication as a treatment for narcolepsy. Since modafinil has not been approved by the FDA for use in multiple sclerosis, there are no precautions specific to MS-related uses of the drug.
- Tell your physician if you have ever had an unusual or allergic reaction to any other nervous system stimulant such as Ritalin® or Dexedrine®.
- This medication may cause some people to become dizzy or confused, or to have blurred vision or difficulty controlling movements. Make sure you know how you react to this medication before driving a car or engaging in any other potentially dangerous activity.
- If you think that the modafinil is not working properly after you have taken it for a few weeks, speak to your physician. Do not increase the dose.
- If you are using a medication for birth control such as birth control pills or implants, the birth control product may not work effectively in combination with modafinil or for one month after you have stopped taking modafinil. During this time, an additional form of birth control should be used.
- Studies of the effects of modafinil in pregnancy have not been done in humans. Studies in animals, however, suggest that the use of modafinil may result in unsuccessful pregnancies or cause birth defects. Before taking this medication, make sure your physician knows if you are pregnant or planning to become pregnant.
- It is not known whether modafinil passes into breast milk. If you are taking modafinil and wish to breastfeed, you should discuss this with your physician.
- When taking modafinil, it is especially important for your physician to know if you are taking any of the following medications that may add to the stimulating effects of modafinil (such as irritability, nervousness, trembling or shaking, insomnia):

  - Amantadine
  - Amphetamines
  - Bupropion (e.g., Wellbutrin®; Zyban®)
  - Medicine for asthma or other breathing problems
  - Medicine for colds, sinus problems, hay fever (including nose drops or sprays)
  - Methylphenidate (e.g., Ritalin®)

  or, any of the following drugs whose action or effectiveness might be affected by the modafinil:

  - Cyclosporine
  - Diazepam (e.g., Valium®)
  - Phenytoin (e.g., Dilantin®)
  - Propranolol (e.g., Inderal®)
  - Warfarin (e.g., Coumadin®)

  or, any of the following drugs that may cause problems when combined with modafinil:

  - Monoamine oxidase (MAO) inhibitors
  - Tricyclic antidepressants (e.g., Elavil®; Anafranil®; Tofranil®; Aventyl®; Pamelor®)

  or the following substance that may add to the stimulating effects of modafinil:

  - Cocaine

## POSSIBLE SIDE EFFECTS

- The side effects listed here pertain to the use of modafinil as a treatment for narcolepsy. There are no reports at the present time of the side effects associated with the use of this drug in the treatment of MS-related fatigue.
- Side effects that may go away as your body adjusts to the medication and do not require medical attention unless they continue or are bothersome: anxiety; headache; nausea; nervousness; trouble sleeping; decrease in appetite; diarrhea; dryness of mouth; flushing or redness of skin; muscle stiffness*; stuffy or runny nose; tingling*; burning, trembling, or shaking*; vomiting.
- Rare side effects that should be reported as soon as possible to your physician: blurred vision* or other vision changes; chills or fever; clumsiness or unsteadiness*, confusion; dizziness or fainting; increased thirst and increased urination; depression; problems with memory*; rapidly changing moods; shortness of breath; difficulty with urination; uncontrolled movements in the face, mouth, or tongue.

*Since it may be difficult to distinguish between certain common symptoms of MS and some side effects of modafinil, be sure to consult your physician if an abrupt change of this type occurs.

**Chemical Name:** Nitrofurantoin (nye-troe-fyoor-*an*-toyn)

*Brand Name:* Macrodantin (U.S. and Canada)

*Generic Available:* No

*Description:* Nitrofurantoin is an anti-infective that is used primarily to treat urinary tract infections.

## PROPER USAGE

- Nitrofurantoin should be taken with food or milk to lessen stomach upset and to promote your body's absorption of the medication.
- Finish the full course of treatment prescribed by your doctor and avoid missing doses. Even if your symptoms disappear after a few days, stopping this medication prematurely may result in a return of the symptoms.
- If you miss a dose of this medication, take it as soon as possible. However, if it is almost time for your next dose, skip the missed dose and go back to your regular dosing schedule. Do not double dose.
- The use of nitrofurantoin may cause your urine to become rust-yellow or brownish. This change does not require medical treatment and does not need to be reported to your physician.

## PRECAUTIONS

- Nitrofurantoin can interact with, or alter the action of, a variety of other medications you may be taking. It is very important to let your physician know about all the medications you are taking so that necessary substitutions or dosage adjustments can be made.
- If you will be taking this medication over an extended period of time, your doctor will need to check your progress at regular visits. If your symptoms do not improve within a few days, or become worse, consult your physician.
- Individuals with diabetes may find that this medication alters the results of some urine sugar tests. Consult with your physician before changing your diet or the dose of your diabetes medicine.
- Certain medical conditions may affect the use of nitrofurantoin. Be sure to alert your physician about any medical conditions you have, especially glucose-6-phosphate dehydrogenase (G6PD) deficiency, kidney disease, or lung disease.
- Because nitrofurantoin may cause problems in infants, it should not be used by

a woman who is within a week or two of her delivery date, or during labor and delivery.

- Nitrofurantoin passes into breast milk in small amounts and may cause problems in nursing babies (especially those with glucose-6-phosphate dehydrogenase [G6PD] deficiency).

POSSIBLE SIDE EFFECTS

- Side effects that may go away as your body adjusts to the medication and do not require medical attention unless they continue or are bothersome: abdominal or stomach pain; diarrhea, loss of appetite, nausea, or vomiting.
- Rare side effects that should be reported to your doctor immediately: chest pain; chills; cough; fever; trouble breathing; dizziness; headache; numbness, tingling, or burning of face or mouth*; unusual weakness or tiredness*; itching; joint pain; skin rash; yellow eyes or skin.

*Since it may be difficult to distinguish between certain common symptoms of MS and some side effects of nitrofurantoin, be sure to consult your healthcare professional if an abrupt change of this type occurs.

**Chemical Name:** Nortriptyline (nor-*trip*-ti-leen)

*Brand Name:* Pamelor (U.S.) Aventyl (Canada)

*Generic Available:* Yes (U.S.)

*Description:* Nortriptyline is a tricyclic antidepressant used to treat mental depression. In multiple sclerosis, it is frequently used to treat painful parsthesias in the arms and legs (e.g., burning sensations, pins and needles, stabbing pains) caused by damage to the pain regulating pathways of the brain and spinal cord.

Note: Other tricyclic antidepressants are also used for the management of neurologic pain symptoms: amitriptyline ( Elavil®—U.S. and Canada), clomipramine (Anafranil®—U.S. and Canada), desipramine (Norpramin®—U.S. and Canada), doxepin (Sinequan®—U.S. and Canada), imipramine (Tofranil®—U.S. and Canada), and trimipramine (U.S. and Canada). Although each of these medications is given in different dosage levels, the precautions and side effects listed here for nortriptyline apply to these other tricyclic medications as well.

PRECAUTIONS

- Nortriptyline will add to the effects of alcohol and other central nervous system depressants (e.g., antihistamines, sedatives, tranquilizers, prescription pain medications, seizure medications, muscle relaxants, or sleeping medications), possibly causing drowsiness. Be sure that your physician knows if you are taking these or any other medications.
- This medication causes dryness of the mouth. Because continuing dryness of the mouth may increase the risk of dental disease, alert your dentist that you are taking nortriptyline.
- This medication may cause your skin to be more sensitive to sunlight than it normally is. Even brief exposure to sunlight may cause a rash, itching, redness or other discoloration of the skin, or severe sunburn.
- This medication may affect blood sugar levels of diabetic individuals. If you notice a change in the results of your blood or urine sugar tests, check with your doctor.
- Do not stop taking this medication without consulting your doctor. The doctor may want you to reduce the amount you are taking gradually in order to reduce the possibility of withdrawal symptoms such as headache, nausea, and/or an overall feeling of discomfort.

- Studies of nortriptyline have not been done in pregnant women. However, there have been reports of newborns suffering from muscle spasms or heart, breathing, or urinary problems when their mothers had taken tricyclic antidepressants immediately before delivery. Studies in animals have indicated the possibility of unwanted effects on the fetus.
- Tricyclics pass into breast milk. Only doxepin (Sinequan®) has been reported to cause drowsiness in the nursing baby.

POSSIBLE SIDE EFFECTS
- Side effects that may go away as your body adjusts to the medication and do not require medical attention unless they continue for more than 2 weeks or are bothersome: dryness of mouth; constipation*; increased appetite and weight gain; dizziness; drowsiness*; decreased sexual ability*; headache; nausea; unusual tiredness or weakness*; unpleasant taste; diarrhea; heartburn; increased sweating; vomiting.
- Uncommon side effects that should be reported to the doctor as soon as possible: blurred vision*; confusion or delirium; difficulty speaking or swallowing*; eye pain*; fainting; hallucinations; loss of balance control*; nervousness or restlessness; problems urinating*; shakiness or trembling; stiffness of arms and legs*.
- Rare side effects that should be reported to the doctor as soon as possible: anxiety; breast enlargement in males and females; hair loss; inappropriate secretion of milk in females; increased sensitivity to sunlight; irritability; muscle twitching; red or brownish spots on the skin; buzzing or other unexplained sounds in the ears; rash; itching; sore throat and fever; swelling of face and tongue; weakness*; yellow skin.
- Symptoms of acute overdose: confusion; convulsions; severe drowsiness*;

enlarged pupils; unusual heartbeat; fever; hallucinations; restlessness and agitation; shortness of breath; unusual tiredness or weakness; vomiting.

*Since it may be difficult to distinguish between certain common symptoms of MS and some side effects of nortriptyline, be sure to consult your healthcare professional if an abrupt change of this type occurs.

**Chemical Name:** Oxybutynin (ox-i-*byoo*-ti-nin)

*Brand Name:* Ditropan (U.S. and Canada)

*Generic Available:* Yes (U.S.)

*Description:* Oxybutynin is an antispasmodic that helps decrease muscle spasms of the bladder and the frequent urge to urinate caused by these spasms.

PROPER USAGE
- This medication is usually taken with water on an empty stomach, but your physician may want you to take it with food or milk to lessen stomach upset.

PRECAUTIONS
- This medication adds to the effects of alcohol and other central nervous system depressants (such as antihistamines, sedatives, tranquilizers, prescription pain medications, seizure medications, and muscle relaxants). Be sure that your physician knows if you are taking these or any other medications.
- This medication may cause your eyes to become more sensitive to light.
- Oxybutynin may cause drying of the mouth. Since continuing dryness of the mouth can increase the risk of dental disease, alert your dentist if you are taking oxybutynin.
- Oxybutynin has not been studied in pregnant women. It has not been shown

to cause birth defects or other problems in animal studies.

- This medication has not been reported to cause problems in nursing babies. However, since it tends to decrease body secretions, oxybutynin may reduce the flow of breast milk.

POSSIBLE SIDE EFFECTS

- Side effects that typically go away as your body adjusts to the medication and do not require medical attention unless they continue for a few weeks or are bothersome: constipation*; decreased sweating; unusual drowsiness*; dryness of mouth, nose, and throat; blurred vision*; decreased flow of breast milk; decreased sexual ability*; difficulty swallowing*; headache; increased light sensitivity; nausea or vomiting; trouble sleeping; unusual tiredness or weakness*.
- Less common side effects that should be reported to your physician immediately: difficulty in urination*.

*Since it may be difficult to distinguish between certain common symptoms of MS and some side effects of oxybutynin, be sure to consult your healthcare professional if an abrupt change of this type occurs.

**Chemical Name:** Oxybutynin (ox-i-*byoo*-ti-nin)

*Brand Name:* Oxytrol (Oxybutynin Transdermal System)

*Generic Available:* Yes (U.S. and Canada)

*Description:* Oxybutynin is an antispasmodic that helps decrease muscle spasms of the bladder and the frequent urge to urinate caused by these spasms. Oxytrol is a skin patch that delivers the active ingredient, oxybutynin, through your skin and into your bloodstream.

PROPER USAGE

- A new patch is applied two times per week (every 3 to 4 days), with each patch worn until it is time to replace it with the next one. Only one patch is worn at a time.
- The patch is placed on clean, dry, and smooth area of the abdomen, hips, or buttocks.
- The patch should not be put at the waistline, where it will be rubbed by tight clothing, or on areas of skin that have been treated with creams or oils that will prevent the patch from sticking.

PRECAUTIONS

- This medication adds to the effects of alcohol and other central nervous system depressants (such as antihistamines, sedatives, tranquilizers, prescription pain medications, seizure medications, and muscle relaxants). Be sure that your physician knows if you are taking these or any other medications.
- This medication may cause your eyes to become more sensitive to light.
- Oxybutynin may cause drying of the mouth. Since continuing dryness of the mouth can increase the risk of dental disease, alert your dentist if you are taking oxybutynin.
- Oxybutynin has not been studied in pregnant women. It has not been shown to cause birth defects or other problems in animal studies. Any woman who wishes to become pregnant while using this medication should discuss it with her physician.
- It is not known whether oxybutynin is excreted in breast milk. Since it tends to decrease body secretions, oxybutynin may reduce the flow of breast milk. Any woman who wishes to breastfeed while using this medication should discuss it with her physician.

POSSIBLE SIDE EFFECTS

- Side effects that typically go away as your body adjusts to the medication and do not require medical attention unless they continue for a few weeks or are bothersome: constipation*; decreased sweating; unusual drowsiness*; dryness of mouth, nose, and throat; blurred vision*; decreased flow of breast milk; decreased sexual ability*; difficulty swallowing*; headache; increased light sensitivity; nausea or vomiting; trouble sleeping; unusual tiredness or weakness*.

- Less common side effects that should be reported to your physician immediately: difficulty in urination*.

*Since it may be difficult to distinguish between certain common symptoms of MS and some side effects of oxybutynin, be sure to consult your healthcare professional if an abrupt change of this type occurs.

**Chemical Name:** Oxybutynin (ox-i-*byoo*-ti-nin) chloride—extended release

*Brand Name:* Ditropan XL (U.S. and Canada)

*Generic Available:* No

*Description:* This form of oxybutynin is an extended-release antispasmodic that is formulated to help decrease muscle spasms of the bladder and the frequent urge to urinate caused by these spasms.

PROPER USAGE

- The tablet is to be swallowed whole, once a day, with liquids. It can be taken with or without food. Because the medication is contained within a nonabsorbable shell that is designed to release the drug at a controlled rate, the tablet should not be chewed, crushed, or divided. The shell is routinely eliminated from the body in the stool.

PRECAUTIONS

- This medication adds to the effects of alcohol and other central nervous sys-

tem depressants (such as antihistamines, sedatives, tranquilizers, prescription pain medications, seizure medications, and muscle relaxants). Be sure that your physician knows if you are taking these or any other medications.

- Oxybytynin, like all anticholinergic medications, can induce drowsiness and/or blurred vision.
- Oxybutynin, like all anticholinergic medications, can cause heat prostration (fever and heat stroke due to decreased sweating) when taken in very hot weather.
- Oxybutynin may cause drying of the mouth. Since continuing dryness of the mouth can increase the risk of dental disease, alert your dentist if you are taking oxybutynin.
- Oxybutynin has not been studied in pregnant women. It has not been shown to cause birth defects or other problems in animal studies. Do not take this medication while pregnant unless specifically instructed to do so by your physician.
- This medication has not been reported to cause problems in nursing babies. However, since it tends to decrease body secretions, oxybutynin may reduce the flow of breast milk. Do not take this medication while nursing without discussing it with your physician.

POSSIBLE SIDE EFFECTS

- Side effects that typically go away as your body adjusts to the medication and do not require medical attention unless they continue for a few weeks or are bothersome: constipation*; decreased sweating; unusual drowsiness*; dryness of mouth, nose, and throat; blurred vision*; decreased flow of breast milk; difficulty swallowing*; headache; increased light sensitivity; nausea or vomiting; unusual tiredness or weakness*.
- Less common side effects that should be reported immediately to your physician

include: urinary retention*, dehydration, cardiac arrhythmia.

*Since it may be difficult to distinguish between certain common symptoms of MS and some side effects of oxybutynin, be sure to consult your healthcare professional if an abrupt change of this type occurs.

**Chemical Name:** Papaverine (pa-*pav*-er-een)

*Brand Name:* None

*Generic Available:* Yes (U.S. and Canada)

*Description:* Papaverine belongs to a group of medicines called vasodilators, which cause blood vessels to expand, thereby increasing blood flow. Papaverine is used in MS to treat erectile dysfunction. When papaverine is injected into the penis, it produces an erection by increasing blood flow to the penis.

PROPER USAGE

- Papaverine should never be used as a sexual aid by men who are not impotent. If improperly used, this medication can cause permanent damage to the penis.
- Papaverine is available by prescription and should be used only as directed by your physician, who will instruct you in the proper way to give yourself an injection so that it is simple and essentially pain-free.

PRECAUTIONS

- Do not use more of this medication or use it more often than it has been prescribed for you. Using too much of this medicine will result in a condition called *priapism*, in which the erection lasts too long and does not resolve when it should. Permanent damage to the penis can occur if blood flow to the penis is cut off for too long a period of time.
- Examine your penis regularly for possible lumps near the injection sites or for

curvature of the penis. These may be signs that unwanted tissue is growing (called fibrosis), which should be examined by your physician.

POSSIBLE SIDE EFFECTS

- Side effects that you should report to your physician so that he or she can adjust the dosage or change the medication: bruising at the injection site; mild burning along the penis; difficulty ejaculating; swelling at the injection site.
- Rare side effect that requires immediate treatment: erection continuing for more than 4 hours. If you cannot be seen immediately by your physician, you should go to the emergency room for prompt treatment.

**Chemical Name:** Paroxetine (pa-*rox*-uh-teen)

*Brand Name:* Paxil (U.S. and Canada)

*Generic Available:* No

*Description:* Paroxetine is used to treat mental depression and some types of anxiety.

PROPER USAGE

- Paroxetine may be taken with or without food, on an empty or full stomach.

PRECAUTIONS

- It may take up to 4 weeks or longer for you to feel the beneficial effects of this medication.
- Your physician should monitor your progress at regularly scheduled visits in order to adjust the dose and help reduce any side effects.
- This medication could add to the effects of alcohol and other central nervous system depressants (e.g., antihistamines, sedatives, tranquilizers, sleeping medicine, prescription pain medicine, barbiturates, seizure medications, and muscle

relaxants). Be sure that your physician knows if you are taking these or any other medications.

- Paroxetine may cause dryness of the mouth. If your mouth continues to feel dry for more than 2 weeks, check with your physician or dentist. Continuing dryness of the mouth may increase the risk of dental disease.
- This medication may cause you to become drowsy.
- Studies have not been done in pregnant women. Studies in animals have shown that paroxetine may cause miscarriages and decreased survival rates when given in doses that are many times higher than the human dose.
- Paroxetine passes into breast milk but has not been shown to cause any problems in nursing infants.

POSSIBLE SIDE EFFECTS

- Side effects that typically go away as your body adjusts to the medication and do not require medical attention unless they continue for several weeks or are bothersome: decrease in sexual drive or ability*; headache; nausea; problems urinating*; decreased or increased appetite; unusual tiredness or weakness*; tremor*; trouble sleeping; anxiety; agitation; nervousness or restlessness; changes in vision, including blurred vision*; fast or irregular heartbeat; tingling, burning, or prickly sensations*; vomiting.
- Unusual side effects that should be discussed with your physician as soon as possible: agitation; lightheadedness or fainting; muscle pain or weakness; skin rash; mood or behavior changes.

*Since it may be difficult to distinguish between certain common symptoms of MS and some side effects of paroxetine, be sure

to consult your healthcare professional if an abrupt change of this type occurs.

**Chemical Name:** Pemoline (*pem*-oh-leen)

*Brand Name:* Cylert (U.S. and Canada)

*Generic Available:* No

*Description:* Pemoline is a mild central nervous system stimulant that has been used primarily to treat children with attention deficit hyperactivity disorder and adults with narcolepsy. It is used in multiple sclerosis to relieve certain types of fatigue.

PROPER USAGE

- As directed by the Food and Drug Administration, Abbott Laboratories, the manufacturer of Cylert, has recommended evaluation of liver function prior to starting this medication, followed by bi-weekly liver function evaluations while the drug is being used. (Note: No liver failure has been reported in anyone with MS; however, extra care should be taken when this medication is used in combination with other drugs that may potentially harm the liver, e.g., the interferons, or carbamazepine [Tegretol®].) The Medical Advisory Board of the National MS Society recognizes the issues raised by the FDA, but also supports the clear benefit of pemoline for many individuals with MS and associated nonexertional fatigue.
- The usual starting dose for the treatment of fatigue in MS is 18.75 mgs each morning for 1 week. If necessary, to manage the fatigue, the dosage can be gradually increased in increments of 18.75 mgs and spread out over the early part of the day. To maximize the medication's effectiveness and minimize sleep disturbance, it should all be taken before mid-afternoon. The maximum dose of this medication is not known. Some individuals feel jittery or uncomfortable taking more than the minimum dose; others tolerate

higher doses without discomfort. Typically, the drug is not prescribed at levels over 100 to 140 mgs per day for MS-related fatigue.

PRECAUTIONS

- Pemoline can increase hypertension. It should not be taken if you have angina and/or known coronary artery disease.
- If you are taking pemoline in large doses for a long time, do not stop taking it without consulting your physician. Your physician may want you to reduce the amount you are taking gradually.
- This drug may interact with the effects of alcohol and other central nervous system depressants (e.g., antihistamines, sedatives, tranquilizers, prescription pain medications, seizure medications, muscle relaxants, and sleeping medications). Be sure your physician knows if you are taking these or any other medications.
- Pemoline may cause some people to become dizzy or less alert than they are normally.
- If you have been using this medicine for a long time and think you may have become mentally or physically dependent on it, check with your physician. Some signs of dependence on pemoline are a strong desire or need to continue taking the medicine; a need to increase the dose to receive the effects of the medicine; withdrawal side effects such as mental depression, unusual behavior, unusual tiredness or weakness after the medication is stopped.
- Pemoline has not been shown to cause birth defects or other problems in humans. Studies in animals given large doses of pemoline have shown that it causes an increase in stillbirths and decreased survival of the offspring.
- It is not known if pemoline is excreted in breast milk.

POSSIBLE SIDE EFFECTS

- Side effects of this medication have not been studied in adults. Side effects that have been reported by some adults in clinical practice include insomnia; elevated heart rate; nervousness; agitation; loss of appetite and weight loss; gastrointestinal upset, including constipation and diarrhea; hallucinations.

**Chemical Name:** Phenazopyridine (fen-*az*-oh-peer-i-deen)

*Brand Name:* Pyridium (U.S. and Canada)

*Generic Available:* Yes (U.S.)

*Description:* Phenazopyridine is used to relieve the pain, burning, and discomfort caused by urinary tract infections. It is not an antibiotic and will not cure the infection itself. This medication is available in the U.S. only with a prescription; it is available in Canada without a prescription. The medication comes in tablet form.

PRECAUTIONS

- The medication causes the urine to turn reddish orange. This effect is harmless and goes away after you stop taking phenazopyridine.
- It is best not to wear soft contact lenses while taking this medication; phenazopyridine may cause permanent discoloration or staining of soft lenses.
- Check with your physician if symptoms such as bloody urine, difficult or painful urination, frequent urge to urinate, or sudden decrease in the amount of urine appear or become worse while you are taking this medication.
- Phenazopyridine has not been studied in pregnant women. It has not been shown to cause birth defects in animal studies.
- It is not known whether this medication passes into breast milk. It has not been reported to cause problems in nursing babies.

POSSIBLE SIDE EFFECTS

- Uncommon side effects that typically go away as your body adjusts to the medication and do not require medical attention unless they continue or are bothersome: dizziness; headache; indigestion; stomach cramps or pain.
- Unusual side effects that should be reported to your physician: blue or blue-purple color of skin; fever and confusion; shortness of breath; skin rash; sudden decrease in amount of urine; swelling of face, fingers, feet and/or lower legs; unusual weakness or tiredness*; weight gain; yellow eyes or skin.

*Since it may be difficult to distinguish between certain common symptoms of MS and some side effects of phenazopyridine, be sure to consult your healthcare professional if an abrupt change of this type occurs.

**Chemical Name:** Phenytoin (*fen*-i-toyn)

*Brand Name:* Dilantin (U.S. and Canada)

*Generic Available:* Yes (U.S.)

*Description:* Phenytoin is one of a group of hydantoin anticonvulsants that are used most commonly in the management of seizures in epilepsy. It is used in MS to manage painful dysesthesias (most commonly trigeminal neuralgia) caused by abnormalities in the sensory pathways in the brain and spinal cord.

PRECAUTIONS

- This drug may interact with the effects of alcohol and other central nervous system depressants (e.g., antihistamines, sedatives, tranquilizers, certain prescription pain medications, seizure medications, muscle relaxants, and sleeping medications). Be sure your physician knows if you are taking these or any other medications.
- Oral contraceptives (birth control pills) that contain estrogen may not be as effective if taken in conjunction with phenytoin. Consult with your physician about using a different or additional form of birth control to avoid unplanned pregnancies.
- This medication may affect the blood sugar levels of diabetic individuals. Check with your physician if you notice any change in the results of your blood or urine sugar level tests while taking phenytoin.
- Antacids or medicines for diarrhea can reduce the effectiveness of phenytoin. Do not take any of these medications within 2 to 3 hours of the phenytoin.
- Before having any type of dental treatment or surgery, be sure to inform your physician or dentist if you are taking phenytoin. Medications commonly used during surgical and dental treatments can increase the side effects of phenytoin.
- There have been reports of increased birth defects when hydantoin anticonvulsants were used for seizure control during pregnancy. It is not definitely known whether these medications were the cause of the problem. Be sure to tell your physician if you are pregnant or considering becoming pregnant.
- Phenytoin passes into breast milk in small amounts.

POSSIBLE SIDE EFFECTS

- Side effects that may go away as your body adjusts to the medication and do not require medical attention unless they continue or are bothersome: constipation*; mild dizziness*; mild drowsiness*.
- Side effects that should be reported to your physician: bleeding or enlarged gums; confusion; enlarged glands in the neck or underarms; mood or mental changes*; muscle weakness or pain*; skin rash or itching; slurred speech or

stuttering; trembling; unusual nervousness or irritability.

- Symptoms of overdose that require immediate attention: sudden blurred or double vision*; sudden severe clumsiness or unsteadiness*; sudden severe dizziness or drowsiness*; staggering walk*; severe confusion or disorientation.

*Since it may be difficult to distinguish between certain common symptoms of MS and some side effects of phenytoin, be sure to consult your healthcare professional if an abrupt change of this type occurs.

**Chemical Name:** Prednisone (*pred*-ni-sone)

*Brand Name:* Deltasone (U.S. and Canada)

*Generic Available:* Yes (U.S. and Canada)

*Description:* Prednisone is one of a group of corticosteroids (cortisone-like medicines) that are used to relieve inflammation in different parts of the body. Corticosteroids are used in MS for the management of acute exacerbations because they have the capacity to close the damaged blood-brain barrier and reduce inflammation in the central nervous system. Although prednisone is among the most commonly used corticosteroids in MS, it is only one of several different possibilities. Other commonly used corticosteroids include dexamethasone; prednisone; betamethasone; and prednisolone. The following information pertains to all of the various corticosteroids.

PROPER USAGE

- Most neurologists treating MS believe that high-dose corticosteroids given intravenously are the most effective treatment for an MS exacerbation, although the exact protocol for the drug's use may differ somewhat from one treating physician to another. Patients generally receive a four-day course of treatment (either in the hospital or as an outpatient), with doses

of the medication spread throughout the day (see methylprednisolone). The high-dose, intravenous dose is typically followed by a gradually tapering dose of an oral corticosteroid (usually ranging in length from 10 days to 5 or 6 weeks). Prednisone is commonly used for this oral taper. Oral prednisone may also be used instead of the high-dose, intravenous treatment if the intravenous treatment is not desired or is medically contraindicated.

PRECAUTIONS

- This medication can cause indigestion and stomach discomfort. Always take it with a meal and/or a glass or milk. Your physician may prescribe an antacid for you to take with this medication.
- Take this medication exactly as prescribed by your physician. Do not stop taking it abruptly; your physician will give you a schedule that gradually tapers the dose before you stop it completely.
- Since corticosteroids can stimulate the appetite and increase water retention, it is advisable to follow a low-salt and/or a potassium-rich diet and watch your caloric intake.
- Corticosteroids can lower your resistance to infection and make any infection that you get more difficult to treat. Contact your physician if you notice any sign of infection, such as sore throat, fever, coughing, or sneezing.
- Avoid close contact with anyone who has chicken pox or measles. Tell your physician immediately if you think you have been exposed to either of these illnesses. Do not have any immunizations after you stop taking this medication until you have consulted your physician. People living in your home should not have the oral polio vaccine while you are being treated with corticosteroids since they might pass the polio virus on to you.

- Corticosteroids may affect the blood sugar levels of diabetic patients. If you notice a change in your blood or urine sugar tests, be sure to discuss it with your physician.
- The risk of birth defects in women taking corticosteroids during pregnancy has not been studied. Overuse of corticosteroids during pregnancy may slow the growth of the infant after birth. Animal studies have demonstrated that corticosteroids cause birth defects.
- Corticosteroids pass into breast milk and may slow the infant's growth. If you are nursing or plan to nurse, be sure to discuss this with your physician. It may be necessary for you to stop nursing while taking this medication.
- Corticosteroids can produce mood changes and/or mood swings of varying intensity. These mood alterations can vary from relatively mild to extremely intense, and can vary in a single individual from one course of treatment to another. Neither the patient nor the physician can predict with any certainty whether the corticosteroids are likely to precipitate these mood alterations. If you have a history of mood disorders (depression or bipolar disorder, for example), be sure to share this information with your physician. If you begin to experience unmanageable mood changes or swings while taking corticosteroids, contact your physician so that a decision can be made whether you need an additional medication to help you until the mood alterations subside.

POSSIBLE SIDE EFFECTS
- Side effects that may go away as your body adjusts to the medication and do not require medical attention unless they continue or are bothersome: increased appetite; indigestion; nervousness or restlessness; trouble sleeping; headache; increased sweating; unusual increase in hair growth on body or face.
- Less common side effects that should be reported as soon as possible to your physician: severe mood changes or mood swings; decreased or blurred vision*; frequent urination*.
- Additional side effects that can result from the prolonged use of corticosteroids and should be reported to your physician: acne or other skin problems; swelling of the face; swelling of the feet or lower legs; rapid weight gain; pain in the hips or other joints (caused by bone cell degeneration); bloody or black, tarry stools; elevated blood pressure; markedly increased thirst (with increased urination indicative of diabetes mellitus); menstrual irregularities; unusual bruising of the skin; thin, shiny skin; hair loss; muscle cramps or pain. Once you stop this medication after taking it for a long period of time, it may take several months for your body to readjust.

*Since it may be difficult to distinguish between certain common symptoms of MS and some side effects of prednisone, be sure to consult your healthcare professional if an abrupt change of this type occurs.

**Chemical Name:** Propantheline (proe-*pan*-the-leen) bromide

*Brand Name:* Pro-Banthine (U.S. and Canada)

*Generic Available:* Yes (U.S.)

*Description:* Propantheline bromide is one of a group of antispasmodic/anticholinergic medications used to relieve cramps or spasms of the stomach, intestines, and bladder. Propantheline is used in the management of neurogenic bladder symptoms to control urination.

PROPER USAGE
- Take this medicine 30 minutes to one

hour before meals unless otherwise directed by your physician.

PRECAUTIONS

- Do not stop this medication abruptly. Stop gradually to avoid possible vomiting, sweating, and dizziness.
- Anticholinergic medications such as propantheline can cause blurred vision and light sensitivity. Make sure you know how you react to this medication before driving.
- Anticholinergic medications may cause dryness of the mouth. If your mouth continues to feel dry for more than 2 weeks, check with your dentist. Continuing dryness of the mouth may increase the chance of dental disease.
- No studies of the effects of this drug in pregnancy have been done in either humans or animals.
- Anticholinergic medications have not been reported to cause problems in nursing babies. The flow of breast milk may be reduced in some women.
- Be sure that your physician knows if you are taking a tricyclic antidepressant or any other anticholinergic medication. Taking propantheline with any of these may increase the anticholinergic effects, resulting in urinary retention.

POSSIBLE SIDE EFFECTS

- Side effects that typically go away as your body adjusts to the medication and do not require medical attention unless they continue for several weeks or are bothersome: constipation*; decreased sweating; dryness of mouth, nose, and throat; bloated feeling; blurred vision*; difficulty swallowing.
- Unusual side effects that require immediate medical attention: inability to urinate; confusion; dizziness*; eye pain*; skin rash or hives.
- Symptoms of overdose that require immediate emergency attention: unusual

blurred vision*; unusual clumsiness or unsteadiness*; unusual dizziness; unusually severe drowsiness*; seizures; hallucinations; confusion; shortness of breath; unusual slurred speech*; nervousness; unusual warmth, dryness, and flushing of skin.

*Since it may be difficult to distinguish between certain common symptoms of MS and some side effects of propantheline, be sure to consult your healthcare professional if an abrupt change of this type occurs.

**Chemical Name:** Psyllium hydrophilic mucilloid (*sill*-i-yum hye-droe-*fill*-ik *myoo*-sill-oid)

*Brand Name:* Metamucil (available in granule form in Canada, in wafer form in the U.S., and in powder or effervescent powder in the U.S. and Canada) is one of several available brands of bulk-forming laxative.

*Generic Available:* No

*Description:* Psyllium hydrophilic mucilloid is a bulk-forming oral laxative. This type of laxative is not digested by the body; it absorbs liquids from the intestines and swells to form a soft, bulky stool. The bowel is then stimulated normally by the presence of the bulky stool.

PROPER USAGE

- Laxatives are to be used to provide short-term relief only, unless otherwise directed by the nurse or physician who is helping you to manage your bowel symptoms. A regimen that includes a healthy diet containing roughage (whole grain breads and cereals, bran, fruit, and green, leafy vegetables), six to eight full glasses of liquids each day, and some form of daily exercise is most important in stimulating healthy bowel function.
- If your physician has recommended this laxative for management of constipation, follow his or her recommendations for

its use. If you are treating yourself for constipation, follow the directions on the package insert. Results are often obtained in 12 hours, but may take as long as 2 or 3 days. Be sure to consult your physician if you experience problems or do not get relief within a week.

- For this type of bulk-forming laxative to work effectively without causing intestinal blockage, it is advisable to drink six to eight glasses (8 ounces) of water each day. Each dose of the laxative should be taken with 8 ounces of cold water or fruit juice. If concerns about loss of bladder control keep you from drinking this amount of water, discuss it with the nurse or physician who is helping you manage your bowel and bladder symptoms.

PRECAUTIONS

- Do not take any type of laxative if you have signs of appendicitis or inflamed bowel (e.g., stomach or lower abdominal pain, cramping, bloating, soreness, nausea, or vomiting). Check with your physician as soon as possible.
- Do not take any laxative for more than 1 week unless you have been told to do so by your physician. Many people tend to overuse laxatives, which often leads to dependence on the laxative action to produce a bowel movement. Discuss the use of laxatives with your healthcare professional to ensure that the laxative is used effectively as part of a comprehensive, healthy bowel management regimen.
- Do not take any laxative within 2 hours of taking another medication because the desired effectiveness of the other medication may be reduced.
- Bulk-forming laxatives are commonly used during pregnancy. Some of them contain a large amount of sodium or sugars, which may have possible

unwanted effects such as increasing blood pressure or causing fluid retention. Look for those that contain lower sodium and sugar.

- Some laxatives pass into breast milk. Although it is unlikely to cause problems for a nursing infant, be sure to let your physician know if you are using a laxative and breastfeeding at the same time.

POSSIBLE SIDE EFFECTS

- Check with your physician as soon as possible if you experience any of the following: difficulty breathing; intestinal blockage; skin rash or itching; swallowing difficulty (feelings of lump in the throat).

**Chemical Name:** Sertraline (*ser*-tra-leen)

*Brand Name:* Zoloft (U.S. and Canada)

*Generic Available:* No

*Description:* Sertraline is used to treat mental depression and certain types of anxiety.

PROPER USAGE

- This medication should always be taken at the same time in relation to meals and snacks to make sure that it is absorbed in the same way. Because sertraline may be given to different individuals at different times of the day, you and your physician should discuss what to do about any missed doses.

PRECAUTIONS

- It may take 4 to 6 weeks for you to feel the beneficial effects of this medication.
- Your physician should monitor your progress at regularly scheduled visits in order to adjust the dose and help reduce any side effects.
- This medication could add to the effects of alcohol and other central nervous system depressants (e.g., antihistamines, sedatives, tranquilizers, sleeping medicine, prescription pain medicine, barbi-

turates, seizure medications, and muscle relaxants). Be sure that your physician knows if you are taking these or any other medications.

- Sertraline may cause dryness of the mouth. If your mouth continues to feel dry for more than 2 weeks, check with your physician or dentist. Continuing dryness of the mouth may increase the risk of dental disease.
- This medication may cause drowsiness.
- Studies have not been done in pregnant women. Studies in animals have shown that sertraline may cause delayed development and decreased survival rates of offspring when given in doses many times the usual human dose.
- It is not known if sertraline passes into breast milk.

POSSIBLE SIDE EFFECTS

- Side effects that typically go away as your body adjusts to the medication and do not require medical attention unless they continue for several weeks or are bothersome: decreased appetite or weight loss; decrease sexual drive or ability*; drowsiness*; dryness of mouth; headache; nausea; stomach or abdominal cramps; tiredness or weakness*; tremor*; trouble sleeping; anxiety; agitation; nervousness or restlessness; changes in vision, including blurred vision*; constipation*; fast or irregular heartbeat; flushing of skin; increased appetite; vomiting.
- Unusual side effects that should be discussed with your physician as soon as possible: fast talking and excited feelings or actions that are out of control; fever; skin rash; hives; itching.

*Since it may be difficult to distinguish between certain common symptoms of MS and some side effects of sertraline, be sure to consult your healthcare professional if an abrupt change of this type occurs.

Chemical Name: Sildenafil (sil-*den*-a-fil)

*Brand Name:* Viagra (U.S.)

*Generic Available:* Yes (Canada)

*Description:* Sildenafil belongs to a group of medicines that delay the action of enzymes called phosphodiesterases that can interfere with erectile function. Sildenafil is used to treat men with erectile dysfunction (also called sexual impotence) because it helps to maintain an erection that is produced when the penis is stroked. Without physical stimulation of the penis, sildenafil will not work to cause an erection. Sildenafil is not indicated for use in women.

PROPER USAGE

- Sildenafil begins to work approximately 30 minutes after it is taken. The medication continues to work for up to 4 hours, although the effect is usually less after 2 hours.
- Sildenafil is available by prescription and should be used only as directed by your physician. The dose of this medication will be different for different patients. Do not take more of this medication than has been prescribed for you.

PRECAUTIONS

- Sildenafil can interact with, or interfere with the action of, other medications you may be taking. Be sure to inform your physician of all other medications you are taking so that appropriate substitutions or dosage adjustments can be made. Sildenafil should not be used by men who are using nitrates such as nitroglycerin (e.g., Nitrostat® or Transderm-Nitro®) to lower their blood pressure; sildenafil can cause the blood pressure to drop too far.
- The presence of certain medical problems can interfere with the use of sildenafil. Be sure to inform your doctor if you have any of the following medical problems: an abnormality of the penis

(including a curved penis or birth defect); bleeding problems; retinitis pigmentosa; any conditions causing thickened blood or slower blood flow (e.g., leukemia, multiple myeloma, polycythemia, sickle cell disease, or thrombocycemia); a history of priapism (erection lasting longer than 4 hours); heart or blood disease; severe kidney problems; severe liver problems.

- Sildenafil has not been studied in combination with other medications that are used in the treatment of erectile dysfunction. At the present time, it is not recommended that these drugs be used together.

POSSIBLE SIDE EFFECTS

- Side effects that you should report to your physician so that he or she can adjust the dosage or change the medication: flushing; headache; nasal congestion; stomach discomfort after meals; diarrhea.
- Rare side effects that should be discussed with your physician: abnormal vision (e.g., blurred vision*, seeing shades of colors differently than before, sensitivity to light); bladder pain; cloudy or bloody urine; dizziness, increased frequency of urination; painful urination.
- **Note:** There are a variety of other, possible side effects that have not yet been definitely shown to be caused by sildenafil. Therefore, if you notice any other effects that cause you concern, be sure to talk them over with your doctor.

*Since it may be difficult to distinguish between certain common symptoms of MS and some side effects of sildenafil, be sure to consult your healthcare professional if an abrupt change of this type occurs.

**Chemical Name:** Sodium phosphate

*Brand Name:* Fleet Enema (U.S. and Canada)

*Generic Available:* No

*Description:* Sodium phosphate enemas are available over-the-counter.

PROPER USAGE

- Rectal enemas are to be used to provide short-term relief only, unless otherwise directed by the nurse or physician who is helping you to manage your bowel symptoms. A regimen that includes a healthy diet containing roughage (whole grain breads and cereals, bran, fruit, and green, leafy vegetables), six to eight full glasses of liquids each day, and some form of daily exercise is most important in stimulating healthy bowel function.
- If your physician has recommended this rectal laxative for management of constipation, follow his or her recommendations for its use. If you are treating yourself for constipation, follow the directions on the package insert.
- Results usually occur within 2 to 5 minutes. Be sure to consult your physician if you notice rectal bleeding, blistering, pain, burning, itching, or other signs of irritation that were not present before you began using a sodium phosphate enema.

PRECAUTIONS

- Do not use any type of laxative if you have signs of appendicitis or inflamed bowel (e.g., stomach or lower abdominal pain, cramping, bloating, soreness, nausea, or vomiting). Check with your physician as soon as possible.
- Do not use any laxative for more than 1 week unless you have been told to do so by your physician. Many people tend to overuse laxatives, which often leads to dependence on the laxative action to produce a bowel movement. Discuss the use of laxatives with your healthcare professional to ensure that the laxative is used effectively as part of a comprehensive, healthy bowel management regimen.

- If you are pregnant, discuss with your physician the most appropriate type of laxative for you to use.

POSSIBLE SIDE EFFECTS
- Side effect that may go away as your body adjusts to the medication and does not require medical attention unless it persists or is bothersome: skin irritation in the rectal area.
- Unusual side effects that should be reported to your physician as soon as possible: rectal bleeding, blistering, burning, or itching.

**Chemical Name:** Solifenacin succinate (sol-i-*fen*-ah-sin *suc*-sin-ate)

*Brand Name:* Vesicare (U.S. and Canada)

*Generic Available:* No

*Description:* Solifenacin succinate is an *antimuscarinic* medication that is used to treat an overactive bladder causing symptoms of frequency, urgency, or incontinence.

PROPER USAGE
- This medication should be taken with liquids and swallowed whole. It may be taken with or without food.
- Take only the amount of this medication that has been prescribed for you by your doctor; taking more than the prescribed amount can cause adverse effects.
- If you miss a dose of this medication, begin taking it again the next day. Do not take two doses of solifenacin succinate in the same day.

PRECAUTIONS
- Individuals with any of the following medical problems should not take this medication: urinary retention, gastric retention, narrow angle or uncontrolled glaucoma, or severe kidney problems. Solifenacin succinate can aggravate each of these conditions.

- Solifenacin succinate may cause blurred vision; do not engage in potentially dangerous activities such as driving until you know the effect of the medication on your vision.
- This medication, like all anticholinergic medications, may cause drying of the mouth. Since continued dryness of the mouth can increase the risk of dental disease, alert your dentist if you are taking this medication.
- Like all anticholinergic medications, solifenacin succinate can cause or worsen constipation.
- Because of decreased sweating, this medication can cause heat prostration when used in a very hot environment.
- This medication has not been studied in pregnant women. However, it has been shown in animal studies to impact pre- and postnatal development. If you are pregnant, or planning to become pregnant, do not start this medication before you have discussed it with your physician.
- It is not known whether solifenacin succinate passes into breast milk. Women who taking this medication and wish to breastfeed should discuss it with their physician.

POSSIBLE SIDE EFFECTS
- Side effects that are expected with this type of medication and do not require medical attention unless they continue or are bothersome: dry mouth; dry eyes; constipation, blurred vision, difficult urination.
- Less common side effect that should be reported to your physician: severe abdominal pain.
- Symptoms of overdose: severe central anticholinergic effects, including blurred vision; clumsiness or unsteadiness; confusion; seizures; severe diarrhea; excessive watering of the mouth; increasing

muscle weakness (especially in the arms, neck, shoulders, and tongue); muscle cramps or twitching; severe nausea or vomiting; shortness of breath; slow heartbeat; slurred speech; unusual irritability, nervousness, or restlessness; unusual tiredness or weakness.

**Chemical Name:** Sulfamethoxazole (sul-fa-meth-*ox*-a-zole) and trimethoprim (try-*meth*-oh-prim) combination

*Brand Name:* Bactrim; Septra (U.S. and Canada)

*Generic Available:* Yes (U.S.)

*Description:* Sulfamethoxazole and trimethoprim combination is used in multiple sclerosis to treat (and sometimes to prevent) urinary tract infections.

PROPER USAGE

- This medication is best taken with a full glass (8 ounces) of water. Additional water should be taken each day to help prevent unwanted effects.
- Finish the full course of treatment prescribed by your physician. Even if your symptoms disappear after a few days, stopping this medication prematurely may result in a return of the symptoms.
- This medication works most effectively when it is maintained at a constant level in your blood or urine. To help keep the amount constant, do not miss any doses. It is best to take the doses at evenly spaced times during the day and night. For maximum effectiveness, four doses per day would be spaced at six-hour intervals.

PRECAUTIONS

- This medication may cause dizziness.
- If taken for a long time, sulfamethoxazole and trimethoprim combination may cause blood problems. It is very important that your physician monitor your progress at regular visits.

- This medication can cause changes in the blood, possibly resulting in a greater chance of certain infections, slow healing, and bleeding of the gums. Be careful with the use of your toothbrush, dental floss, and toothpicks. Delay dental work until your blood counts are completely normal. Check with your dentist if you have questions about oral hygiene during treatment.
- This medication may cause your skin to become more sensitive to sunlight. Stay out of direct sunlight during the midday hours, wear protective clothing, and apply a sun block product that has a skin protection factor (SPF) of at least 15.
- Sulfamethoxazole and trimethoprim combination has not been reported to cause birth defects or other problems in humans. Studies in mice, rats, and rabbits have shown that some sulfonamides cause birth defects, including cleft palate and bone problems. Studies in rabbits have also shown that trimethoprim causes birth defects, as well as a decrease in the number of successful pregnancies.
- Sulfamethoxazole and trimethoprim pass into breast milk. This medication is not recommended for use during breast-feeding. It may cause liver problems, anemia, and other problems in nursing babies.

POSSIBLE SIDE EFFECTS

- Side effects that may go away as your body adjusts to the medication and do not require medical attention unless they continue or are bothersome: diarrhea; dizziness; headache; loss of appetite; nausea or vomiting.
- Less common side effects that should be reported to your physician immediately: itching; skin rash; aching of muscles and joints; difficulty in swallowing; pale skin; redness, blistering, peeling, or loosening of skin; sore throat and fever; unusual bleeding or bruising; unusual tiredness or weakness*; yellow eyes or skin.

*Since it may be difficult to distinguish between certain common symptoms of MS and some side effects of sulfamethoxazole and trimethoprim, be sure to consult your healthcare professional if an abrupt change of this type occurs.

**Chemical Name:** Tadalafil (tah-*dal*-a-fil)

*Brand Name:* Cialis (U.S. and Canada)

*Generic Available:* No

*Description:* Tadalafil belongs to a group of medicines that delay the action of enzymes called phosphodiesterases that can interfere with erectile function. Tadalafil is used to treat men with erectile dysfunction (also called sexual impotence) because it helps to maintain an erection that has been created by stimulation. *Tadalafil will not cause an erection without stimulation of the penis.* Tadalafil is not indicated for use in women.

PROPER USAGE

- Tadalafil, which may be taken up to once per day by most men, remains effective for up to 36 hours.
- Tadalafil is available by prescription and should be used only as directed by your physician. The dose of this medication will be different for different patients. Do not take more of this medication than has been prescribed for you.
- If you are older than 65 or have liver problems, your doctor may start you on a lower dose of this medication.

PRECAUTIONS

- Tadalafil can interact with, or interfere with the action of, other medications you may be taking. Be sure to inform your physician of all other medications you are taking so that appropriate substitutions or dosage adjustments can be made. Tadalafil should not be used by men who are using: nitrates such as nitroglycerin (e.g., Nitrostat or Transderm-Nitro) to lower blood pressure; or alpha blockers (e.g., Hytrin, Flomax, or Cardura) to treat prostate problems or high blood pressure. Tadalafil in combination with these medications can cause the blood pressure to drop too far.
- The presence of certain medical problems can interfere with the use of tadalafil. Be sure to inform your doctor if you have any of the following medical problems: an abnormality of the penis (including a curved penis or birth defect); bleeding problems; retinitis pigmentosa; any conditions causing thickened blood or slower blood flow (e.g., leukemia, multiple myeloma, polycythemia, sickle cell disease, or thrombocycemia); a history of priapism (erection lasting longer than 4 hours); heart or blood disease; severe kidney problems; severe liver problems.
- Tadalafil has not been studied in combination with other medications that are used in the treatment of erectile dysfunction. At the present time, it is not recommended that these drugs be used together.

POSSIBLE SIDE EFFECTS

- Side effects that you should report to your physician so that he or she can adjust the dosage or change the medication: flushing; headache; nasal congestion; stomach discomfort after meals; diarrhea.
- Rare side effects that should be discussed with your physician: abnormal vision (e.g., blurred vision, seeing shades of colors differently than before, sensitivity to light); bladder pain; cloudy or bloody urine; dizziness; increased frequency of urination; painful urination.

**Chemical Name:** Tizanidine hydrochloride (tye-*zan*-i-deen)

*Brand Name:* Zanaflex (U.S. and Canada)

*Generic Available:* No

*Description:* Tizanidine is used in multiple sclerosis to treat the increased muscle tone associated with spasticity. While it does not provide a cure for the problem, it is designed to relieve spasms, cramping, and tightness of muscles.

PROPER USAGE

- Tizanidine is a short-acting drug for the management of spasticity. Its peak effectiveness occurs 1 to 2 hours after dosing and is finished between 3 to 6 hours after dosing. Therefore, your physician will prescribe a dosing schedule that provides maximal relief during activities and periods of time of greatest importance to you.
- To minimize unwanted side effects with this medication, your physician will start you on a low dose and gradually raise it until a well-tolerated and effective level is reached.
- Studies of tizanidine have not been done in pregnant women. Animal studies, using doses significantly higher than those prescribed for humans, have resulted in damage to the offspring. If you are pregnant or planning to become pregnant, discuss this with your physician before starting this medication.
- It is not known whether tizanidine passes into the breast milk. Women should not take this medication while nursing unless told to do so by their physician.

PRECAUTIONS

- Oral contraceptives (birth control pills) may slow the release of tizanidine from the body; women using birth control pills should inform their physician so that the dose level of tizanidine can be reduced accordingly.
- This medication may cause blurred vision*, dizziness, or drowsiness in some people.

- This drug will add to the effects of alcohol and other CNS depressants (such as antihistamines, sedatives, tranquilizers, prescription pain medications, seizure medications, and other muscle relaxants), possibly causing drowsiness. Be sure that your physician knows if you are taking these or any other medications.

POSSIBLE SIDE EFFECTS

- Common side effects that may go away as your body adjusts to the medication and do not require medical attention unless they continue for more than 2 weeks or are bothersome: dryness of mouth; sleepiness or sedation; weakness*, fatigue*, and or tiredness*; dizziness or lightheadedness, especially when getting up from a sitting or lying position; increase in muscle spasms, cramps, or tightness; back pain.
- Common side effects that should be reported to the doctor as soon as possible: burning, prickling, or tingling sensation*; diarrhea; fainting; fever; loss of appetite; nausea; nervousness; pain or burning during urination; sores on skin; stomach pain; vomiting; yellow eyes or skin; blurred vision*.

*Since it may be difficult to distinguish between certain common symptoms of MS and some side effects of tizanidine, be sure to consult your healthcare professional if an abrupt change of this type occurs.

**Chemical Name:** Tolterodine (tole-*tare*-oh-deen) acetate

*Brand Name:* Detrol (U.S.)

*Generic Available:* Yes (Canada)

*Description:* Tolterodine is an *antispasmodic* that is used to treat bladder spasms that cause urinary frequency, urgency, or incontinence.

PROPER USAGE

- Take only the amount of this medication that has been prescribed for you by your doctor; taking more than the prescribed amount can cause adverse effects.
- If you miss a dose of this medication, take it as soon as possible. If, however, it is almost time for your next dose, skip the missed dose and go back to your regular schedule. Do not double dose.

PRECAUTIONS

- Individuals with any of the following medical problems should not take this medication: gastric retention, urinary retention, or narrow-angle or uncontrolled glaucoma. Tolterodine can aggravate each of these conditions.
- Tolterodine may cause dizziness or drowsiness; use caution when driving or doing any activities that require alertness.
- Tolterodine may cause drying of the mouth. Since continued dryness of the mouth can increase the risk of dental disease, alert your dentist if you are taking this medication.
- This medication may interact with fluoxetine (Prozac®) in such a way as to increase the effect of the tolterodine. If you are taking fluoxetine, your physician may start you at a lower dose of tolterodine, gradually raising it to the standard dose if necessary.
- This medication has not been studied in pregnant women. However, it has been shown in animal studies to result in increased embryo deaths, reduced birth weight, and increased incidence of fetal abnormalities. If you are pregnant or planning to become pregnant, do not start this medication before you have discussed it with your physician.
- It is not known whether tolterodine passes into breast milk. Since tolterodine is known to pass into the milk of nursing animals, causing temporary reduction in weight gain in the offspring, women should stop taking this drug as long as they are nursing.

POSSIBLE SIDE EFFECTS

- Side effects that will typically go away as your body adjusts to the medication and do not require medical attention unless they continue for a few weeks or are bothersome: dry mouth; dizziness; headache; fatigue*; gastrointestinal symptoms, including abdominal pain, constipation*, or diarrhea; difficult urination.
- Less common side effects that should be reported to your physician immediately: abnormal vision, including difficulty adjusting to distances; urinary tract infection.
- Symptoms of overdose: severe central anticholinergic effects, including blurred vision*; clumsiness or unsteadiness*; confusion; seizures; severe diarrhea, excessive watering of the mouth; increasing muscle weakness (especially in the arms, neck, shoulders, and tongue); muscle cramps or twitching; severe nausea or vomiting; shortness of breath, slow heartbeat; slurred speech*; unusual irritability, nervousness, or restlessness; unusual tiredness or weakness*.

*Since it may be difficult to distinguish between certain common symptoms of MS and some side effects of tolterodine, be sure to consult your healthcare professional if an abrupt change of this type occurs.

**Chemical Name:** Topiramate (to-*peer*-ah-mate)

*Brand Name:* Topamax (U.S. and Canada)

*Generic Available:* No

*Description:* Topiramate is an antiepileptic used to control some types of seizures in epilepsy. It is used in multiple sclerosis to treat dysesthesias (pain caused by MS lesions) and may also be effective for the treatment of tremor.

PROPER USAGE
- Topiramate may be taken with or without food.
- If you miss a dose of this medication, take it as soon as possible. However, if it is almost time for your next dose, skip the missed dose, then go back to your regular dosing schedule. Do not double dose.
- Drink plenty of fluids every day that you are taking topiramate to help prevent the formation of kidney stones.
- Store away from heat and direct light, and do not refrigerate.

PRECAUTIONS
- This medication may cause some people to have blurred vision; double vision; clumsiness or unsteadiness; to become dizzy or drowsy; or to have trouble thinking. Do not operate heavy machinery or drive a car until you know how this medication affects you.
- Be sure that your physician knows if you are taking acetazolamind (e.g., Diamox®), dichlorphenamide (e.g., Daranide®), carbamazepine (e.g., Tegretol®), phenytoin (e.g., Dilantin®), and/or valproic acid (e.g., Depakote®), as these medications can interact with topiramate.
- Topiramate has not been studied in pregnant women. However, studies in pregnant animals have shown that topirmate may cause birth defects in the offspring as well as adverse effects in the mother. If you are pregnant or planning to become pregnant, discuss this with your physician before starting this medication.
- It is not known whether topiramate passes into breast milk. Women who

wish to breast-feed should consult with their physician.
- Be sure to let your physician know if you have a history of kidney stones, kidney problems, or liver problems.
- Oral contraceptives containing estrogen may not be as effective when used in conjunction with topiramate. Use a different or additional form of birth control while using this medication.

POSSIBLE SIDE EFFECTS
The side effects of this medication can be minimized by starting the medication at a low dose and increasing it gradually.

- Side effects that typically go away as your body adjusts to the medication and do not require medical attention unless they continue for several weeks or are bothersome: breast pain in women; nausea; tremors*; back pain; chest pain; constipation*; heartburn; hot flushes; increased sweating; leg pain*; change in sense of taste.
- Check with your doctor as soon as possible if any of the following side effects occur: blurred vision*; double vision*; eye pain or rapidly decreasing vision*; confusion; dizziness*; drowsiness*; eye redness; generalized slowing of mental and physical activity*; increased eye pressure; memory problems*; menstrual changes; menstrual pain; nervousness; speech or language problems*; trouble concentrating*; unusual tiredness*; weakness*.

*Since it may be difficult to distinguish between certain common symptoms of MS and some side effects of topiramate, be sure to consult your healthcare professional if an abrupt change of this type occurs.

**Chemical Name:** Trospium chloride (*troes-pee-oom chloride*)

*Brand Name:* Sanctura (U.S.)

*Generic Available:* No

*Description:* Trospium chloride is an *antispasmodic, antimuscarinic* medication that is used to treat an overactive bladder causing symptoms of frequency, urgency, or incontinence.

PROPER USAGE

- This medication should be taken 1 hour before meals or on an empty stomach.
- Take only the amount of this medication that has been prescribed for you by your doctor; taking more than the prescribed amount can cause adverse effects.
- If you miss a dose of this medication, take it as soon as possible. However, if it is almost time for your next dose, skip the missed dose and go back to your regular schedule. Do not double dose.

PRECAUTIONS

- Individuals with any of the following medical problems should not take this medication: urinary retention; gastric retention; narrow angle or uncontrolled glaucoma; severe kidney problems. Trospium chloride can aggravate each of these conditions.
- Trospium chloride may cause dizziness or drowsiness; use caution when driving or doing any activities that require alertness.
- This medication, like all anticholinergic medications, may cause drying of the mouth. Since continued dryness of the mouth can increase the risk of dental disease, alert your dentist if you are taking this medication.
- Like all anticholinergic medications, trospium chloride can cause or worsen constipation.
- This medication has not been studied in pregnant women. However, it has been shown in animal studies to result in decreased fetal survival. If you are pregnant or planning to become pregnant,

do not start this medication before you have discussed it with your physician.

- It is not known whether trospium chloride passes into breast milk. Women who are taking this medication and wish to breastfeed should discuss it with their physician.

POSSIBLE SIDE EFFECTS

- Side effects that will typically go away as your body adjusts to the medication and do not require medical attention unless they continue for a few weeks or are bothersome: dry mouth; dry eyes; dizziness; headache; fatigue; gastrointestinal symptoms, including abdominal pain, constipation, or diarrhea; difficult urination.
- Less common side effects that should be reported to your physician immediately: abnormal vision, including difficulty adjusting to distances; urinary tract infection.
- Symptoms of overdose: severe central anticholinergic effects, including blurred vision; clumsiness or unsteadiness; confusion; seizures; severe diarrhea; excessive watering of the mouth; increasing muscle weakness (especially in the arms, neck, shoulders, and tongue); muscle cramps or twitching; severe nausea or vomiting; shortness of breath; slow heartbeat; slurred speech; unusual irritability, nervousness, or restlessness; unusual tiredness or weakness.

**Chemical Name:** Vardenafil (var-*den*-a-fil)

*Brand Name:* Levitra (U.S. and Canada)

*Generic Available:* No

*Description:* Vardenafil belongs to a group of medicines that delay the action of enzymes called phosphodiesterases that can interfere with erectile function. Vardenafil is used to treat men with erectile dysfunction (also called sexual impotence) because it helps to maintain an erection that is produced when the penis is stroked. Without physical stimulation of the penis, vardenafil will not work to cause an erection. Vardenafil is not indicated for use in women.

PROPER USAGE

- Vardenafil should be taken approximately 60 minutes before sexual activity.

- Vardenafil is available by prescription and should be used only as directed by your physician. The dose of this medication will be different for different patients. Do not take more of this medication than has been prescribed for you.

- If you are older than 65 or have liver problems, your doctor may start you on a lower dose of this medication.

PRECAUTIONS

- Vardenafil can interact with, or interfere with the action of, other medications you may be taking. Be sure to inform your physician of all other medications you are taking so that appropriate substitutions or dosage adjustments can be made. Vardenafil should not be used by men who are using: nitrates such as nitroglycerin (e.g., Nitrostat® or Transderm-Nitro®) to lower blood pressure; or alpha blockers (e.g., Hytrin®, Flomax®, or Cardura®) to treat prostate problems or high blood pressure. Vardenafil in combination with these medications can cause the blood pressure to drop too far.

- The presence of certain medical problems can interfere with the use of Vardenafil. Be sure to inform your doctor if you have any of the following medical problems: an abnormality of the penis (including a curved penis or birth defect); bleeding problems; retinitis pigmentosa; any conditions causing thickened blood or slower blood flow (e.g., leukemia, multiple myeloma, poly-cythemia, sickle cell disease, or thrombocycemia); a history of priapism (erection lasting longer than 4 hours); heart or blood disease; severe kidney problems; severe liver problems.

- Vardenafil has not been studied in combination with other medications that are used in the treatment of erectile dysfunction. At the present time, it is not recommended that these drugs be used together.

POSSIBLE SIDE EFFECTS

- Side effects that you should report to your physician so that he or she can adjust the dosage or change the medication: flushing; headache; nasal congestion; stomach discomfort after meals; diarrhea.

- Rare side effects that should be discussed with your physician: abnormal vision (e.g., blurred vision*, seeing shades of colors differently than before, sensitivity to light); bladder pain; cloudy or bloody urine; dizziness, increased frequency of urination; painful urination.

*Since it may be difficult to distinguish between certain common symptoms of MS and some side effects of vardenafil, be sure to consult your healthcare professional if an abrupt change of this type occurs.

**Chemical Name:** Venlafaxine (ven-la-*fax*-een)

*Brand Name:* Effexor (U.S. and Canada)

*Generic Available:* No

*Description:* Venlafaxine is used to treat mental depression and certain types of anxiety.

DOSAGE AND PROPER USAGE

- Unless your physician has instructed otherwise, this medication should be taken with food or on a full stomach to reduce the chances of stomach upset.

- If you miss a dose of this medication, take it as soon as possible. If, however, it is within two hours of your next dose, skip the missed dose and return to your regular schedule. Do not double dose.

PRECAUTIONS

- It may take 4 to 6 weeks for you to feel the beneficial effects of this medication.
- Your physician should monitor your progress at regularly scheduled visits to adjust the dose and help reduce any side effects.
- Do not stop taking this medication without consulting your physician. The doctor may want you to reduce the amount you are taking gradually in order to decrease unwanted side effects.
- This medication could add to the effects of alcohol and other central nervous system depressants (e.g., antihistamines, sedatives, tranquilizers, sleeping medicine, prescription pain medicine, barbiturates, seizure medications, and muscle relaxants). Be sure that you doctor knows if you are taking these or any other medications.
- Venlafaxine may cause dryness of the mouth. If your mouth continues to feel dry for more than two weeks, check with your physician or dentist. Continuing dryness of the mouth may increase the risk of dental disease.
- This medication may cause you to become drowsy or to have double vision.
- Venlafaxine may cause dizziness, light-headedness, or fainting, especially when you stand from a sitting of lying position. If rising slowly from a sitting or lying position does not relieve the problem, consult your physician.
- Studies have not been done in pregnant women. However, studies in animals have shown that venlafaxine may cause decreased survival rates of offspring when given in doses that are many times the usual dose for humans. If you are pregnant, or planning to become pregnant, do not start this medication before you have discussed it with your physician.
- It is not known whether venlafaxine passes into breast milk. Mothers who are taking this medication and wish to breastfeed should discuss this with their doctor.

POSSIBLE SIDE EFFECTS

- Side effects that will typically go away as your body adjusts to the medication and do not require medical attention unless they continue for several weeks or are bothersome: abnormal dreams; anxiety or nervousness; constipation*, dizziness, drowsiness*, dryness of mouth; tingling or burning sensations*; decreased appetite, nausea, stomach or abdominal cramps; trouble sleeping; tiredness*; tremor*.
- Unusual side effects which should be discussed with the doctor as soon as possible: changes in vision or double vision*; changes in sexual desire or ability*; headache, chest pain; fast heartbeat; itching or skin rash; mood or mental changes; problems with urination*; menstrual changes; uncontrolled excitability; high blood pressure.
- Symptoms of overdose include: extreme drowsiness, tiredness, or weakness*.

*Since it may be difficult to distinguish between certain common symptoms of MS and some side effects of venlafaxine, be sure to consult your healthcare professional if an abrupt change of this type occurs.

**Activities of daily living (ADLs)** Activities of daily living include any daily activity a person performs for self-care (feeding, grooming, bathing, dressing), work, home-making, and leisure. The ability to perform ADLs is often used as a measure of ability/disability in MS.

**Acute** Having rapid onset, usually with recovery; not chronic or long-lasting.

**Acute attack** See *Exacerbation*.

**ADLs** See *Activities of daily living*.

**Advance (medical) directive** Advance directives preserve the person's right to accept or reject a course of medical treatment even after the person becomes mentally or physically incapacitated to the point of being unable to communicate those wishes. Advance directives come in two basic forms: 1) a living will, in which the person outlines specific treatment guidelines that are to be followed by healthcare providers; or 2) a healthcare proxy (also called a power of attorney for healthcare decision making), in which the person designates a trusted individual to make medical decisions in the event that he or she becomes too incapacitated to make such decisions. Advance directive requirements vary greatly from one state to another and should therefore be drawn up in consultation with an attorney who is familiar with the laws of the particular state.

**Affective release** Also called pseudo-bulbar affect or pathological laughing and crying; a condition in which episodes of laughing and/or crying occur with no apparent precipitating event. The person's actual mood may be unrelated to the emotion being expressed. This condition is thought to be caused by lesions in the limbic system, a group of brain structures involved in emotional feeling and expression.

**Afferent pupillary defect** An abnormal reflex response to light that is a sign of nerve fiber damage due to optic neuritis. A pupil normally gets smaller when a light is shined either into that eye (direct response) or the other eye (indirect response). In an afferent pupillary defect (also called Marcus Gunn pupil), there is a relative decrease in the direct response. This is most clearly demonstrated by the "swinging flashlight test." When the flashlight is shined first in the abnormal eye, then in the healthy eye, and then again in the eye with the pupillary defect, the affected pupil becomes larger rather than smaller.

**AFO** See *Ankle-foot orthosis*.

**Ankle-foot orthosis (AFO)** An ankle-foot orthosis is a brace, usually plastic, that is worn on the lower leg and foot to support the ankle and correct foot drop. By holding the foot and ankle in the correct position, the AFO promotes correct heel-toe walking. See *Foot drop*.

**Antibody** Protein produced by certain cells of the immune system, which is produced in response to bacteria, viruses, and other types of foreign antigens. See *Antigen*.

**Anticholinergic** Refers to the action of certain medications commonly used in the management of neurogenic bladder dysfunction. These medications inhibit the transmission of certain nerve impulses (parasympathetic) and thereby reduce spasms of smooth muscle in the bladder which can cause urgency, frequency, and other urinary symptoms.

**Antigen** Any substance that triggers the immune system to produce an antibody; generally refers to infectious or toxic substances. See *Antibody*.

**Aspiration** Inhalation of food particles or fluids into the lungs.

**Aspiration pneumonia** Inflammation of the lungs due to aspiration.

**Assistive devices** Any tools that are designed, fabricated, and/or adapted to assist a person in performing a particular task (e.g., cane, walker, shower chair).

**Assistive technology** A term used to describe all of the tools, products, and devices, from the simplest to the most complex, that can make a particular function easier or possible to perform.

**Ataxia** The incoordination and unsteadiness that result from the brain's failure to regulate the body's posture and the strength and direction of limb movements. Ataxia is most often caused by disease activity in the cerebellum.

**Atrophy** A wasting away or decrease in size of a cell, tissue, or organ of the body because of disease or lack of use.

**Autoimmune disease** A process in which the body's immune system causes illness by mistakenly attacking healthy cells, organs, or tissues in the body that are essential for good health. Multiple sclerosis is believed to be an autoimmune disease, along with systemic lupus erythematosus, rheumatoid arthritis, scleroderma, and many others. The precise origin and pathophysiologic processes of these diseases are unknown.

**Autonomic nervous system** The part of the nervous system that regulates involuntary vital functions, including the activity of the cardiac (heart) muscle, smooth muscles

(e.g., of the gut), and glands. The autonomic nervous system has two divisions: the sympathetic nervous system accelerates heart rate, constricts blood vessels, and raises blood pressure; the parasympathetic nervous system slows heart rate, increases intestinal and gland activity, and relaxes sphincter muscles.

**Axon** The extension or prolongation of a nerve cell (neuron) that conducts impulses to other nerve cells or muscles. Axons are generally smaller than 1 micron (1 micron = 1/1,000,000 of a meter) in diameter, but can be as much as a half meter in length.

**Axonal damage** Injury to the axon in the nervous system, generally as a consequence of trauma or disease. This damage may involve temporary, reversible effects or permanent severing of the axon. Axonal damage usually results in short-term changes in nervous system activity, or permanent inability of nerve fibers to send their signals from one part of the nervous system to another or from nerve fibers to muscles. The damage can thus result in a variety of symptoms relating to sensory or motor function.

**B-cell** A type of lymphocyte (white blood cell) manufactured in the bone marrow that makes antibodies.

**Babinski reflex** A pathologic sign in MS in which stroking the outside sole of the foot with a pointed object causes an upward (extensor) movement of the big toe rather than the normal (flexor) bunching and downward movement of the toes. See *Sign*.

**Bell's palsy** A paralysis of the facial nerve (usually on one side of the face), which can occur as a consequence of MS, viral infection, or other infections. It has acute onset and can be transient or permanent.

**Blinding** An attempt to eliminate bias in the interpretation of clinical trial outcomes. It indicates that at least one party involved in the clinical trial is unaware of which patients are receiving the experimental treatment and which are receiving the control substance. Trials may be either single-blind (patients do not know which treatment they are receiving) or double-blind (neither the examining physicians nor the patients know which treatment each patient is receiving).

**Blood-brain barrier** A semipermeable cell layer around blood vessels in the brain and spinal cord that prevents large molecules, immune cells, and potentially damaging substances and disease-causing organisms (e.g., viruses) from passing out of the blood stream into the central nervous system (brain, optic nerves, and spinal cord). A break in the blood-brain barrier may underlie the disease process in MS.

**Brain** That part of the central nervous system that is contained within the cranium (skull).

**Brainstem** The part of the central nervous system that houses the nerve centers of the head as well as the centers for respiration and heart control. It extends from the base of the brain to the spinal cord.

**Catheter** A hollow, flexible tube, made of plastic or rubber, which can be inserted through the urinary opening into the bladder to drain excess urine that cannot be excreted normally.

**Central nervous system** The part of the nervous system that includes the brain, optic nerves, and spinal cord.

**Cerebellum** A part of the brain situated above the brainstem that controls balance and coordination of movement.

**Cerebrospinal fluid (CSF)** A watery, colorless, clear fluid that bathes and protects the brain and spinal cord. The composition of this fluid can be altered by a variety of diseases. Certain changes in CSF that are characteristic of MS can be detected with a lumbar puncture (spinal tap), a test sometimes used to help make the MS diagnosis. See *Lumbar puncture*.

**Cerebrum** The large, upper part of the brain that acts as a master control system and is responsible for initiating thought and motor activity. Its two hemispheres, united by the corpus callosum, form the largest part of the central nervous system.

**Cerebral** Pertaining to the cerebrum.

**Chronic** Of long duration, not acute; a term often used to describe a disease that shows gradual worsening.

**Chronic progressive** A former "catchall" term for progressive forms of MS. See *Primary-progressive MS*, *Secondary-progressive MS*, and *Progressive-relapsing MS*.

**Clinical finding** An observation made during a medical examination indicating change or impairment in a physical or mental function.

**Clinically isolated syndrome (CIS)** A first neurologic event that is suggestive of demyelination, accompanied by multiple, clinically "silent" (asymptomatic) lesions on MRI that are typical of MS. Individuals with this syndrome are at high risk for developing clinically definite MS.

**Clinical trial** Rigorously controlled studies designed to provide extensive data that will allow for statistically valid evaluation of the safety and efficacy of a particular treatment. See also *Double-blind clinical study*; *Placebo*.

**Cognition** High level functions carried out by the human brain, including comprehension and use of speech, visual perception and construction, calculation ability, attention (information processing), memory, and executive functions such as planning, problem-solving, and self-monitoring.

**Cognitive impairment** Changes in cognitive function caused by trauma or disease process. Some degree of cognitive impairment occurs in approximately 50–60 percent of people with MS, with memory, information processing, and executive functions being the most commonly affected functions. See *Cognition*.

**Cognitive rehabilitation** Techniques designed to improve the functioning of individuals whose cognition is impaired because of physical trauma or disease. Rehabilitation strategies are designed to improve the impaired function via repetitive drills or practice, or to compensate for impaired functions that are not likely to improve. Cognitive rehabilitation is provided by psychologists and neuropsychologists, speech/language pathologists, and occupational therapists. While these three types of specialists use different assessment tools and treatment strategies, they share the common goal of improving the individual's ability to function as independently and safely as possible in the home and work environment.

**Combined (bladder) dysfunction** A type of neurogenic bladder dysfunction in MS (also called detrusor-external sphincter dyssynergia [DESD]). Simultaneous contractions of the bladder's detrusor muscle and external sphincter cause urine to be trapped in the bladder, resulting in symptoms of urinary urgency, hesitancy, dribbling, and incontinence.

**Condom catheter** A tube connected to a thin, flexible sheath that is worn over the penis to allow drainage of urine into a collection system; can be used to manage male urinary incontinence.

**Constipation** A condition in which bowel movements happen less frequently than is normal for the particular individual, or the stool is small, hard, and difficult or painful to pass.

**Contraction** A shortening of muscle fibers that results in the movement of a joint.

**Contracture** A permanent shortening of the muscles and tendons adjacent to a joint which can result from severe, untreated spasticity and interferes with normal movement around the affected joint. If left untreated, the affected joint can become frozen in a flexed (bent) position.

**Controlled study** A clinical trial that compares the outcome of a group of randomly assigned patients who receive the experimental treatment to the outcome of a group of randomly assigned patients who receive a standard treatment or inactive placebo.

**Coordination** An organized working together of muscles and groups of muscles aimed at bringing about a purposeful movement such as walking or standing.

**Corpus callosum** The broad band of nerve fiber tissue that connects the two cerebral hemispheres of the brain.

**Cortex** The outer layer of brain tissue.

**Corticosteroid** Any of the natural or synthetic hormones associated with the adrenal cortex (which influences or controls many body processes). Corticosteroids include glucocorticoids, which have an anti-inflammatory and immunosuppressive role in the treatment of MS exacerbations. See also *Glucocorticoids*; *Immunosuppression*; *Exacerbation*.

**Cortisone** A glucocorticoid steroid hormone, produced by the adrenal glands or synthetically, that has anti-inflammatory and immune-system suppressing properties. Prednisone and prednisolone also belong to this group of substances.

**Cranial nerves** Nerves that carry sensory, motor, or parasympathetic fibers to the face and neck. Included among this group of 12 nerves are the optic nerve (vision), trigeminal nerve (sensation along the face), and vagus nerve (pharynx and vocal cords). Evaluation of cranial nerve function is part of the standard neurologic exam.

**Cystoscopy** A diagnostic procedure in which a special viewing device called a cystoscope is inserted into the urethra (a tubular structure that drains urine from the bladder) to examine the inside of the urinary bladder.

**Cystostomy** A surgically created opening through the lower abdomen into the urinary bladder. A rubber or plastic tube inserted into the opening drains urine from the bladder into a plastic collection bag. This relatively simple procedure is done when a person requires an indwelling catheter to drain urine from the bladder, but passage through the urethral opening is not desirable for reasons such as uncontrollable frequency or incontinence.

**Cytokines** Messenger chemicals produced by various cells, particularly those of the immune system, to influence the activity of other cells.

**Decubitus** An ulcer (sore) of the skin resulting from pressure and lack of movement such as occurs when a person is limited to bed or requires a wheelchair for mobility. The ulcers occur most frequently in areas where the bone lies directly under the skin, such as elbow, hip, or over the coccyx (tailbone). A decubitus ulcer may become infected and cause general worsening of the person's health.

**Deep tendon reflexes** The involuntary jerks that are normally produced at certain spots on a limb when the tendons are tapped with a hammer. Reflexes are tested as part of the standard neurologic exam.

**Dementia** A generally profound and progressive loss of intellectual function, sometimes associated with personality change, that results from loss of brain substance and is sufficient to interfere with a person's normal functional activities.

**Demyelination** A loss of myelin in the white matter of the central nervous system (brain, optic nerves, and spinal cord). See *Myelin*.

**DESD** See *Detrusor-external sphincter dyssynergia.*

**Detrusor muscle** The primary muscle of the urinary bladder that contracts and causes the bladder to empty.

**Detrusor-external sphincter dyssynergia (DESD)** See *Combined (bladder) dysfunction.*

**Diplopia** Double vision, or the simultaneous awareness of two images of the same object that results from a failure of the two eyes to work in a coordinated fashion. Covering one eye will erase one of the images.

**Disablement** As defined by the World Health Organization, a disability (resulting from an impairment) is a restriction or lack of ability to perform an activity in the manner or within the range considered normal for a human being.

**Double-blind clinical study** A study in which none of the participants, including experimental subjects, examining doctors, attending nurses, or any other research staff, know who is taking the test drug and who is taking a control or placebo agent. The purpose of this research design is to avoid inadvertent bias of the test results. In all studies, procedures are designed to "break the blind" if medical circumstances require it.

**Dysarthria** Poorly articulated speech resulting from dysfunction of the muscles controlling speech, usually caused by damage to the central nervous system or a peripheral motor nerve. The content and meaning of the spoken words remain normal.

**Dysesthesia** Distorted or unpleasant sensations experienced by a person when the skin is touched, typically caused by abnormalities in the sensory pathways in the brain and spinal cord.

**Dysphagia** Difficulty in swallowing. It is a neurologic or neuromuscular symptom that may result in aspiration (whereby food or saliva enters the airway), slow swallowing (possibly resulting in inadequate nutrition), or both.

**Dysphonia** Disorders of voice quality (including poor pitch control, hoarseness, breathiness, and hypernasality) caused by spasticity, weakness, and incoordination of muscles in the mouth and throat.

**EAE** See *Experimental allergic encephalomyelitis*.

**EEG** See *Electroencephalography*.

**Electroencephalography (EEG)** A diagnostic procedure that records, via electrodes attached to various areas of the person's head, electrical activity generated by brain cells.

**Electromyography (EMG)** Electromyography is a diagnostic procedure that records muscle electrical potentials through a needle or small plate electrodes. The test can also measure the ability of peripheral nerves to conduct impulses.

**EMG** See *Electromyography*.

**Erectile dysfunction** The inability to attain or retain a rigid penile erection.

**Etiology** The study of all factors that may be involved in the development of a disease, including the patient's susceptibility, the nature of the disease-causing agent, and the way in which the person's body is invaded by the agent.

**Euphoria** Unrealistic cheerfulness and optimism, accompanied by a lessening of critical faculties; generally considered to be a result of damage to the brain.

**Evoked potentials (EPs)** EPs are recordings of the nervous system's electrical response to the stimulation of specific sensory pathways (e.g., visual, auditory, general sensory). In tests of evoked potentials, a person's recorded responses are displayed on an oscilloscope and analyzed on a computer that allows comparison with normal response times. Demyelination results in a slowing of response time. EPs can demonstrate lesions along specific nerve pathways whether or not the lesions are producing symptoms, thus making these tests useful in confirming the diagnosis of MS. Visual evoked potentials are considered the most useful in MS. See *Visual evoked potential*.

**Exacerbation** The appearance of new symptoms or the aggravation of old ones, lasting at least 24 hours (synonymous with attack, relapse, flare-up, or worsening); usually associated with inflammation and demyelination in the brain or spinal cord.

**Expanded Disability Status Scale (EDSS)** A part of the Minimal Record of Disability that summarizes the neurologic examination and provides a measure of overall disability. The EDSS is a 20-point scale, ranging from 0 (normal examination) to 10 (death due to MS) by half-points. A person with a score of 4.5 can walk three blocks without stopping; a score of 6.0 means that a cane or a leg brace is needed to walk one block; a score over 7.5 indicates that a person cannot take more than a few steps, even with crutches or help from another person. The EDSS is used for many reasons, including deciding future medical treatment, establishing rehabilitation goals, choosing subjects for participation in clinical trials, and measuring treatment outcomes. This is currently the most widely used scale in clinical trials.

**Experimental allergic encephalomyelitis (EAE)** Experimental allergic encephalomyelitis is an autoimmune disease resembling MS that has been induced in some genetically susceptible research animals. Before testing on humans, a potential treatment for MS may first be tested on laboratory animals with EAE in order to determine the treatment's efficacy and safety.

**Extensor spasm** A symptom of spasticity in which the legs straighten suddenly into a stiff, extended position. These spasms, which typically last for several minutes, occur most commonly in bed at night or on rising from bed.

**Failure to empty (bladder)** A type of neurogenic bladder dysfunction in MS resulting from demyelination in the voiding reflex center of the spinal cord. The bladder tends to overfill and become flaccid, resulting in symptoms of urinary urgency, hesitancy, dribbling, and incontinence.

**Failure to store (bladder)** A type of neurogenic bladder dysfunction in MS resulting from demyelination of the pathways between the spinal cord and brain. Typically seen in a small, spastic bladder, storage failure can cause symptoms of urinary urgency, frequency, incontinence, and nocturia. See *Nocturia*.

**FDA** See *Food and Drug Administration*.

**Finger-to-nose test** The person is asked, with eyes closed, to touch the tip of the nose with the tip of the index finger. This test is part of the standard neurologic exam.

**Flaccid** A decrease in muscle tone resulting in weakened muscles and therefore loose, "floppy" limbs.

**Flexor spasm** Involuntary, sometimes painful contractions of the flexor muscles, which pull the legs upward into a clenched position. These spasms, which last 2 to 3 seconds, are symptoms of spasticity. They often occur during sleep, but can also occur when the person is in a seated position.

**Foley catheter** See *Indwelling catheter*.

**Food and Drug Administration (FDA)** The U.S. federal agency that is responsible for enforcing governmental regulations pertaining to the manufacture and sale of food, drugs, and cosmetics. Its role is to prevent the sale of impure or dangerous substances. Any new drug that is proposed for the treatment of MS in the United States must be approved by the FDA.

**Foot drop** A condition of weakness in the muscles of the foot and ankle, caused by poor nerve conduction, which interferes with a person's ability to flex the ankle and walk with a normal heel-toe pattern. The toes touch the ground before the heel, causing the person to trip or lose balance.

**Frontal lobes** The largest lobes of the brain. The anterior (front) part of each of the cerebral hemispheres makes up the cerebrum. The back part of the frontal lobe is the motor cortex, which controls voluntary movement; the area of the frontal lobe that is further forward is concerned with learning, behavior, judgment, and personality.

**Gadolinium** A chemical compound that can be administered to a person during magnetic resonance imaging (MRI) to help distinguish between new lesions and old lesions.

**Gadolinium-enhancing lesion** A lesion appearing on magnetic resonance imagery (MRI), following injection of the chemical compound gadolinium, that reveals a breakdown in the blood-brain barrier. This breakdown of the blood-brain barrier indicates either a newly active lesion or the re-activation of an old one. See *Gadolinium*.

**Gastrocolic reflex** A mass peristaltic (coordinated, rhythmic, smooth muscle contraction that acts to force food through the digestive tract) movement of the colon that often occurs 15 to 30 minutes after ingesting a meal.

**Gastrostomy** See *Percutaneous endoscopic gastrostomy.*

**Glucocorticoid hormones** Steroid hormones that are produced by the adrenal glands in response to stimulation by adrenocorticotropic hormone (ACTH) from the pituitary. These hormones, which can also be manufactured synthetically (prednisone, prednisolone, methylprednisolone, betamethasone, dexamethasone), serve both an immunosuppressive and an anti-inflammatory role in the treatment of MS exacerbations: they damage or destroy certain types of T-lymphocytes that are involved in the overactive immune response, and interfere with the release of certain inflammation-producing enzymes.

**Healthcare proxy** See *Advance (medical) directive.*

**Heel-knee-shin test** A test of coordination in which the person is asked, with eyes closed, to place one heel on the opposite knee and slide it up and down the shin.

**Helper T-lymphocytes** White blood cells that are a major contributor to the immune system's inflammatory response against myelin.

**Hemiparesis** Weakness of one side of the body, including one arm and one leg.

**Hemiplegia** Paralysis of one side of the body, including one arm and one leg.

**Immune system** A complex network of glands, tissues, circulating cells, and processes that protect the body by identifying abnormal or foreign substances and neutralizing them.

**Immune-mediated disease** A disease in which components of the immune system—T-cells, antibodies, and others—are responsible for the disease either *directly* (as occurs in autoimmunity) or *indirectly* (for example, when damage to the body occurs secondary to an immune assault on a foreign antigen such as a bacteria or virus).

**Immunoglobulin** See *Antibody.*

**Immunology** The science that concerns the body's mechanisms for protecting itself from abnormal or foreign substances.

**Immunosuppression** In MS, a form of treatment that slows or inhibits the body's natural immune responses, including those directed against the body's own tissues. Examples of immunosuppressive treatments in MS include mitoxantrone, cyclosporine, methotrexate, and azathioprine.

**Impairment** Any loss or abnormality of psychological, physiological, or anatomical structure or function. It represents a deviation from the person's usual or expected biomedical state. An impairment is thus any loss of function directly resulting from congenital defect, injury, or disease.

**Incidence** The number of new cases of a disease in a specified population over a defined period of time. The incidence of MS in the United States is approximately 10,000 newly diagnosed people per year.

**Incontinence** Also called spontaneous voiding; the inability to control passage of urine or bowel movements.

**Indwelling catheter** A type of catheter (see *Catheter*) that remains in the bladder on a temporary or permanent basis. It is used only when intermittent catheterization is not possible or is medically contraindicated. The most common type of indwelling catheter is a Foley catheter, which consists of a flexible rubber tube that is inserted into the bladder to allow the urine to flow into an external drainage bag. A small balloon, inflated after insertion, holds the Foley catheter in place.

**Inflammation** A tissue's immunologic response to injury, characterized by mobilization of white blood cells and antibodies, swelling, and fluid accumulation.

**Intention tremor** Rhythmic shaking that occurs in the course of a purposeful movement, such as reaching to pick something up or bringing an outstretched finger in to touch one's nose.

**Interferon** A group of immune system proteins, produced and released by cells infected by a virus, which inhibit viral multiplication and modify the body's immune response. Three interferon-beta medications have been approved by the U.S. Food and Drug Administration (FDA) for treating relapsing forms of MS: IFN beta-1b (Betaseron®); IFN beta-1a (Avonex®); and IFN beta-1a (Rebif®).

**Intermittent self-catheterization (ISC)** A procedure in which the person periodically inserts a catheter into the urinary opening to drain urine from the bladder. ISC is used in the management of bladder dysfunction to drain urine that remains after voiding, in order to prevent bladder distention, prevent kidney damage, and restore bladder function.

**Internuclear ophthalmoplegia** A disturbance of coordinated eye movements in which the eye turned outward to look toward the side develops nystagmus (rapid, involuntary movements) while the other eye simultaneously fails to turn completely inward. This neurologic sign, of which the person is usually unaware, can be detected during the neurologic exam.

**Intrathecal space** The space surrounding the brain and spinal cord that contains cerebrospinal fluid.

**Intravenous** Within a vein; often used in the context of an injection into a vein of medication dissolved in a liquid.

**Lesion** See *Plaque*.

**L'hermitte's sign** An abnormal sensation of electricity or "pins and needles" going down the spine into the arms and legs that occurs when the neck is bent forward so that the chin touches the chest.

**Living will** See *Advance (medical) directive*.

**Loftstrand crutch** A type of crutch with an attached holder for the forearm that provides extra support.

**Lumbar puncture** A diagnostic procedure that uses a hollow needle to penetrate the spinal canal at the level of third–fourth or fourth–fifth lumbar vertebrae to remove cerebrospinal fluid for analysis. This procedure is used to examine the cerebrospinal fluid for changes in composition that are characteristic of MS (e.g., elevated white cell count, elevated protein content, the presence of oligoclonal bands). See *Oligoclonal bands*.

**Lymphocyte** A type of white blood cell that is part of the immune system. Lymphocytes can be subdivided into two main groups: B-lymphocytes, which originate in the bone marrow and produce antibodies; T-lymphocytes, which are produced in the bone marrow and mature in the thymus. Helper T-lymphocytes heighten the production of antibodies by B-lymphocytes; suppressor T-lymphocytes suppress B-lymphocyte activity and seem to be in short supply during an MS exacerbation.

**Macrophage** A white blood cell with scavenger characteristics that has the ability to ingest and destroy foreign substances such as bacteria and cell debris.

**Magnetic resonance imaging (MRI)** A diagnostic procedure that produces visual images of different body parts without the use of X-rays. Nuclei of atoms are influenced by a high frequency electromagnetic impulse inside a strong magnetic field. The nuclei then give off resonating signals that can produce pictures of parts of the body. An important diagnostic tool in MS, MRI makes it possible to visualize and count lesions in the white matter of the brain and spinal cord.

**Marcus Gunn pupil** See *Afferent pupillary defect.*

**Minimal Record of Disability (MRD)** A standardized method for quantifying the clinical status of a person with MS. The MRD is made up of five parts: demographic information; the Neurological Functional Systems (developed by John Kurtzke), which assign scores to clinical findings for each of the various neurologic systems in the brain and spinal cord (pyramidal, cerebellar, brainstem, sensory, visual, mental, bowel, and bladder); the Expanded Disability Status Scale (developed by John Kurtzke), which gives a single composite score for the person's disease; the Incapacity Status Scale, which is an inventory of functional disabilities relating to activities of daily living; and the Environmental Status Scale, which provides an assessment of social handicap resulting from chronic illness. The MRD has two main functions: to assist doctors and other professionals in planning and coordinating the care of persons with MS, and to provide a standardized means of recording repeated clinical evaluations of individuals for research purposes. See *Expanded Disability Status Scale (EDSS).*

**Motor point block** See *Nerve block.*

**MRI** See *Magnetic resonance imaging.*

**Multiple Sclerosis Functional Composite (MSFC)** A three-part, standardized, quantitative assessment instrument for use in clinical trials in MS, that was developed by the Task Force on Clinical Outcomes Assessment appointed by the National MS Society's Advisory Committee on Clinical Trials of New Agents in Multiple Sclerosis. The three components of the MSFC measure leg function/ambulation (Timed 25-Foot Walk), arm/hand function (9-Hole Peg Test), and cognitive function (Paced Auditory Serial Addition Test [PASAT]).

**Muscle tone** A characteristic of a muscle brought about by the constant flow of nerve stimuli to that muscle, which describes its resistance to stretching. Abnormal muscle tone can be defined as: hypertonus (increased muscle tone, as in spasticity); hypotonus (reduced muscle tone); flaccid (paralysis); and atony (loss of muscle tone). Muscle tone is evaluated as part of the standard neurologic exam in MS.

**Myelin** A soft, white coating of nerve fibers in the central nervous system, composed of lipids (fats) and protein. Myelin serves as insulation and as an aid to efficient nerve fiber conduction. When myelin is damaged in MS, nerve fiber conduction is faulty or absent. Impaired bodily functions or altered sensations associated with those demyelinated nerve fibers are identified as symptoms of MS in various parts of the body.

**Myelin basic protein** One of several proteins associated with the myelin of the central nervous system, which may be found in higher than normal concentrations in the cerebrospinal fluid of individuals with MS and other diseases that damage myelin.

**Nerve** A bundle of nerve fibers (axons). The fibers are either afferent (leading toward the brain and serving in the perception of sensory stimuli of the skin, joints, muscles, and inner organs) or efferent (leading away from the brain and mediating contractions of muscles or organs).

**Nerve block** A procedure used to relieve otherwise intractable spasticity, including painful flexor spasms. An injection of phenol into the affected nerve interferes with the function of that nerve for up to 3 months, potentially increasing a person's comfort and mobility.

**Nervous system** Includes all of the neural structures in the body: the *central nervous system* consists of the brain, optic nerves, and spinal cord; the *peripheral nervous system* consists of the nerve roots, nerve plexi, and nerves throughout the body; and the *autonomic nervous system* regulates the internal organs through a balance of the sympathetic and parasympathetic divisions.

**Neurogenic** Related to activity of the nervous system, as in "neurogenic bladder."

**Neurogenic bladder** Bladder dysfunction associated with neurologic malfunction in the spinal cord and characterized by a failure to empty, failure to store, or a combination of the two. Symptoms that result from these three types of dysfunction include urinary urgency, frequency, hesitancy, nocturia, and incontinence. See *Nocturia*.

**Neurologist** Physician who specializes in the diagnosis and treatment of conditions related to the nervous system.

**Neurology** Study of the central, peripheral, and autonomic nervous systems.

**Neuron** The basic nerve cell of the nervous system. A neuron consists of a nucleus within a cell body and one or more processes (extensions) called dendrites and axons.

**Neuropsychologist** A psychologist with specialized training in the evaluation of cognitive functions. Neuropsychologists use a battery of standardized tests to assess specific cognitive functions and identify areas of cognitive impairment. They also provide remediation for individuals with MS-related cognitive impairment. See *Cognition* and *Cognitive impairment.*

**Nocturia** The need to urinate during the night.

**Nystagmus** Rapid, involuntary movements of the eyes in the horizontal or, occasionally, the vertical direction.

**Occupational therapist (OT)** Occupational therapists assess functioning in activities of everyday living, including dressing, bathing, grooming, meal preparation, writing, and driving, which are essential for independent living. In making treatment recommendations, the OT addresses 1) fatigue management; 2) upper body strength, movement, and coordination; 3) adaptations to the home and work environment, including both structural changes and specialized equipment for particular activities; and 4) compensatory strategies for impairments in thinking, sensation, energy, or vision.

**Oligoclonal bands** A diagnostic sign indicating abnormal levels of certain antibodies in the cerebrospinal fluid; seen in approximately 90 percent of people with MS, but not specific to MS.

**Oligodendrocyte** A type of cell in the central nervous system that is responsible for making and supporting myelin.

**Olmstead Decision** The Supreme Court decision in *Olmstead v L.C.* (1999) is an interpretation of Title II of the Americans with Disabilities Act (ADA) that affirms the right of people with disabilities to receive services in the most integrated setting appropriate to their needs. The decision recognizes that unnecessary segregation of persons in long-term care facilities constitutes discrimination under the ADA.

**Ophthalmoscope** An instrument designed for examination of the interior of the eye.

**Optic atrophy** A wasting of the optic disc that results from partial or complete degeneration of optic nerve fibers and is associated with a loss of visual acuity. See *Optic disc.*

**Optic disc** The small blind spot on the surface of the retina where cells of the retina converge to form the optic nerve; the only part of the retina that is insensitive to light.

**Optic neuritis** Inflammation or demyelination of the optic (visual) nerve with transient or permanent impairment of vision and occasionally pain.

**Orthotic** Also called orthosis; a mechanical appliance such as a leg brace or splint that is specially designed to control, correct, or compensate for impaired limb function.

**Orthotist** A person skilled in making mechanical appliances (orthotics) such as leg braces or splints that help to support limb function. See *Orthotic*.

**Oscillopsia** Continuous, involuntary, and chaotic eye movements that result in a visual disturbance in which objects appear to be jumping or bouncing.

**Osteoporosis** Decalcification of the bones, which can result from the lack of mobility experienced by individuals who use wheelchairs or mobility.

**Paralysis** Inability to move a part of the body.

**Paraparesis** A weakness but not total paralysis of the lower extremities (legs).

**Paraplegia** Paralysis of both lower extremities (legs).

**Paresis** Weakness or partial paralysis of a part of the body.

**Paresthesia** A spontaneously occurring sensation of burning, prickling, tingling, or creeping on the skin that may or may not be associated with any physical findings on neurologic examination.

**Paroxysmal spasm** A sudden, uncontrolled limb contraction that occurs intermittently, lasts for a few moments, and then subsides.

**Paroxysmal symptom** Any one of several symptoms that has sudden onset (apparently in response to some kind of movement or sensory stimulation), lasts for a few moments, and then subsides. Paroxysmal symptoms tend to occur frequently in those individuals who have them, and follow a similar pattern from one episode to the next. Examples of paroxysmal symptoms include acute episodes of trigeminal neuralgia (sharp facial pain), tonic seizures (intense spasm of limb or limbs on one side of the body), dysarthria (slurred speech often accompanied by loss of balance and coordination), and various paresthesias (sensory disturbances ranging from tingling to severe pain).

**PEG** See *Percutaneous endoscopic gastrostomy*.

**Percutaneous endoscopic gastrostomy (PEG)** A PEG is a tube inserted into the stomach through the abdominal wall to provide food or other nutrients when eating by mouth is not possible. The tube is inserted in a bedside procedure using an endoscope to guide the tube through a small abdominal incision. An endoscope is a lighted instrument that allows the doctor to see inside the stomach.

**Periventricular region** The area surrounding the four fluid-filled cavities within the brain. MS plaques are commonly found within this region. See *Plaques*.

**Physiatrist** Physicians who specialize in physical medicine and rehabilitation, including the diagnosis and management of musculoskeletal injuries and pain syndromes, electrodiagnostic medicine (e.g., electromyography), and rehabilitation of severe impairments, including those caused by neurologic disease or injury. See *Electromyography (EMG)*.

**Physical therapist (PT)** Physical therapists are trained to evaluate and improve movement and function of the body, with particular attention to physical mobility, balance, posture, fatigue, and pain. The physical therapy program typically involves 1) educating the person with MS about the physical problems caused by the disease, 2) designing an individualized exercise program to address the problems, and 3) enhancing mobility and energy conservation through the use of a variety of mobility aids and adaptive equipment.

**Placebo** An inactive, nondrug compound that is designed to look just like the test drug. It is administered to control group subjects in double-blind clinical trials (in which neither the researchers nor the subjects know who is getting the drug and who is getting the placebo) as a means of assessing the benefits and liabilities of the test drug taken by experimental group subjects.

**Placebo effect** An apparently beneficial result of therapy that occurs because of the patient's expectation that the therapy will help.

**Plantar reflex** A reflex response obtained by drawing a pointed object along the outer border of the sole of the foot from the heel to the little toe. The normal flexor response is a bunching and downward movement of the toes. An upward movement of the big toe is called an extensor response, or Babinski reflex, which is a sensitive indicator of disease in the brain or spinal cord.

**Plaque** An area of inflamed or demyelinated central nervous system tissue.

**Post-void residual test (PVR)** The PVR test determines how much urine is left in the bladder after an attempt to empty the bladder through urination has occurred. It involves passing a catheter into the bladder following urination in order to drain and measure any urine remaining in the bladder. The PVR is a simple, but effective technique for diagnosing bladder dysfunction in MS.

**Postural tremor** Rhythmic shaking that occurs when the muscles are tensed to hold an object or stay in a given position.

**Prevalence** The number of all new and old cases of a disease in a defined population at a particular point in time. The prevalence of MS in the United States at any given time is about 1/750: approximately 400,000 people.

**Primary progressive MS (PPMS)** A clinical course of MS characterized from the beginning by progressive disease, with no plateaus or remissions, or an occasional plateau and very short-lived, minor improvements. See *Remission*.

**Prognosis** Prediction of the future course of the disease.

**Progressive-relapsing MS (PRMS)** A clinical course of MS that shows disease progression from the beginning, but with clear, acute relapses, with or without full recovery from those relapses along the way.

**Pseudo-bulbar affect** See *Affective release*.

**Pseudo-exacerbation** A temporary aggravation of disease symptoms, resulting from an elevation in body temperature or other stressor (e.g., an infection, severe fatigue, constipation), that disappears once the stressor is removed. A pseudo-exacerbation involves symptom flare-up rather than new disease activity or progression.

**Quad cane** A cane that has a broad base on four short "feet," which provide extra stability.

**Quadriplegia** The paralysis of both arms and both legs.

**Recent memory** The ability to remember events, conversations, or content of reading material or television programs from a short time ago (i.e., an hour or two ago or last night). People with MS-related memory impairment typically experience greatest difficulty remembering these types of things in the recent past.

**Reflex** An involuntary response of the nervous system to a stimulus, such as the stretch reflex, which is elicited by tapping a tendon with a reflex hammer, resulting in a contraction. Increased, diminished, or absent reflexes can be indicative of neurologic damage, including MS, and are therefore tested as part of the standard neurologic exam.

**Rehabilitation** Rehabilitation in MS involves the intermittent or ongoing use of multidisciplinary strategies (e.g., physiatry, physical therapy, occupational therapy, speech therapy) to promote functional independence, prevent unnecessary complications, and enhance overall quality of life. It is an active process directed toward helping the person recover and/or maintain the highest possible level of functioning and realize his or her optimal physical, mental, and social potential, given any limitations that exist. Rehabilitation is also an interactive, ongoing process of education and enablement in which people with MS and their care partners are active participants rather than passive recipients.

**Relapsing-remitting MS** A clinical course of MS that is characterized by clearly defined, acute attacks with full or partial recovery and no disease progression between attacks.

**Remission** A lessening in the severity of symptoms or their temporary disappearance during the course of the illness.

**Remote memory** The ability to remember people or events from the distant past. People with MS tend to experience few, if any, problems with their remote memory.

**Remyelination** The repair of damaged myelin. Myelin repair occurs spontaneously in MS, but very slowly. Research is current-

ly underway to find a way to speed the healing process.

**Residual urine** Urine that remains in the bladder following urination.

**Retrobulbar neuritis** See *Optic neuritis.*

**Romberg's sign** The inability to maintain balance in a standing position with feet and legs drawn together and eyes closed.

**Scanning speech** Abnormal speech characterized by staccato-like articulation that sounds clipped because the person unintentionally pauses between syllables and skips some of the sounds.

**Sclerosis** Hardening of tissue. In MS, sclerosis is the body's replacement of lost myelin around CNS nerve cells with scar tissue.

**Scotoma** A gap or blind spot in the visual field.

**Secondary progressive MS (SPMS)** A clinical course of MS that initially is relapsing-remitting and then becomes progressive at a variable rate, possibly with an occasional relapse and minor remission.

**Sensory** Related to bodily sensations such as pain, smell, taste, temperature, vision, hearing, acceleration, and position in space.

**Sign** An objective physical problem or abnormality identified by the physician during the neurologic examination. Neurologic signs may differ significantly from the symptoms reported by the patient because they are identifiable only with specific tests and may cause no overt symptoms. Common neurologic signs in MS include altered eye movements and other changes in the appearance or function of the visual system, altered reflexes, weakness, spasticity, and circumscribed sensory changes.

**Speech/language pathologist** Speech/language pathologists specialize in the diagnosis and treatment of speech and swallowing disorders. A person with MS may be referred to a speech/language pathologist for help with either one or both of these problems. Because of their expertise with speech and language difficulties, these specialists also provide cognitive remediation for individuals with cognitive impairment.

**Sphincter** A circular band of muscle fibers that tightens or closes a natural opening of the body, such as the external anal sphincter, which closes the anus, and the internal and external urinary sphincters, which close the urinary canal.

**Spinal tap** See *Lumbar puncture.*

**Spirometer** An instrument used to assess lung function; it measures the volume and flow rate of inhaled and exhaled air.

**SPMS** See *Secondary progressive MS.*

**Spontaneous voiding** See *Incontinence.*

**Steroids** See *ACTH; Corticosteroid; Glucocorticoid hormones.*

**Suppressor T-lymphocytes** White blood cells that act as part of the immune system and may be in short supply during an MS exacerbation.

**Straight catheter** A straight but flexible, hollow plastic tube of variable length and diameter, which can be inserted through the urinary opening into the bladder to drain excess urine that cannot be excreted normally. The straight catheter is the type used for intermittent self-catheterization (ISC). See *Intermittent self-catheterization.*

**Symptom** A subjectively perceived problem or complaint reported by the patient. In MS, common symptoms include visual problems, fatigue, sensory changes, weakness or paralysis of limbs, tremor, lack of coordination, poor balance, bladder or bowel changes, and psychologic changes.

**T-cell** A lymphocyte (white blood cell) that develops in the bone marrow, matures in the thymus, and works as part of the immune system in the body. See *Thymus.*

**Tandem gait** A test of balance and coordination that involves alternately placing the heel of one foot directly against the toes of the other foot.

**Titubation** A form of tremor, resulting from demyelination in the cerebellum, that manifests itself primarily in the head and neck.

**Transcutaneous electric nerve stimulation (TENS)** TENS is a nonaddictive and noninvasive method of pain control that applies electric impulses to nerve endings via electrodes that are attached to a stimulator by flexible wires and placed on the skin. The electric impulses block the transmission of pain signals to the brain.

**Trigeminal neuralgia** Lightning-like, acute pain in the face caused by demyelination of nerve fibers at the site where the sensory (trigeminal) nerve root for that part of the face enters the brainstem.

**Twins, dizygotic** Also known as fraternal twins, two babies that come from separate, simultaneously fertilized eggs. If one dizygotic twin develops MS, the other has the same genetic risk for MS (approximately 2-5/100) as any other sibling or first-degree relative.

**Twins, monozygotic** Also known as identical twins, two babies that come from a single fertilized egg and share identical genetic makeup. If one monozygotic twin develops MS, the other has a 30/100 risk of developing the disease, indicating that factors other than genetic makeup contribute to the etiology of MS.

**Urethra** Duct or tube that drains the urinary bladder.

**Urinalysis** Screening test to determine whether urinary tract infection, bladder stones, or other abnormality is, or may be, present.

**Urinary frequency** Feeling the urge to urinate even when urination has occurred very recently.

**Urinary hesitancy** The inability to void urine spontaneously even though the urge to do so is present.

**Urinary incontinence** See *Incontinence.*

**Urinary sphincter** The muscle closing the urethra which, in a state of flaccid paralysis, causes urinary incontinence, and in a state of spastic paralysis, results in an inability to urinate.

**Urinary urgency** The inability to postpone urination once the need to void has been felt.

**Urine culture and sensitivity (C & S)** A diagnostic procedure to test for urinary tract infection and identify the appropriate treatment. Bacteria from a mid-stream urine sample are allowed to grow for three days in a laboratory medium and then tested for sensitivity to a variety of antibiotics.

**Urologist** A physician who specializes in the branch of medicine (urology) concerned with the anatomy, physiology, disorders, and care of the male and female urinary tract, as well as the male genital tract.

**Urology** A medical specialty that deals with disturbances of the urinary (male and female) and reproductive (male) organs.

**Vertigo** A dizzying sensation of the environment spinning, often accompanied by nausea and vomiting.

**Vibration sense** The ability to feel vibrations against various parts of the body. Vibration sense is tested (with a tuning fork) as part of the sensory portion of the neurologic exam.

**Videofluoroscopy** A radiographic study of a person's swallowing mechanism that is recorded on videotape. Videofluoroscopy shows the physiology of the pharynx, the location of the swallowing difficulty, and confirms whether or not food particles or fluids are being aspirated into the airway.

**Visual acuity** Clarity of vision. Acuity is measured as a fraction of normal vision. 20/20 vision indicates an eye that sees at 20 feet what a normal eye should see at 20 feet; 20/400 vision indicates an eye that sees at 20 feet what a normal eye sees at 400 feet.

**Visual evoked potential (VEP)** A test in which the brain's electrical activity in response to visual stimuli (e.g., a flashing checkerboard) is recorded by an electroencephalograph and analyzed by computer. Demyelination results in a slowing of response time. Because this test is able to confirm the presence of a suspected brain lesion (area of demyelination) as well as identify the presence of an unsuspected lesion that has produced no symptoms, it is extremely useful in diagnosing MS. VEPs are abnormal in approximately 90 percent of people with MS.

**Vocational rehabilitation (VR)** Vocational rehabilitation is a program of services designed to enable people with disabilities to become or remain employed. Originally mandated by the Rehabilitation Act of 1973, VR programs are carried out by individually created state agencies. In order to be eligible for VR, a person must have a physical or mental disability that results in a substantial handicap to employment. VR programs typically involve evaluation of the disability and need for adaptive equipment or mobility aids, vocational guidance, training, job placement, and followup.

**White matter** The part of the brain that contains myelinated nerve fibers and appears white, in contrast to the cortex of the brain, which contains nerve cell bodies and appears gray.

# Index

NOTE: Boldface numbers indicate illustrations; contributing authors appear in italics.

duloxetine (Cymbalta), 184, 205–206
dysphagia, 101, 112

Effexor. *See* venlafaxine
Elavil. *See* amitriptyline
elbow exercises, 38, **38**
elevators and stair lifts, 142–143
emergency response system (ERS), 167
emotional support, 125
employment agreement form (personal assistant), **171**
enemas, 240–241
Enemeez. *See* docusate
energy conservation, stress management and, 121
energy therapies, 74
entryway access for home, 141–142
epidermis, 51–52, **51**
epididymitis, 86–87, **86**
epilepsy, 90
Equal Employment Opportunity Commission (EEOC), 178
erectile problems, 68–70. *See also* sexual function
ethnic background and risk of MS, 2
evoked potentials, 6
exercise, 14, 34–39, 93–99, 110, 135–137. *See also* joint flexibility and mobility
    adaptive equipment for, 137
    aerobic/cardiorespiratory, 94–95, 135, 136
    balance and, 97, 136–137
    bladder management and, 139
    chair exercises and, 138
    closed and open chain, 96
    deconditioning and, 24
    diet and, 110
    exacerbations and, 88, 139
    exerstriding as, 138
    fatigue and, 24, 138–139
    FITT principle in, 94
    flexibility, 136
    fluid intake during, 139
    handcycling as, 138
    heat and humidity effects of, 88, 139
    horseback riding/hippotherapy, 98
    hydrotherapy (swimming) and, 97–98
    National Center on Physical Activity and Disability (NCPAD) and, 137, 140
    physical fitness and, 135–137
    Pilates, 97
    rate of perceived exercise (RPE) scale in, 94, **94**
    SAM format for, 34
    strength training, 95–96, 136
    stress management and, 120
    stretching and flexibility, 96–97
    t'ai chi as, 98, 138

exercise *(continued)*
    tips for, 140
    vision problems and, 139
    wellness programs and, 98–99
    yoga as, 97, 138
exerstriding, 138

fampridine (4-aminopyridine), 14
Faroe Islands, outbreak of MS, 3
fascia of skin, 52
fatigue, 23–27
    causes of, 23
    characteristics of, versus normal fatigue, 23
    cognitive problems and, 62
    deconditioning and, 24
    demyelination and, 23
    depression and, 23, 24, 25
    diet and, 23, 24
    exercise and, 24, 138–139
    food preparation/eating and, 112
    medications for, 25
    neuromuscular causes of, 24–25
    physical and occupational therapy for, 25
    questionnaire for, Fatigue Severity Scale (FSS), **26**, 27
    rearranging and prioritizing routine to avoid, 25–27
    sexual function and, 70
    sleep disorders and, 23, 24, 25
    types of, 23–24
Fatigue Severity Scale (FSS), **26**, 27
fats in diet and MS, 4
federal resources, 178–180
Federal Trade Commission (FTC), 179
ferry travel, 134
fiber intake, 111
fibromyalgia, 90
financial planning, 125, 149–152. *See also* insurance options
    cost of chronic illness and, 150
    economic consequences and, 150
    living costs in, 149
    medical costs in, 149
    missed opportunity costs in, 149–150
    public benefits programs and, 151–152
finger exercises, 34–35, **34**, 39, **39**
fitness and recreation. *See* exercise; recreation
FITT principle in exercise, 94
Fleet enemas. *See* sodium phosphate
fluid intake, 111
    bladder dysfunction and, 46
    bowel management and, 48
    exercise and, 139
fluoxetine (Prozac), 25, 184, 206–207
*Foley, Frederick W.*, 67